Primary Well-Being: Case Studies for the Growing Child

Deborah Kramer

Primary Well-Being: Case Studies for the Growing Child

Springer

Deborah Kramer
Department of Nursing
College of Mount Saint Vincent
New York
USA

ISBN 978-3-319-56707-5 ISBN 978-3-319-56708-2 (eBook)
DOI 10.1007/978-3-319-56708-2

Library of Congress Control Number: 2017944448

Printed on acid-free paper

This Springer imprint is published by Springer Nature
The registered company is Springer International Publishing AG
The registered company address is: Gewerbestrasse 11, 6330 Cham, Switzerland

This book is dedicated to health professionals and nurse practitioner students who promote wellness in our children and deliver excellent patient care.

This book is also dedicated to my husband, children (and spouses), and my grandchildren, including those who may be born in the future.

This book is also dedicated to the thousands of students I have been privileged to teach for inspiring the awareness of the need for this book.

Preface

Primary Well-Being: Case Studies for the Growing Child fills an urgent need: to emphasize and enhance the normal development of the well child. The primary care provider is the one professional who sees every child and their parent during the early years of life. This is a unique time where the provider can assess the child's health and educate parents on how to provide a healthy environment and important practices to nurture healthy children.

This book will benefit nurse practitioner students as a teaching text and a manual for clinical practice; it will also serve as a guide for nurse practitioners. The book incorporates complementary medicine, professional advocacy, specific development enhancement skills, and parent/provider communication strategies.

The book is unique in providing realistic scenarios of what students will see as they begin their clinical training. It is structured in a question and answer framework to help students and practitioners critically think through the best practices that can be implemented during the well-child visit and develop a plan of action for the family. Each case study describes with sensitivity families from diverse cultural and economic backgrounds. It provides recommendations for broad social policies to help all children succeed.

The case studies help students and nurse practitioners to develop their critical thinking skills while working through typical situations faced by health care providers.

New York, NY

Deborah Kramer

Acknowledgements

To Carole Oshinsky, thank you for generously providing your expertise and time to make this book possible. Working with you in your role as co-president of the New York Zero-to-Three Network and its Infancy Leadership Circles Project helped me gain a greater appreciation of advocacy within the community and across professions that serve children and their families. I have greatly enjoyed working with you and revere your friendship.

To Helen Lerner, thank you for being my professor, mentor, and colleague. You introduced me to the wonderful expanded role of the nurse when you suggested I apply to the nurse practitioner program and my professional life has been forever enhanced. I greatly value you as a colleague and friend.

I would like to thank Ilana Spierer and Shuli Spivak for their generous time and expertise in the field of occupational therapy and recommendations regarding sensory integration for the well child.

I would like to thank my husband, children, my parents, and siblings for their guidance and generosity in enabling and encouraging me to do this work. You gave me the inspiration and support to become a nurse practitioner early in the profession and embrace this once new role.

Contents

Part I

Preparation for the Well-Child Visit

Introduction

1

The purpose of this book is to guide professionals and students of primary care pediatrics in working with children birth to age 18 and teaching their families. These health providers include pediatric care providers, nurse practitioners, medical students, and physician assistants (PAs). Through the use of clinical case studies, questions, and answers, the book will help guide the practitioner in providing comprehensive care and anticipatory guidance during the well-child visit. It has a strong focus on early childhood in fostering health. Research has demonstrated that the 0–3 years are the most important in laying the basis for wellness throughout life (National Research Council and Institute of Medicine 2000; National Scientific Council on the Developing Child 2007). The nurse and the primary care provider are in a unique position to identify health and developmental issues and to teach parenting. They are the professionals that all parents and children interface with from birth (Potts and Mandleco 2012). The well-child visit is the opportune place to teach parents how to parent and nurture healthy children and to offer this information in anticipatory guidance (McInerny et al. 2009).

The plan of health care for children and their families is an integrated one that includes complementary and alternative medicine, reading materials, and other educational resources to help the family choose their own lifestyle approaches. Integrated health can include acupuncture, massage, homeopathy, energy therapies, mind-body medicine, nutritional therapies, chiropractic, and osteopathy. As part of the role of primary health care provider, it is important to identify lifestyle issues that affect health and well-being. This includes not only the foods that we choose to eat but also the toxins that we allow ourselves to be exposed to, whether in the food or our environment, and our relationships. Management of stress and self-care are important in maintaining health for the child, the parent, and the family as a whole. Health care providers offer approaches to stress management and self-care and help the parents become role models and coaches for their families (Culbert and Olness 2009).

This book is written with sensitivity to different families, cultures, and economic backgrounds that must be considered to provide best practice. The questions following the case studies and the discussion answers help the practitioner understand how to think when caring for children. It is also sensitive to the need for parents to be advocates for their children. The health care provider honors the choices of the

D. Kramer, *Primary Well-Being: Case Studies for the Growing Child*,
DOI 10.1007/978-3-319-56708-2_1

family and empowers them to be autonomous over their own care, with the provider being nonjudgmental and respectful.

During the well-child visit, parents are guided to appreciate the challenges and rewards of raising a child. Children grow rapidly—physically, physiologically, and psychologically. Using this book, the primary health care provider will help parents and families to identify normal developmental milestones, foster development, and deal with developmental issues. Diagnostically, using critical thinking skills, the provider will recognize potential problems or red flags that require further follow-up with the parents and specialists.

This book can be used as a teaching text, an adjunct to the basic pediatric text, a manual for clinical practice, and a guide for nursing students by studying the questions and answers after each case description. Each case study will help students to focus on the inclusion of common developmental and behavioral issues within the age group, assessment criteria, and use of assessment tools. The case studies offer suggested dialogue and role playing exercises that can be done quickly in an office setting and suggested follow-up handouts available online to give to families from the Bright Futures initiative of the American Academy of Pediatrics. Unique to this book is the inclusion of alternative and complementary therapies including bibliotherapy. Anticipatory guidance is in each of the chapters, along with checklists and red flags, with a strong focus on socio-emotional development. Advice is offered to guide parents as they grow in their new role.

Also unique are the discussions about the character strengths that children need to navigate childhood and be successful, independent individuals in adulthood that can deal with life's challenges. These discussions can also help parents care for themselves and build a strong relationship with their spouse or other adults in the family as well as nurture their child.

The role of the nurse practitioner in health care includes prevention, promotion, and early intervention. Case studies offer students an appreciation of this role and assist in the integration of assessment, intervention, and development of teaching plans. The case studies use questions that guide the development of a plan of care that includes evidence-based practice, best practice in clinical treatment, teaching plans, and anticipatory guidance. By asking these questions, students and practitioners will be able to critically think through applications for the patients presented in these case studies and develop a plan of care.

Best practices in health care should encompass comprehensive services with diverse professionals located as much as possible in the same facility and helping families with a multitude of issues. These practices include parenting education in the waiting room, assessment and follow-up for depression in the parents, literally taking patients by the hand to another expert (warm hand-off), and doing group well-baby visits to create an atmosphere of parent support. All of these new practices need to be discussed with nursing students and to be considered in a plan of care in clinical practice.

The expanded anticipatory guidance sections include health promotion and wellness and parenting, focusing on how to help children and families handle stress, provide skills for success and nurturing, and incorporating alternative therapies to aid children in their healthy growth and development. Topics include anticipating events such as adaptation to change, stressful family situations, importance of routines, understanding the child's mind, individuality and parenting techniques, appropriate communication, value of toys and play objects, gauging accomplishments and abilities, sibling relationships, and marking milestones and life-cycle events, including planning age-appropriate birthday parties.

References

Culbert T, Olness K (eds) (2009) Integrative pediatrics. Oxford University Press, New York, NY

McInerny TK, Adam HM, Campbell DE, Kamat DM, Kelleher KJ (eds) (2009) Textbook of pediatric care. American Academy of Pediatrics, Elk Grove Village, IL

National Research Council and Institute of Medicine (2000) In: Shonkoff J, Phillips DA (eds) From neurons to neighborhoods: the science of early childhood development. National Academy Press, Washington, DC

National Scientific Council on the Developing Child (2007). The timing and quality of early experiences combine to shape brain architecture (Working Paper No. 5). Boston, MA: Harvard Center for the Developing Child. http://developingchild.harvard.edu/index.php/resources/reports_and_working_papers/working_papers/wp5/. Accessed 18 Nov 2014

Potts NL, Mandleco BL (eds) (2012) Pediatric nursing: caring for children and their families, 3rd edn. Clifton Park, NY, Delmar Cengage Learning

Overview of the Well-Child Visit 2

Primary health care providers assess the physical and emotional development of children during the well-child visit. This is achieved through open and accepting communication as the health care provider obtains a comprehensive history of the child and family and the situation at home. Health care providers often say that 95% of diagnosis comes from listening to the patient and gathering a good history (Segal 2012). This is absolutely true in the well-child visit.

2.1 The Parent/Provider Relationship

Through the well-child visits, the primary health care provider helps parents to learn about their child and to become more knowledgeable, competent, nurturing, observant, empowered, and loving. This is not achieved in one visit, but through the relationship that the primary health care provider establishes over a period of time with the family. Listening to parents and children is the cornerstone to assessing child development and identifying areas that need further observation and assessment.

At each visit, the primary care provider initially responds to the family's questions and concerns based on the current age of their child/children. With the birth of a new baby, especially the first born, parents are anxious and insecure about whether they will be able to care for this child who can't tell them yet what is wrong. The parents are just beginning to establish routines in caring for their new baby. Often parents and other care providers, such as a grandparent, come to the visit with a list of questions. The primary health provider should encourage parents to ask questions and take the time to discuss the questions with the parents with respect, openness, and positive encouragement about their parenting skills.

For each age group, priorities for the visit are established based on expected developmental milestones, and physical and emotional development as outlined in Bright Futures materials published by the American Academy of Pediatrics. In each visit the primary provider should look at family adjustment issues, child adjustment issues, feeding routines and comfort concerns, immunization, safety guidelines and injury prevention, including equipment and toys, using the guidelines developed by the American Academy of Pediatrics Bright Futures Infancy Expert Panel

D. Kramer, *Primary Well-Being: Case Studies for the Growing Child*,
DOI 10.1007/978-3-319-56708-2_2

(Tanski et al. 2010). A recent study of primary care providers discusses the low incidence of conversations around infant care including breastfeeding, immunization, sleep positions, and pacifier use and suggests opportunities for intervention (Eisenberg et al. 2015). The American Academy of Pediatrics recommends that these topics be incorporated in the anticipatory guidance during the well-child visit (Tanski et al. 2010).

2.2 Role of Questions

Asking specific interview questions will facilitate understanding of parents concerns. Specific questions can be asked to assess whether there is maternal depression (Musser et al. 2013), whether the baby is feeding well, participation by the father and others in the family to relieve the mother of care and give her time to rest, how the household is being managed, and any changes anticipated, such as returning to work or school. As the child gets older, interview questions will cover toys and discipline as well.

The primary health provider should observe the interactions between parents or parent and caregiver, and between parent and child, their emotional rapport and interactions, whether one parent is asking all the questions and the other is quiet. By making positive statements about how well the baby is doing and the relationship between parent and child, the primary health provider is empowering the parents in their new role and to speak up about their concerns.

The conclusion of the visit is an opportunity to reinforce how well the parents are doing in caring for their child despite fatigue and other factors in their lives. It is a time for the primary health care provider to ask for additional questions the parents may have, and to talk about other anxieties the parents may be feeling that they might not have expressed. The primary provider should also make sure the parent has set the next appointment and describe what to expect from it.

2.3 Promoting the Parent–Child Relationship

The parent-child relationship is the gift that parents and child give each other. This includes for the baby the gift of constant, unconditional love, self-esteem, values and traditions, joy in life, good health, secure surroundings, and skills and abilities (Shelov 2009). At the same time, children have gifts for their parents: unqualified love, absolute trust, the thrill of discovery, and intense emotions (Shelov 2009). During the well-baby visit, the primary health provider can help the parent/caregiver identify and appreciate these gifts and let them know that displaying loving emotions from birth, such as stating “I love you,” and giving the child hugs and kisses are an important part of parenting and encourage normal development.

The health care practitioner helps the parents to believe in their ability to be good parents, which in turn will help the parents to foster their child’s self-esteem. Over years of parents showing love, listening, praising accomplishments, and believing in their child, children learn to believe in themselves and have a high level of self-respect and self-esteem. When necessary, constructive limit setting in a respectful nonpunitive or nonhurtful manner can help to develop the solid self-esteem that is needed for good emotional health. Even during limit setting as the child gets older, it is important that the primary health provider advise parents to express love for their child and separate the anger the parent may feel over a specific incident or behavior from the child.

Another gift parents give their child is the example they set—whether in their attitudes or behavior, their values, or traditions. This includes showing that parents need to care for themselves and need to be responsible, loving, affectionate, and nurturing in their relationships with all members of the family. When parents provide examples of communicating openly and honestly with one another, and share responsibilities in their household, their children will learn to do the same. Health care providers can explain to parents in their guidance that open communication means expressing feelings in a sensitive way and carefully selecting the words the parents use so as not to hurt the child or other person's feeling. Parents should be encouraged to talk about problems as they arise, and welcome questions and discussion with the health provider and their child. When parents are being open and encouraging of their children's questions and observations, it fosters open, nonjudgmental communication and positive self-esteem for both parents and child.

2.4 Understanding Temperament

Children have different temperaments. Some are more outgoing, some more introspective or quiet, and some more playful. The more joyful the parent is when they are with their child, the more the child will spontaneously embrace joy in life and in their surroundings. The primary health provider can help parents to be more aware of their children's temperament and help the parents foster their child's joy. Some of the ways the primary care provider can do this are helping parents recognize their child as an individual, unique being, identifying their strengths and special needs, their moods, and their joy in play. The more parents appreciate their children's individuality, the more the child's sense of self-esteem and trust is increased.

2.5 Promoting Health and Security

Parents coming for the well-baby visit are encouraging the good health of their child. The primary health provider can empower parents to continue to provide a healthy, nutritious diet for their child, physical exercise, and follow safety protocols to help prevent injuries. Parents need to model these good health habits for their children and their own well-being. This is an opportunity for the primary health provider to help parents review their own health habits and empower them to eliminate unhealthy habits and establish healthy ones, particularly physical activity, reducing alcohol and drug consumption, eliminating smoking, eating healthy, and getting adequate sleep. It is also a time to encourage the parents to foster and nurture their relationship as a couple by finding time for each other and continuing to have date nights and time alone at least 2 h a week.

Secure surroundings help children thrive. This includes physical safety and comfort, preventing emotional distress, and providing consistency and love. The primary health care provider can talk about why it is important for family members to resolve differences within the family or with others. Children can sense conflict; when parents demonstrate they have resolved a problem it gives children the confidence to overcome conflict as well.

2.6 Promoting Learning

The primary health care provider encourages parents to provide infants and children with learning opportunities and diverse activities and experiences with other children and adults. Parents are encouraged to recognize their children's achievements as children enjoy pleasing their parents and gain a great sense of personal satisfaction from their accomplishments. While parents are providing the opportunities, the primary health care provider can point out that children learn at their own rate.

Health care providers teach the parents how to enjoy parenting. Becoming a parent is extremely stressful and parents are often overcome by this stress and lose the joy. The provider can help foster the joy and excitement of parenting by their careful management of the well-child visit. Anticipatory guidance includes helping parents appreciate what they are seeing in their child and sharing the joy of their child's exploration and development.

2.7 Promoting Parent Education

The health provider can encourage the parent to educate themselves about the different developmental issues and problems their child may experience and physical development (McInerny et al. 2009; Potts and Mandleco 2012). One way health care practitioners can reassure parents about children who appear smaller than others their age is to show the parents their child's growth chart. Explain that we are looking for growth curves that are consistent rather than absolute numbers. Providers also help the parents to anticipate the milestones like beginning to smile, rolling over, and walking. These are also indicators of normal development.

As parents are forming a relationship with their child, it is helpful for them to participate in a parent support group, gather resources, and learn how to deal with different situations in a way that fits best with their family. In our information age, using the Internet and other communication resources is available to almost everyone, whether at home or in a library or community setting.

However, information about support services and groups in the community cannot always be easily found. Primary health providers should gather information about these supports for their parents and be knowledgeable about community organizations that provide this information to individual families.

2.8 Parents As Role Models

The healthier and happier parents are, the better it will be for children since children pattern their own habits on their parents. Children notice differences among people. A parent who is tolerant and accepting of others will teach her child act similarly. It is particularly important for a child to observe her parent being respectful and kind to people with disabilities or special needs, people from different ethnic or religious groups, and people who have a different socioeconomic status.

Also remind the family about showing their love for the child by spending time together, showing physical affection, taking time to talk and read, rocking together (not all homes have rocking chairs, but all can do the motion of rocking while the child is on their lap), and making the child feel cherished and secure. Help the parents to understand that children need some quality, special time each day with each parent, and that it is important to include children in everyday activities, such as meal preparation and eating, cleanup time, and shopping trips.

2.9 Promoting Patience and Expressing Emotions

The primary health care provider can help parents nurture growth and change in their child in many ways. They can help guide parents to provide appropriate rules and guidelines and discipline for children at each stage of development so that parents welcome the child's growth. The health care provider can talk about consistency in the home being important with all the care providers that interact with the child. They can remind parents to minimize frustrations and provide opportunities for success for their child using realistic expectations appropriate for the child's age and abilities and his own timetable. Encourage the parents to give their child strategies to cope with frustrations and constructively express their negative feelings. For example, have the parents think about how they handle their own unhappiness and anger, with a clear message that violence is not permissible. Feelings of sadness, anger, hurt, and frustration are all normal feelings that children need to express to have healthy development. Bibliotherapy—using stories and books to help express emotions—can be a resource for helping parents talk with children about their feelings. See Chap. 6 on Complementary Medicine, for an extensive section on bibliotherapy.

2.10 Understanding Parental Stress

The primary health care provider needs to be nonjudgmental and open so that parents feel comfortable presenting problems as they arise with a sense of confidence that the health care provider will help them resolve it and refer them to other supportive providers. Health care providers should be resourceful, accessible, family-centered, and compassionate in helping families to address their specific problems and concerns. For parents who are feeling overloaded or have increased stress in their own life, the primary health care provider should be prepared to make referrals for support services.

As health care providers caring for growing families, you can anticipate that stress is a normal part of growth. Having this perspective and understanding, everyone can develop tools for stress reduction and prevention and how to deal with stress when it occurs—this includes guidance from the health care provider, the parents, and the child. When we understand that stress is a normal part of growth, we are able to deal with it more effectively and be resilient.

2.11 Promoting Resilience

The primary health care provider can guide families to help their children develop resilience. Building resilience in children has been defined as the "capacity to rebound from setbacks" (Shelov et al. 2009). Kenneth Ginsburg, M.D., has identified seven elements called the "7c's" that describe the building blocks of resilience for children that can bolster them in stressful times and help to raise "authentically successful children" (Ginsburg and Jablow 2011). Each stressful occurrence is also an educational opportunity to help teach children skills they can use with their next challenge. The 7c's include competence, confidence, connection, character, contribution, coping, and control. See the Fostering Resilience web site at: www.fosteringresilience.com/7cs_parents.php for guidance on how parents can help children succeed through positive and challenging situations. The web site includes questions parents can use to assess how well their children have been able to develop each of these 7c's and specific sections for parents on signs of trouble, for teens on stress, and details for professionals.

The following are selected national web sites and organizations that provide many useful resources for parents and professionals. There are many other resources too numerous to list. Start with your state's local medical society and early childhood organization for further resources. Local referral services such as 311 or 211 call numbers are also helpful, although some may not include early childhood mental health and other early childhood support services for infants and toddlers and their families. See New York Zero-to-Three Network below for how one organization is addressing this gap.

Bright Futures: www.brightfutures.org provides guidelines and handouts for healthy child development and health practice from the American Academy of Pediatrics, with separate resources for parents.

Center on the Social and Emotional Foundations for Early Learning: http://csefel.vanderbilt.edu promotes the social emotional development and school readiness of young children birth to age 5 using the Pyramid Model for Supporting Social Emotional Competence in Infants and Young Children. Provides user-friendly training materials, videos, and print resources to help early care, health, and education providers implement the Pyramid Model.

Children's Defense Fund: http://www.childrensdefense.org seeks to ensure that every child has a "Healthy Start, a Head Start, a Safe Start and a Moral Start in life" through its "Leave No Child Behind" campaign for preventive investments and its educational activities. It monitors basic data on children's health and well-being in its annual State of America's Children report and other research with particular attention on the status and needs of children of color, children living in poverty, and those with disabilities.

Docs for Tots: www.docsfortots.org encourages pediatricians to promote practices, policies, and investments that will enable young children to thrive, particularly the medical home, developmental screening, high-quality early care and education, social emotional health, and addressing the impacts of poverty.

Harvard Center on the Developing Child: http://developingchild.harvard.edu promotes research-based innovation to enable successful development of children facing multiple risks and adverse life trajectories. Includes videos, working papers, charts on brain architecture, serve and return, toxic stress, executive function, resilience, and innovation. Audience is policymakers, advocates, and general public as well as parents.

National Center for Children in Poverty: www.nccp.org engages in research at the state and national levels to inform public policy and practice to promote family economic security, strong nurturing families, and healthy child development for America's low-income children. It features state-by-state policy profiles and other research aimed at policymakers, practitioners, and advocates, and the media to promote innovative public policies.

National Association for the Education of Young Children: www.naeyc.org is a national membership organization with state and local affiliates of professionals who work with young children to promote high-quality early learning experiences for children birth through age 8. It provides professional accreditation, leadership and professional development, and resources and publications. It works to promote public policies that provide comprehensive equitable access to high-quality early learning programs.

National Education Association: http://www.nea.org/ professional membership organization devoted to public education that offers news, information, and resources.

New York Zero-to-Three Network: www.nyztt.org provides information, networking, professional trainings, and conferences. Its Infancy Leadership Circle Project in counties across the state has mapped resources for infants and toddlers locally and enhanced access via 311 and 211 services as well as working on local issues to enhance quality of services and comprehensive service provision (Infancy Leadership Circle, Niagara 2012).

Zero to Three: National Center for Infants, Toddlers and Families: www.zerotothree.org provides research-based knowledge for professionals and parents on how to nurture early development. It includes advocacy and practice.

References

Eisenberg, S.R., Bair-Merritt, M.H., Colson, E.R., et al (2015). Maternal report of advice received for infant care. Pediatrics, 136(2). http://pediatrics.aappublications.org/content/early/2015/07/21/peds.2015-0551.full.pdf. Accessed 17 Aug 2015

Ginsburg, Kenneth R., Jablow, Martha M. (2011). Building resilience in children and teens: giving kids roots and wings, 2nd. Elk Grove, IL: American Academy of Pediatrics. See http://www.fosteringresilience.com/7cs_parents.php

Infancy Leadership Circle, Niagara. (2012). Niagara County resource directory for new parents. New York, NY: New York Zero-to-Three Network. http://nyztt.org/pdf_NiagaraCountyResource_2012.pdf. Accessed 18 Nov 2014

McInerny TK, Adam HM, Campbell DE, Kamat DM, Kelleher KJ (eds) (2009) Textbook of pediatric care. American Academy of Pediatrics, Elk Grove Village, IL

Musser AK, Ahmed AH, Foli KJ, Coddington JA. (2013). Paternal postpartum depression: What health care providers should know. Journal of Pediatric Health Care 27, 470–485.

Potts NL, Mandleco BL (eds) (2012) Pediatric nursing: caring for children and their families, 3rd edn. Delmar Cengage Learning, Clifton Park, NY

Segal, S. (2012). Diagnosing an illness is an art. *mdpageTODAY's KevinMD.com.* http://www.kevinmd.com/blog/2012/01/diagnosing-illness-art.html. Accessed 21 Jul 2014

Shelov SP, Altmann TR, Hannemann RE (eds) (2009) Caring for your baby and young child, birth to age 5. Bantam Books, New York, NY

Tanski, S., Garfunkel, L.C., Duncan, P.M., Weitzman, M. (Eds.) (2010). Performing preventive services. A Bright Futures handbook. Elk Grove, IL: American Academy of Pediatrics. http://brightfutures.aap.org/pdfs/Preventive%20Services%20PDFs/Forward%20and%20Introduction.pdf. Accessed 12 Jun 2014

Role of Development

3

Evaluating the child's development is an integral part of the primary health care visit. This includes assessing developmental milestones and considering the factors that go into healthy development. These factors include physical and psychosocial growth; gross motor and fine motor coordination; brain development; temperament; family and cultural factors; cognitive, visual, and auditory development; psychosexual development; and language development. Children need to successfully complete one stage of development before they can move to the next stage in any domain.

Play is the universal language of children. It is a form of communication and can be used to assess and treat a child, as well as a way to relate to them. Play is also the way children explore their environment, trying out hypothesis and seeing what happens, such as hitting two blocks together or knocking down a tower of blocks. The child development researcher Alison Gopnik refers to young children as scientists in the crib (Gopnik et al. 2000). Often with the young child, the health provider will do a pretend test on a stuffed animal or doll to relax the child and then complete the examination on the child. Observing the complexity of a child's play will provide information about his physical, intellectual, and social development.

3.1 Developmental Milestones

Assessing developmental milestones is essential for determining the healthy growth of children. Infants in the first year of life grow rapidly. They double their weight by the age of 4 months and triple their weight by a year. They develop from not being able to hold their head up to walking at around 12–18 months.

Age-appropriate developmental milestones can be divided into six categories:

- Gross motor
- Fine motor
- Social and cognitive
- Psychosexual
- Sensory
- Language

D. Kramer, *Primary Well-Being: Case Studies for the Growing Child*,
DOI 10.1007/978-3-319-56708-2_3

These categories are described later in this chapter.

Children's growth and development occur in an orderly sequence. Even if children differ in the time that they present in one stage, they generally follow predictive stages. The pace of growth and development is specific and unique for each individual child. Some children may develop language skills early; others may develop gross motor skills later.

Development occurs from the head down (cephalocaudal) and from close to far extremities (proximodistal). Infants develop motor control starting with head control before being able to sit and walk. They also gain control first from the midline, and then eventually distally to the coordination of the hands. That is why they roll over first, before developing a gross pincer grasp and then a fine pincer grasp.

Over the course of the first year of life, growth and development become increasingly integrated through small changes in progression of skills and behaviors. Children increasingly develop more complex behaviors and are able to organize and differentiate as they continue to mature and experience responses to internal and external cues.

The child's environment plays a major role in his/her ability to achieve milestones. Cultural values, family belief systems, physical environment, and opportunities for play all influence the child's ability for opportunities and experiences that will enhance development. Critical growth periods and development are particularly susceptible to alterations due to internal and external influences throughout the life cycle. Examples include the time period occurring during fetal development and in the attachment process after birth. Understanding of developmental milestones and taking into account of individual factors will help to anticipate times of growth and times of stability and plateaus (Cech and Martin 2011).

Touchpoints is a framework for looking at children and parent's strengths developed by Dr. T. Berry Brazelton. As primary care providers, we are trained to note deficits and delays. Under the Touchpoints model, parents are respected as being the experts on their child's behavior. The primary care provider is the expert in clinical practice. Together they develop a caring, collaborative relationship to foster the child's development. In this relationship parents are more open to share concerns about their child and vulnerabilities. The practitioner is empathetically involved. Development is looked at across multiple dimensions, including motor, cognitive, and emotional. Parents and practitioners revel in the joy of a child striving to do something and glowing with its accomplishment. At each developmental stage, they look for opportunities to promote mastery and development in the child, and focus on the child's strengths instead of deficits (Brazelton 1992; Brazelton and Sparrow 2003).

Assessing delays in milestones or prolongation of milestones is an important factor in the early identification of developmental delays or issues. The health care provider collects data about the child's development and rules out developmental diagnoses using tools such as the Brazelton Neonatal Assessment Scale and others listed in the bibliography below (Ringwalt 2008). These tools are referenced throughout this book. The provider will also provide individual plans of care to the family to promote normal development. When potential developmental delays are found, the provider will want to refer the family to their local government Early Intervention department for an evaluation to determine what services are needed. Gaps in development as the child progresses may also be referred simultaneously for a neuropsychological assessment.

Services that are offered through Early Intervention cover five domains of development: physical, cognitive, communication, social-emotional, and self-help. These services can include occupational and physical therapy; speech, language, and feeding therapy; special education; psychological services; respite services; medical, nursing, and nutrition services; and supportive devices.

3.2 Early Brain Development

Much progress has been made in understanding early brain development. The seminal work, *From Neurons to Neighborhoods*, describes how the experiences of the brain from birth to age 5 are the most important ones for healthy child development (Shonkoff and Phillips 2000). Between conception and age 3, a child's brain size and structure (wiring) grow to 85% of its adult size (Lally 2013). This structure supports the rapid social, emotional, and mental development that children experience in the first 3 years of life. During the rest of childhood and adolescence, the efficiency of the neuronal networks is refined, especially the prefrontal cortex that is responsible for judgment and impulse control. By age 6, the brain is about 95% of its adult size (Shonkoff and Phillips 2000).

Research confirms the fact that early experiences affect the development. Parents' everyday attention to their baby, through activities such as diapering, feeding, talking, holding, playing, calming, and sleep, all influence their baby's brain development. Specifically, health care providers can teach parents that offering predictable, consistent, and loving care helps the infant learn trust, the first stage of psychosocial development according to Erikson. Ongoing stress, including child abuse, neglect, maternal depression, substance abuse, or family violence, can damage the growing brain (McCrory et al. 2010). Health care providers will want to emphasize the importance of positive nurturing and dependable relationships for optimal brain development. Besides positive early stimulation being necessary for optimal brain development, normal brain development requires good nutrition (Shonkoff and Phillips 2000).

3.3 Cultural Influences on Development

Health care providers need to recognize their own cultural biases and how it may affect their approach to certain aspects of the well-child visit. Early milestones, such as eating solid food, weaning from the breast or bottle, sleeping through the night, and toilet training, may occur at different ages and be considered normal in other cultures. Gaining this awareness and understanding will help the health provider to be more effective in serving families during the well-baby visit.

There are tools to help us understand family culture, such as the genogram, eco-map, and family functioning model (Minuchin 1974; Ruperto et al. 2001). These tools can help identify family structure, health history, strengths, resources, and health responses, beliefs, and practices. The childhood health assessment questionnaire (CHAQ) and child health questionnaire (CHQ) have also been adapted to a number of cultural groups (Ruperto et al. 2001).

Parental responses to their children's needs also vary by culture. Using a validated screening tool with high sensitivity, specificity, and reliability will help the provider to better determine which children need referrals. Once the child reaches kindergarten, children from all cultural backgrounds should be at similar development levels (Hagan et al. 2008).

3.4 Gross and Fine Motor Development

Gross and fine motor development occurs in a predictable sequential pattern from simple to more complex, going from general to specific. Infant motor behavior during the first 3 months of life is mostly reflexive. As these reflexes fade, babies use more specific conscious movements to help them explore and manipulate their environment. For example, newborns have their hands tightly fisted; by 2 months their hands are unfisted part of the time, and by 3 months, they are batting at and grabbing objects. Children's physical development allows them to explore their environment and gain strength and coordination. Allowing babies to physically explore their environment is also important for cognitive development.

3.5 Visual and Auditory Development

Visual and auditory development also follows sequential milestones and should be evaluated at each visit.

3.6 Language Development

Language begins with nonverbal behaviors during infancy, starting with vocalizations and crying. Infants have different cries that come to be understood by their parents and primary care providers as they interpret the child's needs (Sharp and Hillenbrand 2008). Language also develops according to a sequential pattern but requires the child to be able to hear and have normal oral and respiratory functioning. Any child with a delay in language should receive a full hearing evaluation. Children with feeding difficulties should also be evaluated for potential language delays.

3.7 Temperament

Infants have different temperaments; some may be very active, some may get easily frustrated, some are observers, and some are fussy. This influences how babies interact with their parents and others (Brazelton and Sparrow 2006; Turecki and Tonner 2000). Frequent infant crying may indicate maternal postpartum depression, or add to a stressed mother/infant bond. The matching or acceptance of the child's temperament with the mother usually leads to a better parent/child relationship. Infant temperament questionnaires can be used to better help parents understand their child's behavior and to provide guidance to parents on how to meet his/her needs.

3.8 Piaget's Theory of Cognitive Development

Jean Piaget developed cognitive learning theory based on his observations of the cognitive development and perceptions of children as they interacted with their environment. Piaget theorized that children are born with inherited potential for intellectual growth and they develop that potential by interacting with their environment. By acquiring information through the senses, processing it, and acting on it, children come to understand the relationships between objects and between themselves and the world. Cognitive development refers to how a person perceives, thinks, and gains understanding of the world through the interaction of genetic and learned factors (Beilin 1994).

Piaget organized his observations into cognitive stages of development from birth to adulthood. By understanding these states of how children learn, the health care provider will be better able to identify cognitive delays. These stages of development include sensorimotor, preoperational, concrete operational, and formal operation. The stages proceed from simple reflexive behavior and learning through the senses to using logic to solve complex problems as an adult (Piaget and Inhelder 1969). Piaget's Cognitive Stages of Development are described in his book: *The psychology of the young child* (Piaget and Inhelder 1969).

Sensorimotor (0–2 Years) Through learning about their senses, starting with reflexes, babies begin to utilize their sensory motor skills and build their cognitive ability to explore their environment. Their growing physical mobility to explore their world leads babies to develop their intellectual abilities.

This period has six substages:

Stage (1) Reflexes (Birth–1 Month)

The infant is focused on his/her own body and learns about the world through his/her sucking, grasping, looking, and other reflexes.

Stage (2) Primary Circular Reactions (1–4 Months)

Infants keep using the same reflexes repeatedly, such as opening and closing their hands or putting their fingers in their months and realizing it feels good.

Stage (3) Secondary Circular Reactions (4–8 Months)

During this stage the infant starts being aware of his/her environment and begins to be able to manipulate it—such as picking something up and dropping it, can make a game of it with a caregiver, and doesn't yet understand consequences of actions.

Stage (4) Coordination of Secondary Circular Reactions (8–12 Months)

Infant begins to see cause and effect when they do an action and may do something specific to get something or gain attention; for example at 8 months infants start to have object permanence, will take a block and put it from one hand into the other, and will play peekaboo with caregiver.

Stage (5) Tertiary Circular Reactions (12–18 Months)

Infant in this substage start to experiment with objects and people, have more physical ability and creativity, and will be better able to experiment within his/her environment.

Stage (6) Mental Representation (18–24 Months)

A toddler in this stage starts to have symbolic thought and can make a plan and formulate actions.

Preoperational (2–7 Years) In this stage problems are solved through representation of objects put into categories, the child's ability to communicate with words is developing (language), thoughts and language tend to be egocentric, and the child at first cannot solve conservation problems.

This stage is divided into two substages.

Preconceptual Thinking (2–4 Years): Child is developing representative thought and can categorize objects.

Intuitive Thinking (4–7 Years): The child starts to understand the concept of conservation.

Concrete Operation (7–11 Years): Child is able to do multiple cognitive operations based on variations in mass, size, and state, and is beginning to understand other people's point of view. Memory is increasing and the child can solve conservation problems.

Formal Operation (11 Years–Adult)**:** Child can think abstractly and use logic to solve problems. In this stage, intelligence is demonstrated through the logical use of symbols related to abstract concepts.

3.9 Erickson's Theory of Psychosocial Development

Eric Erikson, a developmental psychologist and psychoanalyst, observed how children develop socially, needing to successfully complete the task of one age group before moving on to the next task. His theory of five stages of psychosocial development across the life span is used as a major measure of psychosocial development.

Trust **Versus** ***Mistrust Stage (Birth to 1 Year):*** The child learns to trust in others through consistency of care, sucking, being fed and held, and in general having his/her needs met. If the child is not able to establish trust, for example being let cry, he/she develops mistrust, and will not engage with others.

Autonomy* Versus *Shame Stage (Ages 1–3 Years): Toddler learns to develop autonomy and influence the environment directly. Caregiver will want to offer options to the child so the child can be autonomous and consider options on his/her own. If the child is not permitted to develop autonomy, the child will become shy and doubt about himself/herself.

Initiative* Versus *Guilt Stage (3–6 Years): In this stage the child needs praise for his/her accomplishments, including play, art, and behavior. Development is dysfunctional if the child demonstrates fearful or pessimistic behaviors.

Industry* Versus *Inferiority Stage (6–12 Years): The child learns confidence and uses his/her creative energies to influence the environment. The child needs praise from home, school, neighbors, and friends about their accomplishments, industry, and teamwork. Development is dysfunctional if the child demonstrates feelings of inadequacy or mediocrity, and lacks confidence.

Identity* Versus *Role Confusion Stage (12–19 Years): During the teen years, the youngster develops a coherent sense of self and can make plans for his/her future work and education. Development is dysfunctional if he/she is unable to identify his/her perception of self and his/her educational and vocational direction. In this stage, peers and role models provide the child with support (Sanders 2013).

3.10 Freud's Theory of Psychosexual Development

Psychiatrist Sigmund Freud described stages of psychosexual development that are in use today: oral, anal, phallic, latent, and genital. He also postulated that each stage needed to be successfully completed before the child could go on to the next stage of psychosexual development. If any of the stages are fixated on, there is not enough libidinal energy for this stage to develop untroubled (Freud and Brill 1995).

Oral Stage (0–1 Year): During this stage, the infant's pleasure centers are in the mouth and the baby uses his/her mouth to explore his/her word by sucking and tasting.

Anal Stage (1–3 Years): This stage is centered around the rectum, but can also include bladder functions. During this stage children learn to control the expulsion of feces and urine, causing their libidinal energy to become focused in this area.

Phallic Stage (3–6 Years): In this stage the area of gratification comes from the penis for boys and the clitoris for girls. Masturbation is common for both. Boys fall in love with their mothers and girls fall in love with their fathers. Boys note that women have no penis and develop the Oedipal complex, which is fear of castration. Due to this fear, it is important to set guidelines and boundaries around masturbation, limiting it to the bedroom and bathroom. Young girls develop the *Electra* complex, after they come to the realization that they have no penis and look to the father as a substitute for the loss that they perceive. This is termed "penis envy."

Latency Phase (6–12 Years): In this phase, the child begins to make connections to siblings, other children, and adults and it will be a relatively stressless time psychosexually.

Genital Phase (12 Years and Older): Starting at puberty, the child will develop opposite sex relationships.

3.11 Kohlberg's Theory of Moral Development

Psychologist Lawrence Kohlberg developed a six-stage theory of moral development in children, building on Piaget's theory of cognitive development. Kolberg's theory specifies six stages of moral development, arranged in three levels: preconventional/premoral; conventional/role conformity; and postconventional/self-accepted moral principles (Cherry 2014; Davis 2014).

Level I: Preconventional/Premoral

In this stage the child responds to rules and the consequences for following them or not.

Level II: Conventional/Role Conformity

Children want to do behaviors and be seen as good boys and good girls. Reward and punishment guide a child's choices.

Level III: Postconventional/Self-Accepted Moral Principles

Acts are judged by the intentions that prompted it. Rules and judgments become more based on the needs and desires of others. Conflicts will arise between the needs of individuals and those of society.

References

Beilin H (1994) Jean Piaget's enduring contribution to developmental psychology. In: Parke RD, Ornstein PA, Zahn-Waxler C (eds) A century of developmental psychology. American Psychological Association, Washington, DC, pp 257–290

Brazelton TB, Sparrow J (2006) Touchpoints: birth to three, 2nd edn. Da Capo Press, The Perseus Books Group, Boston, MA

Brazelton TB (1992) Touchpoints: emotional and behavioral development. Addison-Wesley, Reading, MA

Brazelton TB, Sparrow J (2003) The touchpoints TM model of development. The Touchpoints Center. http://www.brazeltontouchpoints.org/wp-content/uploads/2011/09/Touchpoints_Model_of_Development_Aug_2007.pdf. Accessed 1 Jun 2015

Cech DJ, Martin ST (eds) (2011) Functional movement development across the life span, 3rd edn. Saunder, Philadelphia, PA

Cherry K (2014) Kohlberg's Theory of moral development: Stages of moral development. About.com Psychology. http://psychology.about.com/od/developmentalpsychology/a/kohlberg.htm. Accessed 24 Jul 2014

Davis D (2014) Kohlberg's moral stages. Haverford College. http://www.haverford.edu/psych/ddavis/p109g/kohlberg.stages.html. Accessed 24 July 2014

Freud S, Brill AA (1995) The basic writings of Freud. Random House, New York, NY

Gopnik A, Meltzoff AN, Kuhl PK (2000) The scientist in the crib: what early learning tells us about the mind. William Morrow Paperbacks, New York, NY

Hagan JF, Shaw JS, Duncan P (eds) (2008) Bright futures: guidelines for health supervision of infants, children, and adolescents, 3rd edn. American Academy of Pediatrics, Elk Grove Village, IL

Lally JR (2013) For our babies: ending the invisible neglect of America's infants. Teachers College Press, New York, NY

McCrory E, De Brito SA, Viding E (2010) Research review: the neurobiology and genetics of maltreatment and adversity. J Child Psychol Psychiatry 51(10):1079–1095

Minuchin S (1974) Families and family therapy. Harvard University Press, Cambridge, MA

Piaget J, Inhelder B (1969) The psychology of the child, 2nd edn. Basic Books, New York, NY

Ringwalt S (2008) Developmental screening and assessment instruments with an emphasis on social and emotional development of young children ages birth through five. National Early Childhood Technical Assistance Center–NECTAC. http://www.nectac.org/~pdfs/pubs/screening.pdf. Accessed 9 Jul 2016

Ruperto N, Ravelli A, Pistorio A et al (2001) Cross-cultural adaptation and psychometric evaluation of the Childhood Health Assessment Questionnaire (CHAQ) and the Child Health Questionnaire (CHQ) in 32 countries. Review of the general methodology. Clin Exp Rheumatol 19(4 Suppl 23):S1–S9

Sanders RA (2013) Adolescent psychosocial, social, and cognitive development. Pediatr Rev 34(8):354–359

Sharp HM, Hillenbrand K (2008) Speech and language development and disorders in children. Pediatr Clin N Am 55(5):1159–1173

Shonkoff JP, Phillips D, Board on Children, Youth and Families (2000) From neurons to neighborhoods: the science of early childhood development. National Academy Press, Washington, DC

Turecki S, Tonner L (2000) The difficult child, rev. ed. Random House, New York, NY

Health History and Physical Exam 4

4.1 Introduction

Taking a complete health history is the health care practitioner's opportunity to establish a relationship with the family and the child, begin to understand the family dynamics, as well as obtain relevant health information. The family-centered approach is demonstrated by asking parents and children about their concerns, having the physical exam that follows reflect these concerns, reviewing appropriate screenings, identifying child and family needs, and developing strength-based approaches to them, including services, preventive strategies, and physical and emotional supports. The health care provider observes if the parents respond to and recognize their children's needs and whether they are comfortable in caring for their child. See the box below, Taking the Health History, for details of the questions to be included in the health history.

While taking the health history, information is gathered regarding all the families' needs. The health care provider assesses what other services the child and family need and how to help obtain them. Usually, this information is discussed near the end of the visit as part of anticipatory guidance and is included in the health care plan. Does the family need food stamps; do they need housing aid? Are there services that do not require legal immigration status for the child? Is a referral sufficient or does the family need a warm handoff (be taken personally to another service provider)? Are there sufficient providers in the community for these services? Do the access rules limit participation of families? Are services colocated in one building or integrated across service systems in different locations? Can the services available in the practice be more comprehensive and coordinated with other service systems such as mental health, early care and education, and child welfare—child abuse and neglect services? These challenges may need to be addressed by joint advocacy efforts with colleagues and organizations in your locality or state. Providers will want to familiarize themselves with the websites for local departments of Health, Education, and Child Welfare and websites for national federal programs such as WIC (Women, Infants, and Children Nutrition Program), Medicaid, Section 8 housing, and SNAP (Supplemental Nutrition Assistance Program (food stamps) and have handouts with this information for families. See

D. Kramer, *Primary Well-Being: Case Studies for the Growing Child*,
DOI 10.1007/978-3-319-56708-2_4

Chap. 5, The Primary Care Provider as Advocate, for a description of this important role of health provider as advocate for families.

During the history and the physical exam, the health care professional incorporates play to establish a relationship with the child. Children can handle real equipment in the office area and play equipment in the waiting area. Stuffed animals can be examined prior to examining the child and the practitioner can talk to the child throughout the examination explaining what they are doing. The physical exam is done with different approaches and sequences based on the age of the child. Be equipped with distracters, like a bright object hanging on your stethoscope or a rattle or small block for the child or mother to hold. Other ways to make the child comfortable are to talk to the child, sing, and make silly noises, smile, and use a soft, gentle voice. For all ages, make sure that the stethoscope is warm and the temperature in the room is warm.

4.1.1 Infant Exam (0–2 Years)

At this age, the child is held on the parent's lap and the examination begins with the heart and lung sounds. Parent or provider needs only to take off the child's shirt or top for the examination to maintain his/her body warmth. As the exam continues, bottom clothes are removed from the lower areas. Leave the diaper on until you are ready to check that area.

Start the exam by listening to the heart and lung sounds. The baby can be feeding during this portion of the exam or distracted by making a clicking sound, having a toy for the infant to look at on the stethoscope or other visual distraction. Then do the abdominal exam. First inspect the abdomen and then auscultate it and then percuss and palpate it. The rest of the examination proceeds from head to toes, beginning with carefully palpating the fontanels. Leave the examination of the eyes, ears, and month until the end because these are the most invasive exams and the baby may be crying. Save testing the Moro reflex for the very last item.

4.1.2 Toddler Exam (2–3 Years)

The exam of the toddler begins in the same way as the infant. Children at around age 18 months are fearful of "white coats" and of the examination. Children this age are best able to cooperate if play is interwoven in the exam. Singing familiar songs such as "head shoulder knees and toes," counting fingers, and offering praise and smiles for cooperation will help the child adjust to the health provider. The exam begins with assessing the heart, lungs, and abdomen. Parents may need to help restrain the child if the child is resisting, especially when the ears are examined.

4.1.3 Preschooler (3–5 Years)

Preschool children usually like standing or sitting alone with the parent next to them. This exam can be done from head to toe incorporating play and manipulating the equipment that are participating in the exam. If the child is not cooperating, make the exam a game as you would with a toddler. Request that the child self-undress, except for underpants which can be kept on. Again, offer equipment for inspection and briefly demonstrate use. Explain what and why you are examining to engage the child as you proceed throughout the exam; for example say "Let's check how strong your muscles are" during the neurological/musculoskeletal exam. Offering children choices when possible such as "do you want me to check your right leg first or your left one?" also promotes cooperation.

4.1.4 School Age (5–12 Years)

School-age children are usually cooperative for the exam and it is done in a head-to-toe manner. It is important to insure privacy for all school-age children. Starting at around age 9, give the child a choice whether they want their parent in the room or not during the history and physical exam. It is important to ask the school-age child if there are any concerns about their body or their health, and about any issues at home or school, or with peers, such as bullying. Open discussion about what is being examined and why it is important will engage the child and also educate the child about their body. Examination of the genitalia is done last and reassuring statements about the child's body should be said throughout the examination.

4.1.5 Adolescent

This exam proceeds from head to toes with the adolescent given the option of parental presence. The teen should be given a gown and only the areas being examined at the time should be exposed. Respect the child's need for privacy and explain your findings during the examination. Especially with adolescents it is important to reassure them on their body image and any normal findings. The breast should be examined as part of the normal health-to-toe sequence. Examine the genitalia as any other body part, but leave till the end. It is important to reinforce confidentiality prior to discussing drug and alcohol use and sexual activity.

The following guide to taking the health history should be used at the initial visit of the provider and family. A form is usually provided to the parent in the waiting room asking for the following information. The provider reviews the information during the exam and may ask follow-up questions.

4.2 Taking the Health History

(Starred items should be included in histories for children of all ages)

1. *Identifying information
   (a) Child's name
   (b) Parents' names (The health care practitioner should refer to the child's father not the mother's husband.)
   (c) Address
   (d) Phone numbers, home, cell
   (e) Child's date and place of birth
   (f) Child's sex
   (g) Child's religion or ethnicity
   (h) Who the informant is
   (i) Date of interview
2. *Reason for visit
   (a) Are there any questions or concerns?
   (b) How is the child feeling?
   (c) How are the parents feeling?
   (d) If they are having any difficulties, when did it start?
   (e) What are the symptoms? (onset, location, duration, associated symptoms, aggravating factors, relieving factors)
   (f) What did they do that worked or didn't work for the symptoms, including complementary therapies?
   (g) What do the parents/caregiver think caused this situation?
   (h) Are there any mind-body interventions you as a parent think would be helpful?
3. Past history
   (a) Prenatal history
      (i) Was it a planned pregnancy?
      (ii) When did prenatal care begin?
      (iii) Were there any complications with the mother during pregnancy?
      (iv) Did the other take any medications, drink alcohol, smoke, or use other drugs or supplements during pregnancy?
   (b) Labor and delivery
      (i) Where was the baby born and who did the delivery?
      (ii) Gestational age, birth weight, length, head circumference, and Apgar score.
      (iii) Was this a vaginal or caesarean delivery?
      (iv) Were there any complications during delivery or after?
      (v) What was baby's weight at discharge from the hospital?
   (c) Feeding of baby
      (i) Is the baby primarily breastfed or bottle-fed?
      (ii) If bottle-fed, what type of formula is used and frequency of eating?
      (iii) Feeding history

1. If currently breastfeeding; how frequently does your child nurse?
   (a) For how long was baby breastfed?
2. If bottle-feeding, what formula, how frequently, and how much at each feeding?
   (a) For how long was your child bottle-fed?

(d) *Is there a history of any past injuries, illness, or operations of the child?
(e) *Are there any allergies in the child (food, medication, or environmental)?
(f) *Is the child taking any medications, including herbs? Why? How much? Is it helping?
(g) *Are there any other medical problems besides the current complaint?
(h) *Is there any current use of alcohol, drugs, or tobacco in the home?
(i) *What is the child's immunization history?
(j) Growth and development history
   (i) *Growth-general
      1. Has the child been consistent on the growth curve in terms of pattern for height, weight, and head circumference?
      2. Is anyone concerned about the child's growth?
   (ii) Milestones of development
      1. Do you remember when your child first:
         (a) Smiled
         (b) Rolled over
         (c) Able to be propped in sitting position
         (d) Sat without support
         (e) Crawled
         (f) Walked
         (g) Got his first tooth
         (h) Said a word, two words, used sentences of 3–4 words
         (i) Fed self
         (j) Drank from cup
         (k) Used fork and spoon
   (iii) Toilet training
      1. At what age was your child toilet trained for urination, both day and night?
      2. At what age was your child toilet trained for bowel movements, both day and night?
      3. If not toilet trained, about how many wet diapers and bowel movements does the child have each day?

(k) *Sleep
   (i) What is the average number of hours your child sleeps?
   (ii) If he/she takes naps, how many and for how long does he/she sleep?
   (iii) Does your child have any nightmares or night awakenings?

(l) *Family history
   (i) Is there a history of any diseases or chronic conditions in family members? (anemia, cardiac disease, diabetes, hypertension, respiratory illness, renal disease, cancer, neurological disorders, sickle cell disease, alcoholism, smoking, mental illness, or substance abuse)

4. *Review of systems
   (a) Skin:
      (i) Are there any rashes or birthmarks?
      (ii) Are there any skin conditions, including the hair and the nails?
   (b) Head:
      (i) Does your child have any headaches or head injuries?
   (c) Eyes:
      (i) Does your child have any vision or eye problems?
      (ii) Has your child had vision test?
      (iii) Does your child wear glasses or contacts?
      (iv) Does your child have trouble seeing the board at front of the classroom?
   (d) Ears:
      (i) Does your child have any hearing or ear problems?
      (ii) Does your infant turn toward sound and to your voice?
      (iii) Has child had a hearing test?
      (iv) Does the child wear headphones to listen to music or other sound recordings?
   (e) Nose:
      (i) Does your child have any discharge or nose bleeding?
      (ii) Does your child have any breathing difficulties?
   (f) Throat:
      (i) Does your child have any throat problems, hoarseness, or infections?
      (ii) Has your child been to the dentist, how often, and any treatments?
   (g) Cardiovascular system:
      (i) Is there any history of cardiac disease or heart murmurs?
      (ii) Is there any history of high cholesterol or high blood pressure in the family?
      (iii) Does your child get any shortness of breath?
   (h) Respiratory system:
      (i) Does the child have any breathing problems or history of respiratory infections?
      (ii) Does the child have any coughing or snoring?
      (iii) Does it seem as if your child stops breathing briefly or is catching their breath in their sleep (sleep apnea)?
      (iv) Does anyone in the house smoke? If so, where do they smoke, i.e., in the house or apartment? If outside, do they change clothes when they return indoors?
   (i) Gastrointestinal system:
      (i) Does your child ever have abdominal pain?
      (ii) Has your child had any recent weight loss?
      (iii) Does your child have any diarrhea, constipation, vomiting, regurgitation or heartburn, or nausea?
      (iv) Does your child wake with a bad taste in his/her month?

   (v) Does your child have any bloody stools, rectal bleeding, anal itching, or fissures?
 (j) Genitourinary system:
   (i) Has your child ever had any urinary tract infections or discharges, or blood in the urine?
   (ii) Does your child have any frequency of burning during urination?
   (iii) What is the urinary stream's appearance?
   (iv) Does your child have any abnormalities of the penis or testes, or sexually transmitted diseases (STI)?
   (v) Beginning from age 9 on, ask the child: are you sexually active?
 (k) Gynecologic:
   (i) What is your child's menstrual history (number of years, how many days, how often)?
   (ii) Does your child experience cramps or have any clots?
   (iii) Does your child have any vaginal discharge, bleeding, or itching?
 (l) Musculoskeletal:
   (i) Does your child have any pain, movement, swelling, or structural problems?
   (ii) Does your child have a history of any strains, sprains, or fractures?
   (iii) Is your child able to engage in outdoor play and sports?
 (m) Neurologic:
   (i) Does your child have any neurological diagnosis or disorder?
   (ii) Does your child have any history of headaches, daydreaming, or seizures?
   (iii) Does your child have a history of any movement disorders?
   (iv) Does your child have a history of loss of consciousness?
   (v) Does your child have any tremors (ticks)?
   (vi) Does your child have any history of ADHD, learning disability, or developmental delay?
   (vii) Does your child have any behavior issues?
     1. Is there any biting, pica (eating nonfood items), head banging, rocking, walking on toes, flapping hands, echolalia, or unusual movements?
     2. Are there frequent temper tantrums?
   (viii) Does your child have any history of mental illness?
 (n) Endocrine:
   (i) Does your child have any endocrine disorders, any problems with growth or sexual maturation?

5. *Psychosocial history
 (a) Who are the family members who live in the home?
 (b) What is their relationship to the child?
 (c) Are the family members working outside of the home?
 (d) Who cares for the child during the day and at night?
 (e) What are your sources of financial support?
 (f) Who do you turn to when you need help?

(g) Do you have someone you can borrow $10 from?
(h) What are the daily exercises and activities the child and family engage in?
(i) What electronic devices with screens are in use in the home and how often is the child using them, a couple of hours daily, once a week, rarely?
(j) Where do family members go for health care?
(k) When was the child's last checkup and dental visit?

6. *Home life
   (a) Ask the child:
      (i) Do you have your own room, own bed, and own toys?
      (ii) Do you share a room?
      (iii) Do you have your own personal space—where you can work, play, sleep, or read?
      (iv) Do you live in a house or an apartment?
      (v) Is there an outdoor play area?
      (vi) What stresses you out?
      (vii) How can people tell that you are stressed out?
      (viii) How do you relax?
      (ix) What do you do for fun?
      (x) Who do you do it with?
      (xi) Tell me about your friends?
      (xii) What things are easy for you and what things are hard?
      (xiii) If you were given three wishes what would they be?
   (b) Ask the parent:
      (i) Is your home in a safe neighborhood?
      (ii) Is there a safe playground near your home where your child can play?
      (iii) Are there things that need repair in your home:
         1. Are their holes in the walls, leaking water, evidence of mold, sighting of insects and rodents, and peeling paint?
         2. Is your home older than 1978?
         3. Has the home been tested for lead paint?
         4. Is your home near a highway or off a major thoroughfare where there are a lot of fumes from traffic?
      (iv) How far away is the school your child attends?
      (v) Is the school safe?
      (vi) How do you discipline your child?
   (c) *School life.
      (i) Questions for the child:
         (a) Tell me what it is like in school?
         (b) Name three friends?
         (c) What are your classes like?
         (d) What subjects do you like best?
         (e) What subjects do you do well in?
         (f) Are there any subjects that you think you need extra help in?
         (g) Are there any bullies at school?
         (h) Do you feel safe at school?

(i) What types of sports or games do you like to play?
(j) What are your favorite activities?

(ii) Questions for the parents
(a) What type of play does your child engage in?
(b) Does he interact well with the children in his daycare, class, and afterschool programs?
(c) Do you have any concerns regarding your child's learning?
(d) Is your child in any special class or program?
(e) What is your child's behavior at school?
(f) Does your child enjoy going to school or does he/she give you a hard time about going to school?
(g) How much time does your child spend using electronic devices, including smartphones, tablets, and computers or television, each day?

7. *Nutritional assessment
(a) What are your favorite foods and what foods do you like least?
(b) Ask the child for a food history for a 24-h period during the week, e.g., what did you eat yesterday morning until night and on one day of the weekend.
(c) Do you skip meals?
(d) Do you argue with your parents over food?
(e) What type of milk do you drink?
(f) What fruits and vegetables are served?
(g) Who is present at mealtimes?
(h) Are you eating in secret?
(i) Are you happy with your current weight?
(j) Have you ever tried to lose weight by vomiting, taking pills, using a laxative, or not eating?

8. Sexual history
(a) For the child: Are you sexually active or do you have any sexual concerns?
(b) Ask the child: are you using birth control and what method are you using?

9. Selective screening guidelines
(a) Overall child development, autism, and behavioral and emotional concerns
(i) Consult the American Academy of Pediatrics, Screening and Assessment web page for recommendations of screening tools and access information at http://www2.aap.org/sections/dbpeds/screening.asp.
(ii) Also see Council on Children With Disabilities; Section on Developmental Behavioral Pediatrics; Bright Futures Steering Committee; Medical Home Initiatives for Children With Special Needs Project Advisory Committee (2006). Identifying infants and young children with developmental disorders in the medical home: An algorithm for developmental surveillance and screening. *Pediatrics, 118*(1), 405–20.
(iii) For actual forms and other recommendations for tools consult McInerny, T.K., Ed. (McInerny 2009). *American Academy of*

Pediatrics Textbook of Pediatric Care: Tools for Practice. Forest Grove, IL: American Academy of Pediatrics and the American Academy of Pediatrics website: www.aap.org.

(iv) Autism:
   1. All children at ages 18 and 24 months should be screened for Autism along with a general developmental screening (Gupta et al. 2007).

(v) Other tools may be appropriate as well. See *American Academy of Pediatrics Textbook of Pediatric Care: Tools for Practice* above and the American Academy of Pediatrics web site: www.aap.org.

(vi) Family relationship assessment
   1. FACES scale (Family Adaptability and Cohesion Scale)
      (a) Use for all families to assess family functioning and stress at first visit (Culbert et al. 2010)
   2. Family Assessment Device (FAD)
      (a) Assesses the interactions between members of the family and its structural and organizational patterns
      (b) It looks at communication, problem solving, roles, effect of responsiveness, effect of involvement, and behavior control as well as general family functioning (Epstein et al. 1983)

(vii) General Development:
   1. All children should have general developmental screens at ages 9, 18, and 30 months (American Academy of Pediatrics 2006).
   2. For children aged 0–6 years, use the Denver Developmental Screening Test.
   3. Ages & Stages Questionnaires (ASQ) has specific scales for individual ages.

(viii) Social-emotional development
   1. At every visit the social-emotional state of the child should be assessed during the health interview and observation and discussion throughout the exam.
   2. If the health care provider has concerns regarding social emotional issues, the appropriate questionnaire should be administered to further assess the concern.
   3. The following tools may be appropriate for further assessment:
      (a) Ages and Stages Questionnaire-Social-Emotional (ASQ:SE)
      (b) Pediatric Symptom Checklist
      (c) Patient Health Questionnaire
      (d) Screen for Child Anxiety-Related Emotional Disorders (SCARED)
      (e) Liebowitz Social Anxiety Scale
      (f) CRAFFT—Brief Screening Test for Adolescent Substance Abuse
      (g) TABS: Temperament and Atypical Behavior Scale
   4. For ADHD:
      (a) NICHQ ADHD Evaluation forms for Parent, Teacher, Informants (National Initiative for Children's Healthcare Quality and American Academy of Pediatrics)

5. For all parents who have a new baby:
   (a) Administer the Edinburgh Postnatal Depression Scale (EPDS)
6. For parents who have expressed the presence of violence in the home:
   (a) Intimate Partner Violence Screening Questionnaire
   (b) Violence History Questionnaire: FISTS

(ix) Speech issues
   1. Use DASE: Denver Articulation Screening Examination

(b) Anemia screening (American Academy of Pediatrics 2004; Centers for Disease Control and Prevention 2011):
   (i) Screen at 4-month visit if baby was premature or had low birth weight
   (ii) Screen if not receiving iron-fortified formula or low iron
   (iii) Screen if early introduction of cow's milk—before one year of age
   (iv) Screen at 18 months; 2-, 3-, 4-, 5-year visit if the child is on a low iron-nonmeat diet, if there are environmental factors (lives in poverty), or if at risk due to special needs
   (v) Screen at 6–10-year visits for children who are on vegetarian diets and not getting iron supplementation
   (vi) Screen adolescents 11–21 years
      1. Screen annually any female with history of menstrual with extensive blood loss, other blood loss, history of iron deficiency, iron-deficient diet
      2. All other nonpregnant adolescents should be screened every 5 years

(c) Dyslipidemia screening (American Academy of Pediatrics, Committee on Nutrition 1998; Hagan et al. 2008)
   (i) Screen if there is a family history of cardiac disease prior to the age of 55 or if you are not able to obtain their history.
   (ii) Screen adolescents who smoke, are overweight, have elevated blood pressure, diabetes mellitus, physical inactivity, and diet high in saturated fats and cholesterol.
   (iii) If the child is overweight, the BMI for age is in the 85–94th percentile with no additional risk factors, do a fasting lipid profile.
   (iv) If BMI for age is in the 85–94th percentile with risk factors, obtain a fasting glucose, aspartate aminotransferase (AST), and alanine aminotransferase (ALT).
   (v) If the child is obese, and the BMI is greater than the 95th percentile, an AST, ALT, blood urea nitrogen (BUN), and creatinine should be done.
   (vi) For a handout of guidelines for cardiovascular health see National Heart, Lung, and Blood Institute (2012). Expert Panel on Integrated Guidelines for Cardiovascular Health and Risk Reduction in Children and Adolescents FULL REPORT: www.nhlbi.nih.gov/files/docs/guidelines/peds_guidelines_full.pdf

(d) *Lead screening
   (i) Screen at ages 6, 9, 12, and 18 months and yearly from 2 to 6 years (American Academy of Pediatrics 1998), especially if family lives in or frequently visits housing built before 1978 or child goes to care or visits regularly in older buildings.

(ii) Screen if child has a sibling diagnosed with lead poisoning.
(iii) Any refugee child from 6 months to 16 years needs to be screened (Centers for Disease Control 2006).

(e) For more details and recommendations on screening for each visit, consult the Bright Futures, American Academy of Pediatrics (2014) Recommendations for Preventive Pediatric Health Care <http://www.aap.org/en-us/professional-resources/practice-support/Periodicity/Periodicity%20Schedule_FINAL.pdf>.

4.3 Pediatric Physical Exam

The pediatric exam differs from the adult exam in a variety of ways. In pediatrics, we measure children's height, weight, head circumference, and body mass index the way it is plotted out on the standard growth chart. Children are growing in a healthy way when they remain in the same percentile over time. Children should be within two standard deviations of each measurement. Generally the average finding of at least two measurements of one site is recorded.

Percentiles: The arm circumference is an indirect measure of muscle mass. The midpoint is measured with a paper tape. Percentiles for arm circumference and triceps skinfolds (body mass index) in children are rated from the 5th to 95th percentiles. These values are plotted on a percentile growth chart.

Children of different families and ethnic backgrounds may fall within different percentiles as compared to the general population. It is important for the health care provider to assess whether the child is continuing to grow within the percentile that they are in, in each of the different measurements. Growth charts that are commonly used are from the National Center for Health Statistics, and range from the 3rd percentile to the 97th percentile (Centers for Disease Control and Prevention 2000). A child is measured according to his/her own growth curve; it is helpful to show the growth chart to parents and explain this during the exam.

Temperature: Body temperature is measured during routine pediatric visits in different ways depended on the age of the child and the situation. For neonates, a core body temperature between 36.5 and 37.6 °C is desirable, taken through the ear (aural) or axillary. A desirable rectal temperature would be 37–37.5 °C. Whenever possible axillary temperature is recommended as it avoids an intrusive procedure and eliminates the risk of rectal perforation.

Body Proportions: Body proportions change during the child's development. The circumference of the chest is less than that of the head at birth by about 2 cm. At around 6 months of age, the head circumference and chest circumference are about equivalent. Lengthening of the lower extremities takes place during the last 6 months of infancy to help foster readiness for walking.

Teeth: Babies' first teeth usually erupt at around 6 months of age, followed by a new one monthly. Children at around 6 years of age lose their first set of teeth and develop their adult teeth.

Pulse: Apical pulse is used in children under 2 years of age, counted for one full minute. Pulses can be taken radially after 2 years of age.

Respiration: One counts the respiratory rate in children by observing the infant's abdominal movements, since respirations are primarily diaphragmatic. Respiratory rates in older children can be measured like adults; both are measured for a full minute.

Ears: To position for visualizing the eardrum, the health care provider should pull the pinna down and back if the child is below 3 years of age and pull the pinna up and back after the exam.

4.4 Adolescent Exam

When doing a history on the adolescent patient, the provider will have additional considerations. Speak to the teen and the parent separately as well as together and establish a relationship of respect with both. Explain the role of a health care provider and that the primary goal is the health of the adolescent. Tell both parent and adolescent that information is needed separately from them and time will be spent asking the teen about his/her concerns. Know your state's confidentially and consent laws and describe how they are met in the health practice. Also explain the limits on confidentiality if the adolescent or anyone else can be physically harmed by homicide, suicide, or sexual abuse. Emphasize that the information the teen is sharing with the health provider is very personal but it is important for understanding the adolescent's health and will not be shared with his/her parents.

It is especially important with adolescents for the health care provider to listen carefully and show interest in their concerns. Note hesitations in speech and the body language of the teen, and try to articulate the nonverbal messages you perceive as well as show that you have heard the verbal messages. Strive to be nonjudgmental in gathering all the information needed to understand and help with the teen's concerns before offering advice and referrals. It will be helpful to know about community resources and have a supply of clear and informative fact sheets and booklets that address the typical issues of concern to adolescents, such as facts on substance abuse, sexuality, contraception, menstruation, sexually transmitted diseases, and coping with stress and depression.

Ask the parents what advice they would give on typical teen concerns, such as substance abuse and sex. Watching how the parent(s) and adolescent interact during the visit will help you understand what is discussed at home and how open they are with each other. Encourage the parent and teen to talk about these concerns together.

One important area to ask about is what responsibilities the teen has at home. Many parents make teens carry out specific chores in the home in order to get privileges. This method can also be used to ensure fair negotiations among family members.

The health care provider can use a framework tool to interview the adolescent to ensure review of all systems. The most popular tool is the HEEADSSS (Goldenring and Rosen 2004). The letters stand for:

H—household and home
E—Eating
A—Activities
D—Drugs
S—Sexuality
S—Suicide/depression
S—Safety/history of violence

The health care provider can use this tool to ask open-ended questions about the topics covered (see box below). The answers will give a snapshot of the teen's life and identify problem areas to focus on. If an undesired behavior is identified through the screening and it can be dealt with during the visit, the health care provider should state the desired behavior, offer health information on the behavior's negative effects, and talk about the benefit of change, and alternatives to the behavior. The aim is to have the teen commit to change, and set a goal and timeframe. The provider should offer support and resources, and set up a follow-up time.

HEADSSS Questionnaire

Household and Home:

Where do you live?
Who lives with you? What are relationships like?
Are there recent changes in living conditions? Do you have your own room?
Who can you talk to at home?
Is there anyone new living in the house? Has anyone left recently?
Have you ever lived away from home? Why?

Education and Employment:

What are your favorite subjects at school? What do you like least?
Are there any recent changes in your school performance, or learning issues, especially during transition points in sixth or ninth grade?
Plans for future employment?
Employment history—number of jobs, working conditions
Are there difficulties with reading or math?
Was there a need to change schools?
How does adolescent get along with teachers?
How does the adolescent feel that his/her life at school is?
What are future educational goals or employment plans?
Are you working and how much?

Where do you work?
What is it like to work there?

Eating:
What do you like or not like about your body?
Have there been any recent changes in your weight?
Have you dieted in the past year? How and how often?
Have you done anything else to manage your weight?
How much exercise do you get in a day? Week?
What do you think is a healthy diet?
How does that compare to the way you eat now?

Activities:
What do you and your friends do for fun?
What do you and your family do for fun?
Do you participate in any sports?
Do you regularly attend a group or club?
How much reading do you do outside of school?
How much TV do you watch each day?—could be escape—inactivity leads to obesity
If driving, do they own a car

Drugs:
Do you take any over-the-counter or other drugs regularly?
Do any of your friends use drugs at parties or when "hanging out"? Have your friends tried to get you to do drugs?
Have you used alcohol, tobacco, or drugs? How often and how much?
Does anyone in your family use tobacco, alcohol, or other drugs?
Do you drive after you have been drinking?
Have you ever ridden with someone who was intoxicated?

Sexuality:
Have you ever been in a romantic relationship?
Tell me about people you have dated or tell me about your sex life?
Do you have a boyfriend or girlfriend
Have you ever thought about having sex
What would go into your decision to have sex with someone or become sexually active?
Have any of your relationships been sexual relationships?
What does the term "safe sex" mean to you?

Suicide/Depression:
How do you feel your life is going? Note if adolescent has severe problems, sudden changes in friends, or preoccupation with death.
Is there a family history of psychological problems or suicide?
Is there a history of suicide in friends?

Are there eating or sleeping difficulties? How long does it take you to fall asleep?—amount of sleep may increase or decrease
Overeating or poor appetite? May be precursor to suicidal behavior
Is adolescent bored with life? depression
Safety/Violence:
Family history of violence—number of fights and yelling within the last 3 months
Were there any episodes of pushing, shoving, or hitting—was injury incurred?
How does the parent discipline child?
Does the adolescent know how to avoid fights?
Violence Prevention:
What are the consequences of fighting in the street or at home? What are some ways to avoid fights?
How can children avoid conflicts? If you have a problem with me, let's talk about it. Walking away from a fight.
Ask for solutions to potential violence.
Hypothetical situations what would child do?
How do you seek out help?
How can you solve a disagreement in a nonviolent manner?
What are the consequences of violence?
Sources: *Goldenring, J.M. and Rosen, D.S. (2004). Getting into adolescent heads: An essential update.* Contemporary Pediatrics *21(4), 64–90.*
Gupta, VB, Hyman, SL, and Jackson, CP (2007). Identifying children with autism early? *Pediatrics 119,* 152–153.

Another behavioral screening tool for use with adolescents up to age 21 is the CRAFFT Screening Tool, available from Children's Hospital, in Boston, Massachusetts. CRAFFT is a mnemonic acronym of first letters of key words in six screening questions. The questions should be asked exactly as written. The CRAFFT is recommended by the American Academy of Pediatrics' Committee on Substance Abuse. It consists of a series of six questions developed to screen adolescents for high-risk alcohol and other drug-use disorders simultaneously. It is a short, effective screening tool meant to assess whether a longer conversation about alcohol and other drug use is warranted.

Screening using the CRAFFT begins by asking the adolescent to "Please answer these next questions honestly"; telling him "Your answers will be kept confidential"; and then asking three opening questions. If the adolescent answers "No" to all three opening questions, the provider only needs to ask the adolescent the first of the six questions—the CAR question (see box). If the adolescent answers "Yes" to any one or more of the three opening questions, the provider asks all six CRAFFT questions. A pocket card with the CRAFFT questions is available for clinical use. The CRAFFT screen comes in a format for clinicians and a self-administered format for adolescents. The questions have been translated into several languages. Go to http://www.ceasar-boston.org/CRAFFT/index.php to learn more about CRAFFT.

The CRAFFT Screening Tool

C—Have you ever ridden in a CAR driven by someone (including yourself) who was "high" or had been using alcohol or drugs?

R–Do you ever use alcohol or drugs to RELAX, feel better about yourself, or fit in?

A–Do you ever use alcohol/drugs while you are by yourself, ALONE?

F—Do you ever FORGET things you did while using alcohol or drugs?

F—Do your family or FRIENDS ever tell you that you should cut down on your drinking or drug use?

T—Have you gotten into TROUBLE while you were using alcohol or drugs?

Sources: *The Center for Adolescent Substance Abuse Research. (2009)* The CRAFFT Screening Tool. *Accessed March 20, 2015 at:* http://www.ceasar-boston.org/CRAFFT/screenCRAFFT.php.

It is important to continuously review with parents their child's ongoing developmental milestones and assessments with safety in mind. Aspiration, falling, suffocation, drowning, poisoning, and burns are all preventable. Teach parents to childproof their home and to be aware of choking hazards and safety precautions as their child grows and becomes more mobile. This includes using gates; not leaving bathroom doors open; not leaving children unattended in bathtubs; not leaving washing pails in reach of children; storing poisons and choking hazards including plastic bags, Band-Aids, and balloons in a locked cabinet; storing wires and cords away from children's reach; and other precautions. Remind the parents that children put everything in their mouths as a way of learning. As the child starts rolling and moving to further explore his/her environment, childproofing the house becomes essential.

4.5 Using Teaching Plans for the Well-Child Visit

To best use the well-child visit to think about how the child and family are doing, it is good to have a teaching plan developed in advance. The plan will reflect the wide range of topics needed for optimal child health and development, strong families, and positive early learning.

Teaching Topics for Anticipatory Guidance

Note: We have included the following topics in our case studies throughout the book. At the end of each case study, which corresponds with a pediatric visit, the Bright Futures teaching plan for parents and for health professionals will be an excellent resource as well as your own additional teaching plans. All topics in this box are based on fostering development and wellness in the child and the family.

- Developmental Milestones and Celebrations
  - Early Intervention and Prevention
- Physical Development
- Cognitive Development
- Psychosocial Development
  - Play
  - Behavior appropriateness
  - Role of sports and teams
- Psychosexual Development
- Moral Development
- Building Good Mental Health—Parent(s) and Child
  - Temperament
  - Self-esteem
    Positive affirmations
    Heart math
    Emotional freedom technique (EFT)
    Parents expressing love
  - Depression screening in parents and other caregivers
  - What constitutes successful child rearing: building character, values, resilience, self-satisfaction
  - Developmental health
    Sense of personhood
    Interface in the world around them
- Nutrition, obesity, and brain development
- Safety
  - Physical and emotional
  - Bullying prevention
  - Violence, media, and technology
- Cultural Factors—Religion, Race, Ethnicity
- Family Factors—Economic, Social, Relationships, Empowerment
  - Impact of poverty and low income
  - Impact of privilege
  - Strengthening families

What are they empowered to do already/their strengths
What are their challenges and how can we turn them into strengths

Resources: *See the Bright Futures Tool and Resource Kit for parent handouts, assessment tools, and healthy living prescription pads at*: http://brightfutures.aap.org/tool_and_resource_kit.html

References

American Academy of Pediatrics. Committee on Environmental Health (1998) Screening for elevated blood lead levels. Pediatrics 101:1072–1078

American Academy of Pediatrics, Committee on Nutrition (2004) Iron deficiency. In: Kleinman RE (ed) Pediatrics nutrition handbook. Elk Grove, IL, American Academy of Pediatrics, pp 299–312

American Academy of Pediatrics, Committee on Nutrition (1998) Cholesterol in childhood. Pediatrics 101:141–147

American Academy of Pediatrics, Council on Children with Disabilities, Section on Developmental Behavioral Pediatrics, Bright Futures Steering Committee and Medical Home Initiatives for Children with Special Needs Project Advisory Committee (2006) Identifying infants and young children with developmental disorders in the medical home: an algorithm for developmental surveillance and screening. Pediatrics 118:405–420

Bright Futures, American Academy of Pediatrics (2014) Recommendations for preventive pediatric health care. http://www.aap.org/en-us/professional-resources/practice-support/Periodicity/Periodicity%20Schedule_FINAL.pdf. Accessed 24 July 2014

Binkley LS (2012) Bates' guide to physical examination and history taking, 11th edn. Lippincott, Williams & Wilkins, Philadelphia, PA

Burns CE et al (2009) Pediatric primary care: a handbook for nurse practitioners, 4th edn. W.B. Saunders, Philadelphia, PA

Centers for Disease Control and Prevention (2006) CDC lead poisoning prevention and treatment recommendations for refugee children. In: Lead poisoning prevention in newly arrived refugee children: tool kit. Centers for Disease Control and Prevention, Atlanta, GA. http://www.cdc.gov/nceh/lead/publications/refugeetoolkit/refugee_tool_kit.htm. Accessed 20 Mar 2014

Centers for Disease Control and Prevention. (2011). Iron and iron deficiency. Recommendations to prevent and control iron deficiency in the United States. http://www.cdc.gov/nutrition/everyone/basics/vitamins/iron.html. Accessed 17 Mar 2015

Centers for Disease Control and Prevention, National Center for Health Statistics (2000) CDC growth charts for the United States. Washington, DC, U.S. Centers for Disease Control. http://www.cdc.gov/growthcharts/clinical_charts.htm. Accessed 24 July 2014

Council on Children With Disabilities; Section on Developmental Behavioral Pediatrics; Bright Futures Steering Committee; Medical Home Initiatives for Children With Special Needs Project Advisory Committee (2006) Identifying infants and young children with developmental disorders in the medical home: an algorithm for developmental surveillance and screening. Pediatrics 118(1):405–420

Culbert TP, Maizes V, Mendenhall T, Becker DK (2010) Assessment and treatment planning in integrative pediatric practice. In: Culbert TP, Olness K (eds) Integrative pediatrics. Oxford University Press, New York, NY, pp 13–29. Chapter 2

Duderstadt K (2006) Pediatric physical examination. Elsevier, St. Louis, MO

Epstein NB, Bishop LM, Bishop D (1983) The McMaster Model view of healthy family functioning. J Marital Fam Ther 9:171–118

Goldenring JM, Rosen DS (2004) Getting into adolescent hears: an essential update. Contemp Pediatr 21(4):64–90

Gupta VB, Hyman SL, Jackson CP (2007) Identifying children with autism early? Pediatrics 119:152–153

Hagan JF, Shaw JS, Duncan P (eds) (2008) Bright futures: guidelines for health supervision of infants, children, and adolescents, 3rd edn. American Academy of Pediatrics, Elk Grove Village, IL

Harlor AD, Bower C, The Committee on Practice and Ambulatory Medicine, The Section on Otolaryngology-Head and Neck Surgery (2009) Clinical report—hearing assessment in infants and children: Recommendations beyond neonatal screening. Pediatrics 124(4):1252–1263

Hockenberry MJ, Wilson DW (2011) Wong's nursing care of infants and children, 9th edn. Elsevier/Mosby, New York, NY

Jarvis C (2012) Physical examination & health assessment, 6th edn. Elsevier, New York, NY

Kleinsorge C, Covitz LM (2012) Impact of divorce on children: developmental considerations. Pediatr Rev 33:147–155

McInerny TK (ed) (2009) American Academy of Pediatrics Textbook of pediatric care: tools for practice. American Academy of Pediatrics, Forest Grove, IL

Richardson B (ed) (2011) Pediatric primary care: practice guidelines for nurses. Jones & Bartlett Learning, Burlington, MA

Sanders RA (2013) Adolescent psychosocial, social, and cognitive development. Pediatr Rev 34(8):354–359

Seith D, Isakson E (2011) Who are America's poor children? Examining health disparities among children in the United States. Columbia University, School of Public Health, National Center for Children in Poverty, New York, NY

5 The Primary Care Provider as Advocate

Primary care providers in pediatrics are in the unique situation of being able to tell the real-life stories that would promote advocacy in support of specific legislative policies to benefit children. These providers are greatly concerned about creating a safe environment to nurture children's healthy growth and development. This includes making essential preventive services available to all children, such as immunization and developmental screenings, and providing follow-up with referrals to make sure that families get the services they need, and that public policy reflects the needs of infants, toddlers, and children across their developmental stages, especially those children that face additional challenges. The health profession is an important first responder and expert in the community and is an appropriate messenger to advocate for policies that promote child and family health and well-being (American Academy of Pediatrics 2015a).

The American Academy of Pediatrics has developed a legislative policy agenda that will enable a healthy start for children and their families and provides many tools on its website for pediatric providers. It also periodically updates its recommendations on many issues related to child well-being and family health (American Academy of Pediatrics 2015b). The AAP agenda includes the following:

1. All children have a Medical Home covered by insurance—a medical office with high-quality services that provide a range of supports for children and their families with coordination of care across health systems, and attention to social and emotional health and development including maternal depression.
2. Raising the minimum wage to address community poverty and expand access to poverty reduction programs such as food stamps, housing, and child care subsidies.
3. Instituting a Paid Family Leave Program in every state.
4. Integrating pediatric health and mental health in the primary care office.
5. Expanding access to a full range of immunizations, including meningococcal, HPV, and influenza.
6. Creating pediatric standards for urgent care centers.
7. Integrating children's socio-emotional well-being into physical health care and working with child care education programs to expand screening and health services.

D. Kramer, *Primary Well-Being: Case Studies for the Growing Child*,
DOI 10.1007/978-3-319-56708-2_5

8. Support for Early Literacy programs in the medical office, in libraries, and in other community settings, such as Reach Out and Read where providers distribute free books during office visits and have volunteers reading to children in the waiting room.
9. Ensure a healthy environment with lead testing, reducing air pollution, cleaning up chemical emissions, safe storage of guns and ammunition.
10. Promote good nutrition practices at home, at school, and in the community with laws that promote breastfeeding and require labeling of sugar content, reducing beverage size and access to sweetened snacks, having green gardens and fresh food carts in supermarket-poor neighborhoods.
11. Preventing human trafficking and treating its victims.

The key ingredient to successful advocacy is your passion. Also needed is commitment to change over time and patience to see the agenda passed and implemented. Think about the issues that your clients bring up when you are taking the health history. What stands out as the most challenging or needy? What could be remedied quickly; what will need a long-term program of advocacy? Choose what you care the most about and devote your advocacy efforts to that issue. Find colleagues who share your concerns about the issue or educate colleagues to join in advocating for change. Reach out to organizations that should be concerned about the issue. Engage the local chapter of the American Association of Pediatrics.

Look at the data and indicators of well-being available in your state and locality that show how your community or state is doing on the issue you select—its strengths and needs. For issues that do not have sufficient data, such as social-emotional development, you may need to start by advocating to develop an initial set of indicators to be able to chart progress (Isakson et al. 2011). Think about the different service systems and how they can provide screening and preventive services that impact your issue: health care promotion and prevention system; early care and education; and child welfare system; look for data collected by these systems that could become indicators of how these systems are doing in your state on the issue (Isakson et al. 2011). Data may come from federal data collection sources, e.g., information from national programs such as Head Start, from national surveys, from state or local departments of epidemiology, from universities and nonprofit organizations, or from research projects and foundations (Isakson et al. 2011).

Plan to make phone calls, send e-mails, and meet with local elected officials and statewide ones as well. Share your personal experiences related to the issues you are concerned about; tell the dramatic stories. Gather the facts in written material and leave it with the people you visit or send materials afterwards with a thank-you note.

A few basic rules to remember when meeting with policymakers (Ward 2015):

1. Be consistent.
2. Stick to one agenda item at the meeting.
3. Know your issue thoroughly and have your talking points organized beforehand.

4. Know your legislators and what interests them. What policies and laws have they supported in the past or currently?
5. Be passionate when you talk to policymakers and other constituents.
6. Learn to laugh when you win as well as loose.
7. Focus on the issue, not personalities—the issue doesn't go away; personnel change and need reminding about your issues.
8. Team up with other primary care providers and reach across to other service systems to gain wider support for the issues, both regional and statewide, such as children's associations, local and statewide professional organizations, early care and learning coalitions, and public or private state child-focused organizations. And don't forget about business leaders—they have children too and want to keep their employees productive and happy.
9. Reach out to top officials in your state as well as local elected ones.
10. Bring in diverse sectors of the community to advocate together and be sensitive to ethnic and cultural needs to reduce racial disparities (Bruner and Schor 2009).
11. Recognize that children in different age groups have particular needs and policy requirements.

In addition to the issues of concern to you as primary pediatric providers, get to know the services for children and the people who provide them (Docs for Tots 2015). Beyond knowing about the application process for Medicaid and health insurance options and programs available to children of undocumented immigrants as well as citizens (Children's Aid Society undated), providers should also visit a sampling of programs in the community that are geared to low-income families and children. Spend a few hours at a Head Start program or do a visit with an Early Head Start teacher or as a Nurse-Family Partnership home visitor. Go to an afterschool center in a low-income neighborhood and see the challenges the children face. Speak with youth about their dreams and frustrations. In other words, you are a part of the community and by making yourself available to the community you will better be able to advocate for its needs. Good advocacy and programs start where families are and build on community strengths (Bruner 2015).

References

American Academy of Pediatrics (2015a) Advocacy and policy: AAP policy. https://www.aap.org/en-us/advocacy-and-policy/pages/advocacy-and-policy.aspx. Accessed 27 March 2015

American Academy of Pediatrics (2015b) AAP health initiatives. https://www.aap.org/en-us/advocacy-and-policy/aap-health-initiatives/Pages/AAP-Health-Initiatives.aspx. Accessed 28 March 2015

Bruner C (2015) Health, equity and young children: pediatric roles. In: Talk presented at ground rounds, Thursday, March 19th at NYS pediatric advocacy conference. Icahn School of Medicine at Mount Sinai, New York, NY

Bruner C, Schor E (2009) Clinical health care practices and community building: addressing racial disparities in healthy child development. Ames, IA: National Center for Service Integration

(NCSI) Clearinghouse and The Child and Family Policy Center. http://www.finebynine.org/uploaded/Clinical%20Health%20Care%20Practices%20and%20Community%20Building.pdf. Accessed 28 March 2015

Children's Aid Society (undated) Know your rights: benefits for undocumented immigrants. http://www.childrensaidsociety.org/files/upload-docs/11-Benefits_for_Immigrants-1.pdf. Accessed 28 May 2015

Docs for Tots (2015) Medical home. http://docsfortots.org/what-we-do/medical-home. Accessed 28 March 2015

Isakson EA, Davidson LL, Higgins LB, Cooper JL (2011) State-level indicators for social-emotional development: building better systems. National Center for Children in Poverty, Columbia University Mailman School of Public Health, New York, NY

Ward E (2015) Legislative updates. Thursday, March 19th at NYS pediatric advocacy conference. Icahn School of Medicine at Mount Sinai, New York, NY

6 Complementary Medicine

Complementary and alternative therapy (CAM) in health care has been a topic of interest in the literature for a number of years. Many health care providers have found these alternative techniques helpful in their personal and professional lives as well as in their clinical practice (Lie and Boker 2006; Chaterji et al. 2007). Yet many health care providers have chosen not to incorporate complementary and alternative therapies into their practice. This may be because of the lack of sufficient evidence-based studies about CAM. In a large children's hospital study, 67% of pediatric staff recommended CAM to their patients, but those who used CAM personally were more likely to recommend the techniques (76% versus 45%) (Kundu et al. 2011). The study also showed very little communication between the CAM provider and the pediatrician. Health care providers need to be given tools to evaluate these therapies and integrate them in their own practice if they choose.

Using CAM in a health practice is not purely about managing an illness. CAM is about developing an understanding concerning the etiology of the illness. A CAM practitioner looks at their client's lifestyle for the physical, emotional, and spiritual components that promote wellness. They look at the adverse childhood experiences that research tells us create levels of toxic stress in the body and make chronic disease in adulthood and shorter life spans more likely (Anda et al. 2006; Felitti 2009; Shonkoff et al. 2012). CAM also incorporates many concepts from traditional Chinese medicine that center around energetic flow and clearing of blockages. While Western medicine incorporates the use of diet and exercise, CAM also looks at connecting different places on the body that often correlate with Chinese medicine energy pathways called meridian lines. These lines are used to promote healing and calmness in Chinese medicine, such as in acupuncture. These modalities that are included in this case study book can help decrease stress in children and are very important in thinking about their overall health and decreasing morbidity.

Part of practicing CAM includes being an active listener and being present for the client during the visit. The provider needs to find out if the client has ever used complementary and alternative methods, assess their development and behavior, and consider lifestyle factors (including spiritual and emotional practices), as well as the conventional assessment data. CAM practitioners can use the FACES scale (Family Adaptability and Cohesion Scale) to assess family functioning, since children's families have great impact on their health. From the perspective of the

D. Kramer, *Primary Well-Being: Case Studies for the Growing Child*,
DOI 10.1007/978-3-319-56708-2_6

integrative pediatric provider, the assessment encompasses all aspects of the child's life, and will provide the key elements to create a comprehensive and integrative plan (Culbert et al. 2010).

Components of CAM which are especially relevant for children are described in this chapter. These include exercises and activities to integrate the child neurologically and activate the sensory and motor systems to function better together, exercises to promote right and left brain activity (for example Brain Gym), strategies to promote a sense of calm (such as Heart Math and Emotional Freedom Technique), self-regulation techniques that help manage moods and energy levels throughout the day (such as the Alert Program, Take Five, and How to Make Your Engine Run), play-enhancing activities, and food and supplements for health maintenance. Energy medicine and touch techniques such as Reiki, infant massage, and Healing Touch have also been found helpful in calming children and also parents (Ott et al. 2010; Glover et al. 2002; Galicia-Connolly et al. 2011). Individuals and parents can take classes to learn how to do these therapies. This chapter, in addition, provides bibliotherapy suggestions parents can use to promote dialog with their children about issues of concern.

6.1 Environmental Stress

Today's children are growing up in toxic environments that include dangerous levels of chemicals such as lead, air pollution, inadequate sanitary conditions, as well as emotional stress from community and domestic violence, family dysfunction, and low-quality educational settings. There are high rates of asthma among children in low-income, crowded urban neighborhoods, where roach droppings are prevalent (Landrigan et al. 2001; Kang 1990; Etzel 2003; Crain et al. 2002).

A prime prevention of illness is hand washing with plain liquid soap and water. Children should be encouraged to wash certainly before mealtimes, but also when coming in from outdoors, after using the bathroom, after blowing their nose, after playing with pets, and after rolling around on the floor. Anytime these activities are done, hand washing should be routine. Child and/or parent should sing "Happy birthday to you" at least two times for a total of 30 s as they lather their hands and rub them together (Landrigan et al. 2001).

Another key element is eliminating lead from the environment at home and in school. Children should be tested for lead using a blood sample during the well-child visit as infants and again at age 3 and then annually until age 6 (Ness 2013). Especially during the first 3 years, lead can affect the developing brain. Assess drinking water for lead levels, and in areas with lead in the water, use bottled water for drinking and cooking at home and in school. Scrape off lead paint and remove it using the proper precautions. Pots and dinnerware should be lead free. Other sources of lead can be from spices stored in glazed pots, toys, imported cosmetics, candy, and art supplies. For example, toys and crayons made in China may contain lead, and also painted toys from Mexico. Before purchasing toys, ceramics, candy, or cosmetics, look to see that they are lead free. During lead abatement in homes and schools, children and pregnant women need to relocate temporarily as the removal process kicks up more lead particles in the air and the home will need to be cleaned thoroughly before the child and parent return to remove the lead dust (Landrigan et al. 2001).

Try to use products around the home without pesticides in them, since many pesticides have not been tested for their effects on children (American Academy of Pediatrics 2010). Similarly, try to use organic produce or at least scrub fruits and vegetable and peel before using. The 1993 report *Pesticides in the Diets of Infants and Children,* from the National Academy of Sciences, states that traces of pesticides in food can negatively affect the health and development of children and their hormone function (National Research Council 1993). Pesticides interfere with child development, and growth of the brain and hormones that regulate growth and development. Chemicals that are neurotoxins interfere with brain growth. Endocrine disruptors interfere with hormones (Bevacqua 2013; Landrigan et al. 2001). Children who are placed on the floor or crawling are more exposed to pesticides and other chemicals in the home (Bevacqua 2013).

Other environmental strategies for raising healthy children are:

- Eliminate wall-to-wall carpeting as carpets contain dust and mold.
- Install smoke detector in baby's room as well as in all other bedrooms and hallways in the house.
- Install carbon monoxide detector in the home.
- Remove mold and conditions that promote mold, such as leaky pipes and inadequate ventilation.
- Quit smoking. Raising children is a good motivation for quitting smoking and making the environment smoke free.

6.2 Food as Alternative Medicine

Food is also medicine. If we are feeding our bodies toxic food, we are promoting unhealthy development. While nutrition is discussed as appropriate in each case study to meet the physical needs of the body using the guidelines of the American Academy of Pediatrics, food can also be viewed as a vehicle to fortify the body's defenses and healing capacity (Weill 2000). Nutrition training is often lacking or minimal during health care training, and available information can be conflicting or go to extremes (Weill 2000).

The health care provider can help parents understand the importance of good food choices prenatally and for their developing child. The standard recommendation is that mothers breastfeed for a year with the first 6 months being only breast milk and then introduce solid foods. Research supports that breastfeeding is the best choice for babies; it leads to reduced risk for asthma, atopic dermatitis, food allergies, and respiratory allergies (Klingler and Scott 2010).

Food choices for infants and young children are important in physical and brain development. The basic food needs can be found at the web site ChooseMyPlate.gov/kids. Benefits have been demonstrated for cognitive development when mothers take fish oil during pregnancy and while breastfeeding (Nyardi et al. 2013). Children can receive fish oil from early ages when there are no longer concerns about aspiration, between 2 and 3 years. Fish consumption for children needs to be limited due to mercury toxicity. Current recommendations include choosing wild caught instead of farmed fish, using smaller fish such as sardines, and consulting a safe fish chart such as the one put out by the Dept. of Health, Washington State, which can be downloaded at http://www.doh.wa.gov/CommunityandEnvironment/Food/Fish/HealthyFishGuide. The U.S.

The Food and Drug Administration is in the process of revising its 2004 fish recommendations as of June 2014. A draft document can be found at http://www.fda.gov/Food/FoodborneIllnessContaminants/Metals/ucm393070.htm.

Research also supports the choice of organic or locally grown foods when possible. This not only has health benefits to the family but also will maintain a safe and clean environment. Organophosphate pesticides contain compounds that can affect child development by changing the release of neurotransmitters (Shetreat-Klein 2012, 2015). Studies point to a link between pesticide use and increasing risk of ADHD diagnosis (Bouchard et al. 2010; Sagiv et al. 2010), and a link between neurobehavioral deficits and increased blood pressure in children prenatally exposed to pesticides (Harari et al. 2010). Each year lists are developed of the ten most important fruits and vegetables that prominent organizations recommend to buy organic versions for. These items include peaches, apples, pears, winter squash, green beans, grapes, strawberries, raspberries, spinach, and potatoes (Klingler and Scott 2010). Know the top ten fruits and vegetables each year that have the greatest and least amounts of pesticides on them and choose for your family the least as much as possible. If certified organic produce is not available, buying locally in season produce, especially from farmer's markets, usually means less pesticide on the produce.

Choosing organic dairy products is also recommended. Dairy products that are not organic contain hormones that cows are given to increase milk production. Hormone IGF-1 and RBST (Recombinent Bovine Somatatrophin) have been linked to breast cancer, osteogenic sarcoma, colon cancer, and lung cancer (Landrigan et al. 2001).

Other recommended nutrition strategies that ensure toxic-free foods include (1) choosing livestock and poultry that are not given hormones, and are grass fed or organically fed; (2) using eggs from hens that are hormone free and fed organic feed; and (3) staying away from food additives, such as artificial colors, stabilizers, preservatives, and artificial flavoring.

Sugars: While naturally occurring sugar in foods is part of a balanced diet, such as fruits and vegetables and dairy products, adding processed sugar and artificial sweeteners are not beneficial to brain health (Weill 2000; Shetreat-Klein 2012, 2015). Refined sugars increase the risk of obesity and diabetes and have effects on brain cells (Shetreat-Klein 2012, 2015). Many processed foods contain added sugar and/or artificial sweeteners as well as MSG (Herbert and Weintraub 2012). Reading the label does not always help identify the sugars as many names are given to them. Usually artificial sweeteners are made from aspartame (Equal) or saccharine (Sweet and Low). Saccharine has been demonstrated to cause cancer in laboratory animals.

Aspartame and/or "Splenda," used in many sodas, alters the nervous system by affecting brain receptors and overstimulating the brain (Abou-Donia et al. 2008).

Probiotic supplements can also be used safely in children to promote good flora in the intestine that research shows supports a healthy immune system (Flock and Kim 2010; Kleinman 2009). Probiotics are intestinal microbes that are helpful to animals and humans. They are manufactured in a supplement form to promote intestinal health. The microflora of the intestine needs to be filled with certain helpful bacteria to help maintain healthy maturation and functioning of the intestinal and immune systems. Probiotics help by stimulating the growth of beneficial bacteria (Saavedra and Dattilo 2010). Prebiotics are raw foods that help stimulate the growth of probiotics, such as leaves, spinach, broccoli, or cabbage. Probiotics have a role in pediatrics (Machail and Sherman 2009). Using probiotics on a regular basis maintains health and, when illness occurs, provides microbes in the gut to help support the immune response. Increased research and documentation on this topic is being done. While we know much about probiotics, further progress in terms of quality control and regulation is needed, including rigorous testing and ensuring that the probiotic product is therapeutic (Quigley 2009). In the future, it is predicted that pharmaprobiotics will be available (Quigley 2009).

6.3 Bibliotherapy as Alternative Medicine

Reading to children is a key element to their development. Books are a safe format for children to explore different concepts, feelings, and attitudes while allowing them to better understand their environment, community, and societal expectations. Reading to children increases self-esteem, gives comfort, and may aid children in coping with difficult situations. This modality is dependent on the child having someone who is able to read to them. Many libraries offer literacy classes and/or have story hours that may focus on particular issues in the books selected. See American's Literacy Directory at www.literacydirectory.org for a guide to programs in your area.

Bibliotherapy is the "use of written materials to gain understanding and engage in problem solving relevant to the person's therapeutic needs" (Goddard 2012). It has been used successfully to communicate illness to children. Stories chosen where the child can identify with the characters that are facing similar issues will be good jumping off points for the child and parent or child and provider to start talking about the issues involved in their illness or concerns (Marrs 1995; Thibault 2004).

The health care provider can offer the names of books related to specific topics that parents can read to their child. Books can help the child relate to characters that are coping with similar problems. This may help children in dealing with difficult situations as they realize that they are not alone. Hearing the story, the child may share their feelings about being in a similar situation. Spending time in reading to children is a safe way to explore feelings and attitudes, increases children's self-esteem, and provides comfort (Goddard 2012). Topics appropriate for bibliotherapy include sibling rivalry, bullying, self-esteem, death, feeling sad, parental depression, visit to the hospital, doctor or dentist, sleepovers, fear of the dark, taking a trip, learning to be potty trained, bed wetting, being seriously ill, experiencing having disabilities and raising sensitivity to others with disabilities, taking medicine, over-eating, and more.

6.4 Books to Share with Children

6.4.1 Books to Help Children Self-Regulate

6.4.1.1 Learning to Get Along Series

Written by Cheri J. Meiners, books in this series explore young children's feelings and behavior. Each book covers an essential social skill such as empathy, respect, cooperation, and kindness. The books help children visualize how their appropriate behavior positively impacts themselves and others. Each book has a parent guide and uses colorful pictures to illustrate behaviors and activities to reinforce the ideas in the book. Suggested for ages 4–8. Reading level 1. Some titles are available in Spanish. Titles include

Accept and Value Each Person
Be Careful and Stay Safe
Be Honest and Tell the Truth
Be Polite and Kind
Cool Down and Work Through Anger
Join In and Play
Know and Follow Rules
Listen and Learn
Reach Out and Give
Respect and Take Care of Things
Share and Take Turns
Talk and Work It Out
Try and Stick with It
Understand and Care
When I Feel Afraid

6.4.1.2 Being the Best Me! Series

This is another series from author and educator Cheri J. Meiners that focus on attitudes, attributes, and character traits that help children be resilient and control their behavior. Each book also contains activities that parents can do with their child to foster appropriate behavior in different situations. Published by Free Spirit Press, the titles include

Be Positive!
Bounce Back!
Feel Confident!
Forgive and Let Go!
Have Courage!
Stand Tall!

6.4.1.3 Best Behavior Series

This collection of board books and paperbacks by Elizabeth Verdick helps guide children to behave in positive ways in everyday situations. Books suitable for ages 1–4 come as durable board books; titles for ages 4–7 come as paperbacks. Some titles are available in bilingual and English/Spanish editions.

Titles for ages 1–4 years include
Diapers Are Not Forever (2008)
Feet Are Not for Kicking (2004)
Germs Are Not for Sharing (2006)
Hands Are Not for Hitting (2006)
Noses Are Not for Picking (2014)
Pacifiers Are Not Forever 2007)
Tails Are Not for Pulling (2005)
Teeth Are Not for Biting (2003)
Voices Are Not for Yelling (2015)
Words Are Not for Hurting (2004)
Expanded paperbacks for ages 4–7 years include
Hands Are Not for Hitting (2006)
Germs Are Not for Sharing (2006)
Tails Are Not for Pulling (2005)
Words Are Not for Hurting (2004)
Voices Are Not for Yelling (2015)

6.4.2 Books and Resources for Parents on Self-Regulation

Parentingsimply.com is a site founded by Adina Soclof, MS, CCC-SLP, a parent educator and certified speech pathologist who offers 7 days of free parenting tips on behavior management and building self-esteem via e-mail as well as advice on common topics in blog and video formats. Ideas for parenting babies, preschoolers, school-age children, and teens are simply stated with sample dialogue for parents to use with their children. Based on ideas in two books by Adele Faber and Elaine Mazlish (*How to Talk So Kids Will Listen & Listen So Kids Will Talk* and *Siblings Without Rivalry: How to Help Your Children Live Together So You Can Live Too*) and in Mary Sheedy Kurcinka's book *Raising Your Spirited Child, Third Edition: A Guide for Parents Whose Child Is More Intense, Sensitive, Perceptive, Persistent, and Energetic*.

No More Meltdowns: Positive Strategies for Managing and Preventing Out-Of-Control Behavior by Jed Baker; foreword by Carol Kranowitz, author of *The Out-of-Sync Child*: This book provides tools to understand and help the out-of-control child calm in the face of four typical meltdown situations: where demands are being made; when the child is required to wait; when there are threats to his or her self-image; or when the child has unmet wishes for attention. It offers strategies and suggests a prevention plan that parents can use to reduce and eliminate meltdowns.

What Angry Kids Need: Parenting Your Angry Child Without Going Mad by Jennifer Anne Brown and Pam Provonsha Hopkins: This practical guide helps parents understand why their child may be angry and offers effective strategies to prevent and reduce anger and improve quality of life by helping children with their feelings and behavior.

Emotional Intensity in Gifted Students: Helping Kids Cope with Explosive Feelings by Christine Fonseca: Using case studies and role play, this book particularly helps parents with gifted children have a greater understanding of how to help their children regulate and monitor their behavior. All parents will benefit by reading it.

A Volcano in My Tummy: Helping Children to Handle Anger by Eliane Whitehouse and Warwick Pudney: Aimed at children aged 6–12, this book contains stories and lessons to help them reduce and manage their anger, as well as activities that parents, teachers, or caregivers can do with children.

How to Take the Grrrr Out of Anger by Elizabeth Verdick and Marjorie Lisovskis: This book, geared toward children aged 8–13 and their parents, describes the many faces of anger and offers five steps for taming the anger as well as a six-step strategy to solve the problems that might be causing an individual to feel angry.

6.4.3 Books About Self-Esteem for Children

Best Friends by Miriam Cohen (1989): This 1971 classic, first published in 1971, is the story of a friendship in nursery school, complete with hurt feelings and eventual reconciliation. For ages 3–6.

Beautiful Girl: Celebrating the Wonders of Your Body by Christiane Northrup, Kristina Tracy, and Aurelie Blanz (2013): This provides positive powerful messages about a little girl's body to give her self-confidence and "set the stage for her physical and mental health throughout her life." Helps girls view their bodies as "perfect and miraculous" and enables parents to start a conversation with their daughter to help her internalize a positive body image and give her confidence as she grows. Beautiful illustrations enhance the text. Appropriate for girls aged 4 and up.

I Want Your Moo: A Story for Children About Self-Esteem by Marcella Bakur Weiner and Jill Neimark (2009): Toodles, a turkey, dislikes her appearance and sound and tries to trade her gobbling noise with other barnyard animals until her gobble is needed for an emergency.

6.4.3.1 The Best Me I Can Be Series

Written by David Parker and published by Scholastic Press, this series covers character traits such as friendship, cooperation, self-control, respect, honesty, responsibility, acceptance of everyone, and generosity. Recommended for pre-k through first grade, ages 4–7. Titles include

I Accept You As You Are (2004)
I Am a Leader (2005)
I Am Creative (2005)

I Am Responsible (2004)
I Can Cooperate (2004)
I Show Respect! (2004)
I'm a Good Friend! (2004)
I'm in Charge of Me (2004)
I Make Good Choices (2004)
Our Class Works Together (First Chapter Book, 2007)

6.4.3.2 First Experience Series

Mister Fred Rogers, the beloved host of the PBS show, "Mister Rogers' Neighborhood," wrote a number of books for young children to help them deal with everyday experiences that may seem frightening or overwhelming at times. Series titles include the following:

Going to Day Care (1987)

Helps children understand the typical activities and emotions they will experience in day care settings and reassures them of their parents' love and going home at the end of the day.

Making Friends (1987)

Describes what friendship is and the importance of learning to share and compromise.

6.4.3.3 Books by Dr. Wayne W. Dyer

Dr. Dyer is a well-known new-age motivational speaker and writer. His books for children, written with Kristina Tracy, talk about values and present maxims in simple language and beautiful illustrations with parent discussion guides. The publisher is Hay House in Carlsbad, California.

Incredible You! 10 Ways to Let Your Greatness Shine Through (2005)

Formulated to make children feel that nothing is impossible for them. Colorful illustration and suggested questions will stimulate dialogue with your children and help them make up their own stories to match the drawings. Good bedtime reading. Concepts include sharing goodness, finding what you love, being loving, finding your inner quiet, making each day great, having positive thoughts, picturing what you want, and taking care of yourself. Appropriate for ages 4 and up.

It's Not What You've Got: Lessons for Kids on Money and Abundance (2007)

Through rhymed verse and colorful illustrations, it teaches children a positive, spiritual approach to money, emphasizing that abundance comes in many forms and money does not define a person. For ages 4–10.

No Excuses!: How What You Say Can Get In Your Way (2009)

Shows how excuses stop children from reaching their goals and helps them stop making them. Uses story of a farm boy's fascination with sea turtles and his family's less than enthusiastic support of his ambition to be a marine biologist to show where excuses come from, why we make excuses, and how to stop making them. Colorful illustrations and guidance to distinguish between excuses and positive words. Appropriate for ages 6 and up.

Unstoppable Me!: 10 Ways to Soar Through Life (2006)

Uses rhyming introductions and stories of everyday life to explain and illustrate guidance for children on how to lead a fulfilling and happy life. Based on his book for adults, *What Do You Really Want for Your Children?* Concepts include developing self-confidence, being persistent, welcoming the unknown, making choices, worrying less, being calm, living in the present, being healthy, being creative, and giving to others. Appropriate for ages 4 and up.

6.4.4 Books That Help Parents and Children Explore Feelings

6.4.4.1 The Way I Feel Series

These books by Cornelia Maud Spellman and others help children understand and explore and manage their emotions in a positive way. Some titles have links to a web site enabling read-alongs. Published by Albert Whitman & Company, titles include the following:

When I Feel Angry (2000)

This title distinguishes between feeling an emotion and acting on it to help children manage their emotions without hurting others.

When I Feel Scared (2002)

A young bear helps children identify their fears such as loud noises, bad dreams, mother going away, and being hurt or for no reason, and helps them articulate how they feel—like crying, hiding, running away, wanting to be held, or stop being scared. The child bear receives acknowledgment, understanding, and comfort from a caring adult and learns how to manage his fears.

When I Miss You (2004)

A young guinea pig describes situations that would make a child miss his parents, how it feels to miss them, and what he can do to feel better. The book validates the child's feelings and then suggests activities the child can do to distract and relax, such as self-soothing, playing, laughing, or drawing a picture to show the parent. It also reminds children that there are always others around to help when parents leave.

Other titles in the series include

When I Care About Others (2002)

When I Feel Good About Myself (2003)

When I Feel Jealous (2003)

When I Feel Sad (2002)

6.4.5 Books About Common Childhood Issues

My Body Belongs to Me: A Book about Body Safety by Jill Starishevsky (2014)

Describes in rhyme about setting boundaries and saying no to unhealthy touch and defines private parts. Suitable for ages 3–8.

What to Do When You Dread Your Bed: A Kid's Guide to Overcoming Problems With Sleep by Dawn Huebner (2008)

Part of the What to Do Guides for Kids series, this book teaches school-age children cognitive-behavioral techniques to treat problems with bedtime and sleep. Includes introduction for parents. Teaches children how to play games with themselves, like monster time apart from bedtime, and provides other planning strategies to overcome fears of sleep by acknowledging different concerns a child might have.

6.4.5.1 Books by Julia Cook

This former teacher and school guidance counselor uses creative, funny stories with delightful illustrations to involve the reader and help children become "better." Most have introduction or section for parents and others on using the material and helping children with the specific problem the book addresses. Published by National Center for Youth Issues in Chattanooga, TN. For ages 2–12.

Personal Space Camp (2013)

Uses a fun story to help children understand personal space and how it impacts other children's reactions to them.

Melvin the Magnificent Molar (2010)

Written from the tooth's point of view, this book on the importance of taking care of your teeth gives readers an overview of what to expect when going to the dentist. It makes taking care of teeth fun, including a visit from the tooth fairy. Includes ten tips.

How to be Comfortable in Your Own Feathers (2013)

Uses a bluebird influenced by a hummingbird to be unhappy with her feathers to creatively speak to children who may be struggling with body-image concerns and unhealthy eating. The writing style gives children an opportunity to apply the characters' experiences to their own lives and shows appropriate adult responses to encourage healthy eating habits and promote positive self-esteem. Has "live it" tips for parents. For ages 5–12.

It's Hard to be a Verb! (2008)

Uses heart and humor in the story of Louis who has a hard time keeping still. Provides strategies for any child who can't stay focused, including children with ADHD.

Ricky Sticky Fingers (2012)

A story about ownership and how it feels when someone does not respect your things. Ricky is a child who takes things until he learns to empathize with others when his bicycle is missing and decides to use the "good" in him to overtake the "bad" by returning all the items he has stolen.

The Bubble Wrap Queen (2008)

Uses humor to disseminate messages about how to live and play safely. In the story, a mother goes crazy bubble wrapping everything, including the playground, to keep her child safe until there is no more bubble wrap in the stores and she has to go back to the "Basics": Be Aware and Safe in Common Situations.

Cell Phoney (2012)

In this delightful story Joanie learns she has to take a Cell Phone Safety Course and master the six rules of cell phone usage that will keep them safe and keep them from hurting others, thus avoiding becoming a "cell phoney."

My Mouth is a Volcano! (2005)

Uses humor and the story of Louis to help children learn how to manage their thoughts and words without interrupting others. Louis thinks all his thoughts are important and they erupt from his tummy like a volcano until he learns how to respectfully wait his turn. Ages 4 and up.

Blueloon (2012)

A book with humor and sensitivity about depression for children of all ages to understand what is happening to them. Uses the image of a blue partially deflated balloon with a string tied in knots to talk about depression and what it feels like to children. Shows how the balloon "bounces back" to being its bright, round, and full self after encountering a wise rock. Includes note to parents and educators. For ages 6 and up.

Soda Pop Head! (2011)

Lester has a hard time controlling his anger when he is stressed or frustrated and blows up. His father helps him manage his anger in practical, fun, and creative ways. Uses humor and empathy to explore a difficult but common behavior. Appropriate for ages 6 and up.

Smarter Than the SCOOPERS: Keeping Your Child Safe from Predators! (2012)

Uses empathetic storytelling to help children gain the skills and confidence they need to make wise choices in daily social interactions and prevent child abduction. Offers five personal safety strategies using SCOOP as an acronym: be *S*mart, use your *C*all list, zer*O* talking to strangers, keep strangers *O*ut of your personal space, and always *P*air up.

Straight from the Horse's Mouth (2012)

Story told by a horse about how he helps people heal on the inside using the analogy of getting rid of flies and overcome difficult struggles in their lives. Based on the professional mental health treatment called equine-assisted psychotherapy.

Bully B.e.a.n.s. (2009)

Mother gives her child magic jelly beans and the courage to use effective strategies to prevent and stop bullying. Story helps understand why bullying happens and what children and adults can do about it.

The Kid Trapper (2010)

Presents the topic of child sexual abuse in a sensitive way using the analogy of a butterfly caught in a spider's web. Story will empower and strengthen victims and make the innocent aware of how to keep themselves from being "trapped." Can be used to teach children and adults how to recognize and prevent the traps child molesters set as well as a diagnostic tool to assess if abuse is taking place. Often the molesters are acquaintances in their community and children fear they won't be believed if they try to speak up.

I am a Booger … Treat me with Respect (2007)

Uses a humorous story told by a booger demanding respect to teach children about the dangers of picking their nose, the role of boogers in preventing illness, and the hygienic way to blow one's nose.

Grief is Like a Snowflake (2011)

Story for grieving children focuses on how a Little Tree learns to cope with the death of his father pine tree with the help and support of other trees—family and friends—in the woodland nursery. Little Tree sees eventually that his father's memory lives on and what is important is what you give in life, not what you get.

It's You and Me Against the Pee … and the Poop too! (2011)

Three-year-old Stanley is having trouble remembering to use the potty until he learns a new game to help him become a "potty expert" and his parents realize it takes a team effort to be successful. Coauthored with Dr. Laura Jana, pediatrician and award-winning parenting book author.

The D (divorce) word (2011)

Otis thought his family was perfect until his parents announced they were getting divorced. Otis describes what it is like to live through the divorce process, first blaming himself and then with the help of his grandmother, coming to understand the three Cs of divorce: " I didn't CAUSE IT, I CAN'T control it, so I'm going to have to learn to COPE with it!" These are good guides for any stressful situation outside one's control. Ages 4 and up.

A Bad Case of Tattle Tongue (2006)

Uses a visit from the Tattle Prince to help Josh learn the rules to keep from tattling in school and at home. Helps children develop life skills to tell what their needs are as opposed to tattling on others. Appropriate for children aged 6 and up.

Wilma Jean the Worry Machine (2012)

Uses story form to help children deal with excessive worry and fear using humor. Provides strategies for parents to help their anxious children.

Don't be Afraid to Drop (2008)

Uses the story of a rain drop that is afraid to leave his cloud to help children talk about their fear of change and understand that change can be rewarding and bring happiness. Appropriate for ages 4 and up.

My Mom Thinks She's My Volleyball Coach … But She's Not! (2007)

Told from the daughter's point of view about a hovering mother pushing her daughter to excel in a sport. Based on interviews with coaches about what parents do that drives them crazy and what a good volleyball parent would look like. Uses humor and colorful illustrations to make the point that parents shouldn't be coaches.

6.4.5.2 Toddler Tools Series

These rhyming board books by Elizabeth Verdick use gentle humor and are suitable for children aged 2 and up. Stories include tips for parents and caregivers on being good role models, and strategies for reinforcing the lessons in the book. Series titles include

Bedtime (2010)
Bye-Bye Time (2008)
Calm-Down Time (2010)
Germs Are Not for Sharing (2006)
Clean-Up Time (2008)
Listening Time (2008)

Manners Time (2008)
Mealtime (2011)
Naptime (2008)
On-the-Go Time (2011)
Sharing Time (2009)

6.4.6 Books About Children with Special Needs

Arnie and His School Tools: Simple Sensory Solutions That Build Success by Jennifer Veenendall (2008)

A children's book that presents in story form how Arnie uses a variety of tools and materials to give his nervous system the additional stimulation it needs through movement, touch, oral, and heavy work to make Arnie more successful and tools that reduce distracting stimulation such as auditory sounds. Arnie's "Tools for Learning" include sitting on a ball or soft cushion instead of a seat so he can move around, holding a fidget during listening time to help focus, chewing on a special piece of plastic at the end of his pencil or crunchy food to concentrate, placing a heavy blanket in his lap or wearing a heavy vest to help relax to work better, taking breaks frequently, having a designated work area, or wearing head phones or ear plugs to block out distracting noise. Other strategies include exercise breaks, having movement tasks that are chores to smooth transitions such as sweeping, pushing a cart with mail, or playing, taking exercise breaks every 10 min while doing homework, or wrapping a band around his legs to push on when they are restless at his desk while doing an assignment.

Why Does Izzy Cover Her Ears? Dealing with Sensory Overload by Jennifer Veenendall (2009)

Uses story form to show how children can overcome sensory overload, especially unpleasant and loud noises, too many visual distractions, being bumped, and standing too close at home and school to function and learn more successfully. Strategies include anticipating the loud noise, wearing earplugs, moving to another location, sitting at the end of a row for more space, and being with quieter children. Other ideas are taking breaks in a "motor" room, using a heavy blanket, using anti-fidget tools, using daylight and floor lamps instead of florescent light, and taking a quiet-room break. Also see www.asperger.net.

6.5 Sensory Motor Integration as Alternative Medicine

Sensory motor integration is an important developmental function that all children need, not only children with disabilities but neurotypical children as well. The primary health care provider can recommend books and resources to parents that will help integrate their child's sensory and motor functions to enhance physical, emotional, and cognitive development. In general it is helpful to have other family members participate in as many of these activities as possible to make it more fun to the child. Below we list individual books as well as activities that would be helpful to parents, teachers, and health care providers to help promote sensory motor integration in all children.

6.5.1 Brain Gym

Brain Gym: Simple Activities for Whole Brain Learning, by Paul Dennison and Gail E. Dennison (2010), is a set of 26 exercises based on mounting evidence "that each person's capacity to master new and remember old information is improved by biological changes in the brain brought on by physical activity" (Ratey 2010). The teacher's edition contains detailed instructions for performing the exercises: *Brain Gym, Teacher's Edition: A Companion Guide to Brain Gym: Simple Activities for Whole Brain Learning* (1986).

The exercises teach parents how to enhance their child's ability to self-regulate, concentrate, maintain their energy level, and calm down. It teaches children to be aware of how they are feeling and provides tools and exercises to help them function at their optimal levels. It will help with problem solving, social interactions, cognitive learning, and physical activity.

6.5.2 Tools for Tots

A resource to help with normal toddler behaviors that are difficult for parents and the child is *Tools for Tots: Sensory Strategies for Toddlers and Preschoolers* by Diana A. Henry, Maureen Kane-Wineland, and Susan Swindeman (2007).

Often common sensory behaviors of children are not addressed by the health care provider. It is extremely helpful for the health professional to share this information with parents and explain that although these wonderful recommendations are written in books categorized as for individual with sensory issues, we all have sensory issues on different levels and these books have invaluable strategies to make our lives easier. *Tools for Tots* describes certain children's normal behaviors and how parents can, through the use of play, provide tools to modify the behavior to help the child. A parent might observe that "my child sits while going down the stairs," "my child is cautious," "my child is very clean and doesn't like getting dirty," "my child is a picky eater," my child is afraid of the vacuum cleaner," "my child screams when their nails are being cut, my child doesn't like having her hair brushed," "he doesn't notice when his diaper is soiled," or "my child has difficulty going to sleep." The tools in this book allow parents to respect their child's normal response and, through the use of games and specific strategies, help diminish the difficulty the child and family are experiencing to make it more tolerable, easier for the parent and child and even fun.

For example, the child may experience a comb or brush or scissors on their hair as dangerous or perhaps they are sensitive to touch on their hair. Suggestions include distraction with a video, allowing the tot to bush their own hair, having them sit on your lap while brushing, or having them brush a doll's hair first. It is important for the health care provider, in doing their overall assessment of the child, to consider whether an early intervention referral in sensory motor integration is needed (see box "Parenting Strategies from Tools for Tots"). Parents can also prepare a sensory backpack to take while away from home or use in school when the child needs to maintain self-control (see box "Creating a Sensory Backpack").

Parenting Strategies from Tools for Tots

Sensory Integration

- Help children to prepare for potentially overwhelming situations by creating a story to discuss the event before it occurs, such as a fire drill in school or a visit to the doctor.
- Teach children to take several breaths before working on a difficult project or transitioning to another activity, especially in a busy environment.
- Use songs to help younger children transition from one activity to another, such as when it's time to clean up. One web site with suggestions and lyrics is Songs for Teaching, http://www.songsforteaching.com/.
- Marching is another activity that can help children, particularly young children, with transitions. Children like the rhythm and the alternate foot motions in marching. This movement seems to help organize the child for the next activity.

Organize/Focus

- In describing how to do a task, give the child step-by-step directions and then model the activity for him or her. Let the child try and practice several times.
- In planning to do an activity, ask the child what materials he or she will need and what will he or she do first.
- Have a consistent place to store materials. This will help children develop the organizational skills of knowing where to put items when they are finished and get items when they want to start using them.
- Offer suggestions for projects or school assignments to help the child formulate what they want to do or organize a brainstorming group with the child's peers.
- Help the child organize for class by suggesting the use of color-coded notebooks and book covers. Green for science; yellow for English, blue for geography, red for math.
- Play classical music such as Mozart's Sonata in D major for Two Pianos, K488 and Vivaldi pieces such as "The Four Seasons," in the background when working independently; such music is thought to assist learning.

- Provide water bottles or chewy, crunchy snacks for the child at his desk or table. This will stimulate focus and organization.
- Have younger children pretend to push the walls down or hold up the walls when waiting in line for something to reduce fidgeting. Older children can do push-ups in their seats using their hands when they fidget.
- Handle or "fiddle" a small object such as an eraser or a paper clip. Depending on circumstances, the child should be allowed to "fiddle" with objects during "listening activities."
- Take a movement break in which the child stands and stretches between. The child who can't seat still can be assigned to give out supplies or other chores to keep her moving around the classroom but still be engaged.

Sources:

Henry, D.A., Kane-Wineland, M., and Swindeman, S. (2007). Tools for tots: Sensory strategies for toddlers and preschoolers. *Glendale, AZ: Henry Occupational Therapy Services.*

6.5.3 Getting in Touch with Feelings

Two books in particular talk about sensory integration and getting in touch with feelings, and provide activities and games to help parents and children articulate their feelings and sensitivities:

Starting Sensory Therapy: Fun Activities for the Home and Classroom by Bonnie Arnwine (2011).

No Longer a Secret: Unique Common Sense Strategies for Children with Sensory or Motor Challenges by Doreit Sarah Bialer and Lucy Jane Miller (2011).

Both books suggest that parents who can describe their own feelings to their child model how the child can understand his or her own feelings and regulate them. One activity is to go around the dinner table and ask everyone to describe their emotional state. Another approach if the child cannot yet express their emotions is to make educated guesses and ask them to say if you are right or wrong. Point out to the child the importance of learning to interpret facial expressions, body language, and the tone in which things are said. Cutting out pictures from magazines or family photographs, you can discuss what the expression on each face is. Having pictures of happiness or sadness can sometimes trigger the child's expressing their own emotional state. When the child is in a calm state, model for him or her lying on the floor, breathe normally in and out, put a stuffed animal on your stomach, and watch how the inhalations and exhalations are calming and soothing; then have the child try it and express how they feel.

6.6 Staying in Control

Children don't like surprises. They need predictability to feel in control. Parents can provide children with a daily schedule of the plan for the day, breaking it down into smaller steps, like getting up, getting dressed, playing, doing homework, going to school, chores, and preparing for bedtime. See box for more recommendations to help parents and child stay in control (see boxes "Staying in Control" and "Self-Regulation Training").

Staying in Control

- Give children 10-min warnings to prepare them for the transition to the next activity/setting and then a 1-min countdown to prepare for the change.
- Stay calm. It is important for the parent or caregiver to approach children when we are in a calm state to discuss anything that has occurred that is stressful.
- Give the child crunchy or chewy foods to focus attention and stimulate arousal. Crunchy foods, such as cut-up fruits and vegetables, are alerting and arousing. Chewy foods, such as raisins and other dried fruits, increase organization.
- Put the child's distress, temper tantrum, or meltdown into words. Say: "I see you are having a hard time. Let's put you in a special calm down place." "I'll be around as long as you are here and you can cry as long as you want." Arrange the place ahead of time—it can be a room, or a corner, as long as it is quiet and not stimulating.

Sources:

Arnwine, Bonnie. (2011). Starting sensory therapy: Fun activities for the home and classroom. *Arlington, TX: Sensory World.*

Bialer, D.S. and Miller, L.J. (2011). No longer a secret: Unique common sense strategies for children with sensory or motor challenges. *Arlington, TX: Sensory World, Future Horizons.*

6.6.1 Encouraging Movement and Inner Reflection

All children sometimes crave sensation, spin, bump into objects, or like messy stimuli. Create relay races to allow for different types of gross motor activities (Connell and McCarthy 2013). These could include:

- Walk, run freeze
- Spinning in one direction for a set amount of time and then the other direction
- Jumping
- Playing games with repetitive song or movement such as "Duck, Duck Goose," "Musical chairs," "Ring Around the Rosy"

Providing more description in play and activities helps add richness to the child's understanding of the world and his or her inner life. Talk about the way things can be classified such as "let's find things that are blue," or "let's find things that we can smell." Take turns in naming objects. This also helps the child understand what is the same and what is different. Use the Sesame Street song: "Guess which thing is not like the other" to make the game fun.

Help the child to visualize details about what they are thinking and to differentiate objects. For example, put a box in a bag and ask the child to guess what it is. Write a large letter or number in the air and then draw it on paper. Have the child describe what they see before writing the letter down. Or have the child make their body into the shape of what they see. The child can also say, "I'm thinking of …" and the adult has to guess what it is by asking questions.

In communication, encourage details about how the child feels. For example, when he or she expresses an emotion such as impatience, encourage details, such as "You feel impatient because you are so tired." When children need to express anger, try having them pound clay or play dough to help them express this feeling. See box "Reinforcing Positive Behaviors."

Reinforcing Positive Behaviors

- Catch your children doing positive behaviors and complement them at the time.
- Use simple charts to track positive behavior and offer meaningful rewards for reaching a specified amount of gold stars or checks.
- A special object or time alone with a parent can be a reward, such as going to the park together or having an ice cream treat out rather than at home.

Sources:

Arnwine, Bonnie. (2011). Starting sensory therapy: Fun activities for the home and classroom. *Arlington, TX: Sensory World.*

Bialer, D. S. and Miller, L. J. (2011). No longer a secret: Unique common sense strategies for children with sensory or motor challenges. *Arlington, TX: Sensory World, Future Horizons.*

Out in Public: Predictable Tasks

- When standing on line in the grocery store, when waiting to take a turn, or when riding in a car, play games such as I Spy, sing familiar songs such as the Itsy, Bitsy Spider (http://www.grandparents.com/grandkids/activities-games-and-crafts/itsy-bitsy-spider), or play Bingo (see: http://www.songsforteaching.com/folk/BINGO.php).

- Parents can carry soft, squeezable items in a bag that the child can play with.
- Make use of the game and video capacity on cell phone to amuse the child, including games such as concentration, and drawing games.

Sources:

Arnwine, Bonnie. (2011). Starting sensory therapy: Fun activities for the home and classroom. *Arlington, TX: Sensory World.*

Bialer, D. S. and Miller, L. J. (2011). No longer a secret: Unique common sense strategies for children with sensory or motor challenges. *Arlington, TX: Sensory World, Future Horizons.*

6.7 Specific Games/Activities

6.7.1 Sensory Wrestling Game

This is a form of deep pressure, referred to as "heavy work." Through the use of this game, the child increases their awareness of their body position. This is an activity that can be done 15 min before a sport's game to help increase body awareness and improve motor skills. The game is played by the child pushing against the parent as hard as they can with their body while the parent is mostly still. The parent holds the child down while the child pushes back hard and eventually escapes the parent's grasp (Arnwine 2011; Bialer and Miller 2011).

6.7.2 Jumping on a Trampoline

Trampoline jumping while playing catch can be done 15 min before a sports activity to help the child get warmed up. The child jump up and down while an adult throw a ball and the child tries to match their jump to the toss so they can catch the ball. This game increases the child's spatial awareness and vestibular stimulation and helps improve motor skills (Arnwine 2011; Bialer and Miller 2011).

6.7.3 Doing Heavy Work

Any activity that works the muscles and joints such as lifting a heavy object provides proprioceptive input. This is helpful when a child has difficulty focusing on a given task and needs help with sensory organization as the child is feeling overloaded (Arnwine 2011; Bialer and Miller 2011).

6.7.4 Noodle Kidoodle Movement

This exercise uses a pool noodle to help the child develop his or her core muscles. Start by having the child hold the noodle above his or her head while on his or her back on the floor. He or she then rolls over to his or her stomach, still holding the noodle, which is now on the floor. Then the head and upper torso are raised from the knees with the noodle still on the floor. For the final position, the child places the noodle behind his or her bent knees and pulls the noodle forward between his or her ankles and toes, holding the ends in his or her fists with bent arms as he or she raises his or her head off the ground (Bialer and Miller 2011.

6.7.5 Stop-Light Bracelet Game

This game uses red, green, and yellow bracelets to represent feelings. The green bracelet represents a positive state—the green light, such as happiness, confidence, or satisfaction. The yellow bracelet represents becoming unhappy, frustrated, or upset. The red bracelet represents anger and frustration. Family members can play this game together by putting on a bracelet and taking turns acting out the feelings it represents or family members can choose a bracelet to express their current "feeling" state. This game can help children recognize their feelings and slow down the shift of feeling from green to yellow and from yellow to red. This is a cognitive technique to help move the child away from the automatic fight or flight response to a cognitively mediated response, thinking their way through the situation, eliminating red altogether and providing more emotional control and greater internal awareness (Arnwine 2011; Bialer and Miller 2011).

6.7.6 Find It, Feel It, Show It Wheel Game

This school-age game is a version of 20 questions and can be played by one or more children. Divide a large circle drawn on heavy paper up into eight sections. Each section contains a specific question the child can answer based on an object someone else has chosen and hides from the players: size (big, little), shape (square, round, triangle, rectangle), smell (sweet, sour), color (light, dark, bright, dim), weight (light or heavy), and taste (sweet, sour, salty). Fasten the wheel to a cardboard or another heavy piece of paper with a small brad fastener to allow it to spin (for younger children, an older child or parent can read the questions).

Questions can include: What size am I? What do I smell like? What do I taste like? Am I heavy or light? What shape am I? What color am I? How do you use me? What am I the same as? (Arnwine 2011; Bialer and Miller 2011).

Body awareness games, such as playing Simon Says, or Twister, or Hokey, Pokey, or If you are Happy and You Know it Clap Your Hands … and having the child describe what they did will help increase body sense and self-awareness (Arnwine 2011; Bialer and Miller 2011).

6.7.7 Snap and Clap

In this game, every time you say a designated word in a story the child is supposed to snap or clap. This helps the child have better auditory attention.

6.7.8 Say It, Play It with Clay

Child A writes down on a paper the name of an object that they will create out of play dough or clay. Another child is asked to guess what the object is once it is finished. The second child needs to use as many descriptive words as possible to describe the object such as big, small, color, shape, of the whole or any part, e.g., "you created long floppy ears. Is it a bunny?"; or "you created a round nose and long tale, is it a dog?" (Arnwine 2011; Bialer and Miller 2011).

6.7.9 What's in Your Hand Sensory Game

This game uses the sense of touch to enhance tactile stimulation and can be played with one or more children or an adult. An adult or a child picks out common objects around the house and places them on a table. The child then holds one object under the table and has to describe what she feels—texture, shape, and size. If an object is unfamiliar, two of them can be used—one to look at and another to describe. The game can also be played by putting objects in a bag and having to pick out one without looking to describe under the table and then guessing what it is. Use objects such as a crayon, eraser, salt shaker, ball, pot holder, paper clip, tube of cream, or wash cloth (Arnwine 2011; Bialer and Miller 2011).

A game like Charades lets the child use discriminators, give clues to other children, be a leader, use descriptors, and also demand self-control in playing (Arnwine 2011; Bialer and Miller 2011).

6.7.10 Listening to Music

Listening to CDs can be helpful emotionally in many situations, such as preparing for a sporting event, getting to sleep, relieving stress over schoolwork, and learning to relax. Some recommended recordings are:

- Betty Mehling's Magic Island, recommended for ages 5–12 which empowers the child through a guided meditation.
- Deb Weiss-Gelmi's Sing-song Yoga DVD, which helps with energy, strength, and flexibility.
- Dr. Rox's Grain of Sand CD, which has songs and stories to teach stress management, self-acceptance, and a positive approach to challenges.

Preparing a Sensory Backpack

Fill a backpack with objects that engage children's senses and can calm them in stressful situations. Include the following types of items:

- Sports bottle with a straw
- A soft fleece jacket
- Small squishy toys that make sounds
- A favorite cloth doll or stuffed animal
- Books
- Small puzzles
- An aroma bracelet (gauze pad infused with essential oil placed within a folded sports band)
- Interconnected play rings
- Soft paintbrushes to swab themselves with
- Bottle of bubbles and stick to blow with
- Small weighted lap pillow that can be placed on shoulders or held in a hand
- Weighted sock snakes (put beans in large sock and close up)
- Chewy snacks such as dried raisins or dried cranberries or dried apples

Sources:

Arnwine, Be. (2011). Starting sensory therapy: Fun activities for the home and classroom. *Arlington, TX: Sensory World.*

Bialer, D.S., and Miller, L.J. (2011). No longer a secret: Unique common sense strategies for children with sensory or motor challenges. *Arlington, TX: Sensory World, Future Horizons.*

Another helpful resource for parents as well as teachers is *Answers to Questions Teachers Ask About Sensory Integration: Forms, Checklists, and Practical Tools for Teachers and Parents,* 2nd ed., by Carol Stock Kranowitz, Stacy Szkut, Lynn Balzer-Martin, Elizabeth Haber, and Deanna Iris Sava (2001). The authors have many suggestions that parents and teachers can incorporate into their daily routines to further sensory motor integration. For example, to handle schedule/changes/transitions: every morning, outline the schedule of the day with your child and highlight any changes from the typical routine that will occur.

The book *Helping Hyperactive Kids—A Sensory Integration Approach: Techniques and Tips for Parents and Professionals* by Lynn J. Horowitz and Cecile Rost (2004) offers many ways to calm down that utilize taste, movement, touch, or sight (see box "Ways to Calm Down").

Ways to Calm Down

- Whole body:
  - Do slow, deep breathing in through the nose and gently out through pursed lips.
  - Stretch both hands high above the head reaching for the sky and counting to 10.
- Use the taste buds:
  - Drink cold water slowly through a straw. The slow repetitive sips are calming.
  - Eat a sweet fruit.
  - Drink a liquid that is half frozen.
- Use physical exertion
  - Playing outside.
  - Do sports.
  - Dance.
  - Run up and down steps.
  - Ride a bike.
- Use touch
  - Message the ear from the bottom to the top, using a slight pressure.
  - Snuggle by lying down on or holding tightly to cushions.
  - Cuddle a pet.
  - Find a corner of the room to gently wedge your back into, to simulate being hugged.
- Use tactile stimulation
  - Hold a paper clip, ball, or toy.
  - Touch or play with a pet.
  - Wash face with cold water.
  - Take a bath.
- Use visual calming
  - Watch fish in an aquarium.
  - Dim the lights.
  - Read.

- Use auditory calming
  - Listen to classical music with a soothing rhythm (e.g., by Mozart).
  - Turn all sound off and be in a quiet room.

Sources:

Arnwine, Bonnie. (2011). Starting sensory therapy: Fun activities for the home and classroom. *Arlington, TX: Sensory World.*

Bialer, D. S. and Miller, L. J. (2011). No longer a secret: Unique common sense strategies for children with sensory or motor challenges. *Arlington, TX: Sensory World, Future Horizons.*

Horowitz, L. J. and Rost, C. (2004). Helping hyperactive kids—A sensory integration approach: Techniques and tips for parents and professionals. *Berkeley, CA: Hunter House Publishers.*

Drawing on the taste stimuli, the authors suggest drinking through a straw, eating a sweet fruit, or drinking a liquid that is half frozen. Physical exertions, such as playing outside, sports, dancing, running up and down steps, or riding a bike, can also promote calmness. Snuggling by lying down on or holding tightly to cushions or cuddling a pet is also recommended. For tactile stimulation for calming, they suggest holding a paper clip, ball, or toy, or touch or play with a pet, wash the face with cold water, or take a bath. Visual calming can also be achieved by watching fish in an aquarium or dimming the lights or reading. Auditory calming includes listening to classical music with a soothing rhythm (e.g., by Mozart) or turning all sound off and being in a quiet room.

Barbara Sher, in her 2009 book *Early Intervention Games: Fun, Joyful Ways to Develop Social and Motor Skills in Children with Autism Spectrum or Sensory Processing Disorders*, suggests games to teach children about group social dynamics. Playing games can also help children learn about taking turns, following the rules, getting brief attention, tolerate being the center of attention, and realizing that the enjoyment of social activities takes many forms and can be modified for particular children. Remember to make it easy at the beginning to promote self-confidence. Some samples from the book include the following:

Hide and go seek: Have two players do the counting as a way to include the child who is learning to count or has trouble patiently waiting until the count is up (Sher 2009).

Blanket ride: One child sits on a blanket. An adult and another child gently pull the blanket in different directions. Switch children. This game teaches children that they can be the source of another child's pleasure (Sher 2009).

Box ride: Get a clean box from a grocery or liquor store, large enough to fit a small child. Have children take turns sitting in it and being pushed by their friends or adults (Sher 2009).

I am here: This game enhances name recognition and social responsiveness in a playful, nonthreatening situation. Put a box on the floor and have the child pretend to hide behind a box. Someone calls the child's name, saying, "Jonny, where are you?"

Jonny responds by appearing and saying "I am here." Everyone claps and smiles and says "Hi, Jonny." Each child takes a turn hiding behind the box (Sher 2009).

Jump to colors: Put pieces of different colors of construction paper on the floor, leaving an inch between each sheet. Children have to jump on different colors as the leader (either an adult or a child, taking turns) says, "Jump!" (Sher 2009).

Messages: This game assists the mind and body to self-organize and helps children pay attention. The adult sits on the floor with the child between his or her legs. The adult makes long, firm strokes on the child's arms, legs, and back. The adult sings as he or she massages the child: "This is the way we rub our arms, rub our arms, this is the way we rub our arms, early in the morning." Repeat, substituting different body parts (Sher 2009).

Throwing the balls into the box: This game uses the element of surprise to learn about anticipating results, eye/hand coordination, and understanding concepts of place—inside, outside, and behind. Take a medium-size cardboard box and two balls per player (can be made from scrunched up newspaper held together with tape). Remove the tape from the bottom flaps of the box and open them; also open the top flaps of the box. Sing a song to the tune of "Mary had a Little Lamb": Throw the balls into the box, into the box, into the box, throw the balls into the box, where did the balls go? Then ask the children, "Where are the balls? Are they in front of the box? Behind the box? Under the box? Inside the box?" Then dump the balls, have the kids pick them up, and play again (Sher 2009).

Marching game: This game practices following instructions, listening to verbal cues, imitating motor elements, and being part of a group. Children sing a song as they act out the words:

Marching, marching, marching, marching
Hop, hop, hop
Hop, hop, hop
Running, running, running
Running, running, running
Then we stop! (Hold out your hand as you stop)
(Sher 2009)

Drawing faces: A child and adult draw together on a piece of paper. The adult draws the shape of a face. The child fills in the expression, e.g., a happy face, or a sad face. This teaches the child how to read facial expressions and be aware of other's feelings (Sher 2009).

6.8 Focus, Organization and Self-Regulation

The Alert Program called Take Five, created by Mary Sue Williams and Sherry Shellenberger, is described in a set of two books they wrote based on their "How to Make Your Engine Run" program for regulating alertness levels: *Take Five, Staying*

Alert at Home and in School (2001) and *How Does Your Engine Run: A Leader's Guide to the Alert Program for Self-Regulation* (1996).

The Alert Program theorizes that our bodies and brains were not made to be sitting in classrooms or in front of computers for long periods of time. After a period of time at these tasks our brains become less efficient. By taking a break we can gain more productive time. The program is centered around five concepts for regulating alertness levels: tasting, moving, touching, looking, and listening. *Take Five* offers adults and children practical kid-tested activities to remain productive and attentive. It enables children to know when they need to be more alert and they can eventually be independent in regulating themselves. In the program, parts of the brain are stimulated by heavy work that involves pulling, pushing, climbing, tugging, or hanging.

The program uses engine terminology to describe how alert a person is, for example, when Jonny's engine needs a boost he is in low gear. Adults can help preschoolers in identifying when their engines are low and when they need a boost to be ready to learn so that their engines can run just right. This will set up children's nervous system for success. When engines are participating in heavy work they are in high gear and send a message to the rest of the brain and body that says "we are not in danger here, we can relax, calm down, and focus." If an engine is in low gear and the child participates in heavy work, the brain and body say "be alert, wake up, we need to focus." Heavy work helps whether the engine is in high or low gear. High gear can be achieved by doing whole-body heavy work, i.e., gross physical activity, such as tug-of-war, wrestling, or sweeping the floor; by working the hands, such as playing with putty; and by working the mouth, such as chewing gum.

Parents can start their children's day off with "heavy" work, such as physical exercise, before going to school to prepare them to be fully alert. In the evening, wrestling and doing heavy work before going to sleep can benefit muscles and joints and allow the child to be ready to sleep and not be restless. Strategies to change alert levels when engines are not running just right are divided into five sensory categories that take 5 min, 1 h, or 5 h or more. This sensory diet includes activities that stimulate the touch, sight, hearing, taste, smell, and movement. Parents need to think about their child's sensory motor preferences and help their child find activities that will help keep him or her alert and rejuvenate him or her. Sometimes these strategies will include sipping and sucking using food items, straws, or exercise water bottles. The child can blow a cotton ball with a straw and move it across the desk while sitting upright. He can also use musical instruments that involve blowing, like kazoos or harmonicas, or a wind instrument like the tuba or clarinet or flute or make one with wax paper over a comb, and take a music break. Young children can also do deep breathing and make different sounds such as barking, neighing, or quaking (see box "Helping Your Child Using the Alert Program: Take Five").

Helping Your Child Using the Alert Program: Take Five

Questions to ask:

- What do you do in a small subtle way to maintain your appropriate alert level that a child may need to do in a larger more intense way?
- Notice which types of sensory input give your child comfort and which bother him? Do they fall under a particular type of sensory input, such as touch?
- How frequently, how long, how intense, and with what rhythm does your child use these techniques to change his or her alertness?
- What sensory input does your child prefer when he or she is at his or her workspace to concentrate more efficiently:
  - In or around your mouth, e.g., food, drink, chews
  - Touch, e.g., clothing texture, holding object
  - Movement, e.g., rocking, stretching breaking, walking breaks
  - Visual preferences, e.g., lighting, pictures, bright colors, papers files high, clear desk
  - Auditory, e.g., music, beat, talking to self or others, quiet, noise

Source:

Reprinted from Williams, M.S. and Shellenberger, S. (1996). *How does your engine run? A leader's guide to the alert program for self-regulation.* Albuquerque, NM: Therapy Works

Raising a Sensory Smart Child: The Definitive Handbook for Helping Your Child with Sensory Processing Issues by Lindsey Biel and Nancy Peske (2005) helps parents and health practitioners to identify sensory-motor integration issues such as "when does your child have sensory overload?" It provides practical, easy solutions for what sometimes can be difficult to deal with. It helps children to get organized, focus, deal with overload at school, decrease stress, and address other issues that every child and parent deal with.

The Out-of-Sync Child: Recognizing and Coping with Sensory Processing Disorder by Carol Stock Kranowitz (2005) has an excellent chapter titled, "Looking at Your Child in a New Light: A Parent's Epiphany." This chapter discusses healthy ways to deal with difficult emotions, organization challenges, and tactile and auditory sensitivities. Kranowitz's tips offer ways to make difficult experiences, such as dressing and mealtimes, easier, less stressful, and more enjoyable.

In *Squirmy Wormy* (2009), author Lynda Farrington Wilson raises awareness of sensory issues and offers activities that parents can use to meet their child's sensory needs. For example, parents often complain that their child is playing with their food, trying to touch things, or licking, chewing, or sucking on their clothing. Many neurotypical children can benefit when the health care provider helps parents to recognize their children's sensory needs, and this book has fun and easy activities to provide sensory stimulation.

For example, a child can dip toy cars and other objects in shaving cream (best done in an empty bathtub or on a tray to contain the mess) or use shaving cream and food coloring to paint with their toes on a cookie sheet. Another activity uses vanilla pudding or plain yogurt, food coloring, and a muffin tin to create "edible" finger paint. After the ingredients are combined in each cup of the tin, the child can dip his or her fingers and "paint" a cookie sheet as if it were art paper. If the child doesn't like touching the paint directly, he or she can use a paintbrush (Wilson 2009).

6.8.1 Normal Child Behaviors That Are Difficult for Parents and the Child

6.8.1.1 Self-Regulation

The following books will help parents encourage self-esteem and self-regulation in their children.

104 Activities that Build Self-Esteem, Teamwork, Communication, Anger Management, Self-Discovery and Coping Skills by Alanna Jones (1998) contains instructions for a variety of therapeutic problem-solving games and activities that will make teaching, learning, growing, and changing emotionally fun. The games help participants see their problems from a different perspective and enable them to heal and be emotionally healthy throughout their lives. The text provides discussion prompts and suggestions for using the same game in different ways depending on the goal, for example, raising self-esteem or managing anger.

Parenting a Child Who Has Intense Emotions: Dialectical Behavior Therapy Skills to Help Your Child Regulate Emotional Outbursts & Aggressive Behaviors by Pat Harvey and Jeanine A. Penzo (2009) suggests specific strategies to address a child's intense feelings and behaviors. The authors first focus on the parent's emotional and behavioral stability. Once a parent can heal and grow, he or she will be better able to give support to his or her challenging children. The authors use dialectical behavior therapy principles to improve family interaction and communication skills and promote emotional stability.

Emotional Intensity in Gifted Students: Helping Kids Cope with Explosive Feelings by Christine Fonseca (2011) is aimed at teachers and parents. A particularly useful chapter is about how parents can act as coaches for their children to help them deal with their feelings. Strategies include looking at the child, doing active listening, and developing an emotional vocabulary to assist in your child in communicating his or her feelings. The author also discusses ways to deal with difficult situations and challenging relationships, and ways to become more resilient.

Children Learn What They Live: Parenting to Inspire Values by Dorothy Law Nolte and Rachel Harris (1998) presents positive parenting messages using brief stories and scenarios to instill values and self-esteem in children as they grow.

6.8.1.2 Relaxation Tapes

Still Quiet Place: Mindfulness for Teens: A Place to Chill and Be Yourself narrated by Amy Saltzman (2010) promotes internal power and peace that the teen can carry with him or her in daily stressors and challenging situations through the use of mindfulness training and daily practice. Can help with situations that invoke strong emotions such as struggling with homework, hanging with friends, arguing with parents, or feeling upset, heartbroken, happy, angry, afraid, bored, or stupid. Promotes kindness and curiosity about one's life.

Still Quiet Place: Mindfulness for Young Children, Playful Practices to Promote Health and Happiness narrated by Amy Saltzman (2004): This tape helps children achieve inner awareness to reduce stress and enhance their physical health, social relations, academic abilities, and sense of well-being. It is based on the use of mindfulness to develop moment-to-moment inner awareness. The narration helps children find the "special place inside of you that you can visit anytime," especially if they are angry, sad, afraid, or upset.

6.8.1.3 Energy Therapies

In more recent years, the use of energy therapies for stress management and pain has become more well known and used in conjunction with Western medicine (Ott et al. 2010; Glover et al. 2002). Two such techniques applicable to children are Heart Math and the Emotional Freedom Technique (tapping).

Emotional Freedom Technique

Susan Jeffrey Busen explores an emotional freedom technique that parents can use with their children in *Tap into Joy: A Guide to Emotional Freedom Techniques for Kids and Their Parents* (2007). This technique, sometimes referred to as an energy therapy tool, can empower children to help themselves resolve inner emotional distress by validating the child's experience and helping the child to release the emotional energy associated with the experience. The book is a practical reference guide about using specific points on the body that a person taps to release the emotional energy associated with the experience or task at hand. Sources of this energy include how one feels about oneself, homework, being bullied, or dealing with a potentially stressful situation. The book is written in a clear, usable format to enable the parent to apply the techniques. The *Tap into Joy* DVD is available at www.TapIntoBalance.com.

Busen also wrote *Tap into Success: A Guide to Thriving in College Using Emotional Freedom Techniques*, which is for older children as they move through middle school, high school, and college (2007).

HeartMath

The HeartMath Institute in Boulder Creek, California, has developed research-based tools to reduce stress and help people manage their emotions using their own body's "heart intelligence" and ability to heal itself. The tools are based on activating the heart and the body's natural rhythms and connections to brain function to enable one to achieve a state of "coherence" or "being in the zone." HearthMath promotes positive connections among the immune system, cognitive function, communication, creativity, intuition, and other aspects of ourselves to improve our emotional stability and sense of well-being. For more information, go to www.heartmath.org/free-services/tools-for-well-being/tools-for-well-being-home.html.

Heart Feelings

Shift and Shine is a free tool developed by The HeartMath Institute for children aged 3–6 years. Text and audio versions can be found at www.heartmath.org/free-services/tools-for-well-being/shift-and-shine-age-3-to-6.html. Shift and Shine uses the concept of shifting from one emotion to another by progressing from physical exercises to emotional exercises to sense and activate change. The short audio clip can be used by parents to help their young child develop positive emotions, control their impulsive behaviors, and understand the loving qualities of the heart. The tool is based on focusing attention to the area around the heart and using special heart breathing, sensing warm feelings in the heart, and sending the feeling to someone else.

The Heart Shift tool is for ages 7–11 years and comes in text and audio versions. This tool helps older children shift from experiencing uncomfortable feelings such as anger and frustration to more comfortable ones such as joy and satisfaction. Children will notice what they are feeling when they have these emotions and learn to do heart shift to calm them down and feel better fast. Exercises start with sensing different body parts and then the heart to help focus in three easy steps. The first step is to notice what you feel during the day—all the various emotions—happy, fear, and boredom, for example, and saying them out loud. Step 2 shifts to the heart as the center of focus, taking the fingers from head to heart. Step 3 is slow, deep breathing to feel calm, taking three special breaths. Step 4 is noticing changes. Available for free at www.heartmath.org/free-services/tools-for-well-being/heartshift-age-7-to-11.html.

The Quick Coherence tool comes in text and audio versions for ages 12–18 and adults. It is useful for quick relief from stress and negative emotions and to engender calm and improved focus. It is based on focusing on the heart, using special heart breathing to reduce and release negative thoughts, and thinking about and experiencing positive feelings while continuing to breathe through the heart. The tool can be used anytime or any place unobtrusively:

www.heartmath.org/free-services/tools-for-well-being/quick-coherence-age-12-to-18.html

www.heartmath.org/free-services/tools-for-well-being/quick-coherence-adult.html.

References

Abou-Donia MB, El-Masry EM, Abdel-Rahman AA et al (2008) Splenda alters gut microflora and increases intestinal p-glycoprotein and cytochrome p-450 in male rats. J Toxicol Environ Health A 71(21):1415–1429

American Academy of Pediatrics, Committee on Environmental Health (2010) Policy statement: Chemical-management policy: prioritizing children's health. Pediatrics 127(5):938–990

Anda RF, Felitti VJ, Bremner JD et al (2006) The enduring effects of abuse and related adverse experiences in childhood. A convergence of evidence from neurobiology and epidemiology. Eur Arch Psychiatry Clin Neurosci 256((3)):174–186

Arnwine B (2011) Starting sensory therapy: fun activities for the home and classroom. Sensory World, Arlington, TX

Bevacqua J (2013) Manufactured environmental toxins and children's health: an evidence-based review and anticipatory guidance. J Pediatr Health Care 27:13–22

Bialer DS, Miller LJ (2011) No longer a secret: unique common sense strategies for children with sensory or motor challenges. Sensory World, Future Horizons, Arlington, TX

Bouchard MF, Bellinger DC, Wright RO, Weisskopf MG (2010) Attention deficit/hyperactivity disorder and urinary metabolites of organophosphate pesticides in U.S. children 8–15 years. Pediatrics 125:e1270–e1277

Chaterji R, Tractenberg RE, Amri H et al (2007) A large-sample survey of first- and second-year medical student attitudes toward complementary and alternative medicine in the curriculum and in practice. Altern Ther Health Med 13:30–35

Connell G, McCarthy C (2013) A moving child is a learning child: how the body teaches the brain to think. Free Spirit Press, Minneapolis, MN

Crain EF, Walter M, O'Connor GT et al (2002) Home and allergic characteristics of children with asthma in seven U.S. urban communities and design of an environmental intervention: the inner-city asthma study. Environ Health Perspect 110(9):939–945

Culbert TP, Maizes V, Mendenhall T, Becker DK (2010) Assessment and treatment planning in integrative pediatric practice. In: Culbert TP, Olness K (eds) Integrative pediatrics. Oxford University Press, New York, NY, pp 13–29; Chapter 2

Dennison PE, Dennison GE (2010) Brain gym: teacher's edition: a companion guide to brain gym, simple activities for the whole brain. Hearts at Play, Inc., A division of Edu-Kinesthetics, Ventura, CA

Ratey, J. (2010). Quoted in Dennison, P.E. Dennison, G.E., Brain gym: teacher's edition: a companion guide to brain gym, simple activities for the whole brain. Ventura, CA: Hearts at Play, Inc., A division of Edu-Kinesthetics.

Etzel RA (2003) How environmental exposures influence the development and exacerbation of asthma. Pediatrics 112(Suppl 1):233–239

Felitti VJ (2009) Adverse childhood experiences and adult health. Academics 9(3):131–132

Flock MH, Kim AS (2010) Probiotics: a clinical guide. Slack, Thorofare, NJ

Galicia-Connolly EZ, Shamseer L, Vohra S (2011) Disabilities: complementary, holistic, and integrative medicine: therapies for learning. Pediatr Rev 32(2):e18–e24

Glover V, Onozawa K, Hodgkinson A (2002) Benefits of infant massage for mothers with postnatal depression. Semin Neonatol 7(6):495–500

Goddard AT (2012) Children's books for use in bibliotherapy. J Pediatr Health Care 25:57–61

Harari R, Julvez J, Murata K, Barr D, Bellinger DC, Debes F, Grandjean P (2010) Neurobehavioral deficits and increased blood pressure in school-age children prenatally exposed to pesticides. Environ Health Perspect 118(6):890–896

Henry DA, Kane-Wineland M, Swindeman S (2007) Tools for tots: sensory strategies for toddlers and preschoolers. Henry Occupational Therapy Services, Glendale, AZ

Herbert M, Weintraub K (2012) The autism revolution: whole-body strategies for making life all that it can be. Ballantine Books, New York, NY

Kang BC (1990) Cockroach allergy. Clin Rev Allergy 8(1):87–93

Kleinman R (ed) (2009) Pediatric nutrition hand book (Policy of the American Academy of Pediatrics), 6th edn. American Academy of Pediatrics, Elk Grove Village, IL

Klingler B, Scott E (2010) A pediatric perspective on nutritional therapeutics. In: Culbert TP, Olness K (eds) Integrative pediatrics. Oxford University Press, New York, NY, pp 314–339; Chapter 9

Kundu A, Tassone RF, Jimenez N et al (2011) Attitudes, patterns of recommendation, and communication of pediatric providers about complementary and alternative medicine in a large metropolitan children's hospital. Clin Pediatr 50(2):153–158

Landrigan PJ, Needleman HL, Landrigan M (2001) Raising healthy children in a toxic world: 101 smart solutions for every family. Rodale Press, Emmaus, PA

Lie DA, Boker J (2006) Comparative survey of complementary and alternative medicine (CAM) attitudes, use, and information-seeking behaviour among medical students, residents & faculty. BMC Med Educ 6:58

Machail S, Sherman M (eds) (2009) Probiotics in pediatric medicine. Humana, Totowa, NJ

Marrs R (1995) A meta-analysis of bibliotherapy studies. Am J Comm Psychol 23:843–870

National Research Council, Committee on Pesticides in the Diets of Infants and Children, Board on Agriculture and Board on Environmental Studies and Toxicology, Commission on Life Sciences (1993) Pesticides in the diets of infants and children. National Academy Press, Washington, DC

Ness R (2013) Practice guidelines for childhood lead screening in primary care. J Pediatr Health Care 27:395–399

Nyardi A, Li J, Hickling S et al (2013) The role of nutrition in children's neurocognitive development, from pregnancy through childhood. Front Hum Neurosci 7:97–169

Ott MJ, Bossi L, Colbath J (2010) A pediatric perspective on energy therapies. In: Culbert TP, Olness K (eds) Integrative pediatrics. Oxford University Press, New York, NY, pp 180–203; Chapter 9

Quigley EM (2009) The future of probiotics. In: Machail S, Sherman M (eds) Probiotics in pediatric medicine. Humana, Totowa, NJ, pp 323–329; Chapter 23

Saavedra JMM, Dattilo AM (2010) Use of probiotics and prebiotics in children. In: Flock MH, Kim AS (eds) Probiotics: a clinical guide. Thorofare, NJ, Slack Inc, pp 141–180; Chapter 11

Sagiv SK, Thurston SW, Bellinger DC, Tolbert PE, Altshul LM, Korrick SA (2010) Prenatal organochlorine exposure and behaviors associated with attention deficit hyperactivity disorder in school-aged children. Am J Epidemiol 171(5):593–601

Sher B (2009) Early intervention games: fun, joyful ways to develop social and motor skills in children with Autism Spectrum or sensory processing disorders. Jossey-Bass, San Francisco, CA

Shetreat-Klein, M. (2012). Brainmending: using food to heal the brain. Slide talk presented at the Sigma Theta Tau International, Chapter 184 Eta Sigma Conference: Opening your mind to alternative modalities in health care, College of Mount Saint Vincent, Bronx, NY, April 25

Shetreat-Klein M (2015) The dirt cure: a whole food, whole planet guide to growing healthy kids in a processed world. Simon & Schuster, New York, NY

Shonkoff JP, Garner AS, Committee on Psychosocial Aspects of Child and Family Health, American Academy of Pediatrics, 2010–2011 (2012) The lifelong effects of early childhood adversity and toxic stress (technical report). Pediatrics 129(1). http://m.pediatrics.aappublications.org/content/129/1/e232. Accessed 23 March 2015

Thibault M (2004) Children's literature promotes understanding. University of North Carolina, School of Education. K-12 Teaching and Learning, Chapel Hill, NC. www.learnnc.org/lp/pages/635. Retrieved 31 Oct 2014

Weill A (2000) Eating well for optimum health: the essential guide to bringing health and pleasure back to eating. Quill, HarperCollins/Publishers, New York, NY

Wilson LF (2009) Squirmy wormy. Sensory World, Future Horizons, Arlington, TX

Part II

Case Studies

7 Newborn Visit

Note: The newborn is the beginning of establishing a long-term relationship between the family and the health provider. Many topics will be discussed and the new parents will probably have many questions and concerns but some may be feeling so overwhelmed or anxious that they have no questions. In this case study we have chosen to describe what happens during a typical newborn rather than posing individual questions for study or guidance.

Mrs. Hernandez has just delivered a baby boy in a major medical center at 39 weeks' gestation as a result of in vitro fertilization. The delivery lasted 6 h with transition phase lasting 45 min. It was a normal vaginal delivery with no complications. This is Mrs. Hernandez' first child born alive after three miscarriages and she has long anticipated the birth of a child. She had no complications during pregnancy, no hypertension, and no urinary tract infections. She does not smoke and abstained from alcohol during the pregnancy and conception. She tested negative for HIV, hepatitis B, and group B streptococcus. She is feeling tired but could not be happier with the birth of her baby boy Juan. The baby's Apgar score at birth was 9 at 1 min and 10 at 5 min. The Apgar evaluated baby Juan's heart rate, reflexes, respiratory function, muscle tone, and color. A score of 10 is perfect. Baby Juan weighed 3.4 kg (7.48 lb) and was 49.5 cm (19.8 in.) long at birth, placing him in the 40th percentile for weight and height. His head circumference is 35 cm (14 in.), also in the 40th percentile. Right after delivery the Dubowitz Scale was administered to assess baby Juan's actual gestational age, which is 39 weeks. This scale uses physical flexibility to assess neuromuscular and physical maturity. See Dubowitz/Ballard Exam for Gestational Age: www.carteret.edu/...P/DubowitzBallard%20Exam.doc. At birth, baby Juan's skin was red, puffy, and smooth. There were no café au lait spots. No hemorrhage or ecchymosis was noted.

The primary care provider invites Mrs. Hernandez to the nursery for an examination of her baby. This visit commonly takes place in the hospital or at a birthing center within hours of a child's birth; occasionally it occurs after a home delivery. Sometimes the examination is done without the parent in the nursery, and sometimes at the bedside of the mother. It is important to include parents in this assessment because it increases their sense of power.

The primary care provider will include the Brazelton Neonatal Assessment Scale to assess baby Juan's infant state and certain categories of behavior. This assessment

D. Kramer, *Primary Well-Being: Case Studies for the Growing Child*,
DOI 10.1007/978-3-319-56708-2_7

is usually done in the first 6–8 h after birth known as the first period of reactivity—when the baby is alert. It is redone in the second period of reactivity after the baby has had his first deep sleep. Mrs. Hernandez had been attending childbirth education classes that were provided by the hospital throughout her pregnancy and was able to breastfeed Juan after delivery and the placenta was delivered intact. Juan was alert and latched on immediately, and suckled for 5 min on each side.

Both parents are present for baby Juan's exam. During the physical exam, the nurse tells Mrs. Hernandez what she is finding and confirming that the observations are normal.

Head

His head is soft. The anterior fontanel is diamond shaped and flat and measures 4 cm. The posterior fontanel is triangular, and measures 0.5 cm and is flat. His head is round.

Eyes, Ears, Nose, and Throat

The baby's eyelids are edematous. The red reflex is present. The blink reflex is present. There is an absence of tears and baby Juan is able to fixate on another's face and follow objects to midline. The sclera is white. His ears are able to recoil. The ears are horizontal with the outer canthus and shaped similarly to his mother's. Baby Juan's response to sudden noise demonstrates the Moro reflex. His nasal patency shows thin, white nasal discharge, and there was no nasal flaring. His uvula is midline; his palette is intact. His tongue is not protruding and there is no salivation or drooling. The sucking reflex is strong and coordinated. The rooting, gag, and extrusion reflexes are intact, and baby Juan demonstrates vigorous crying. His neck is short with skin folds and tonic neck reflexes present.

Chest and Respiratory

The baby's chest shows slight sternal retractions during inspiration, xiphoid process is evident, and there is slight breast enlargement. The lateral and anteroposterior diameter is equal. His lungs and abdominal respirations equal bronchial breath sounds. His heart sounds are normal. His heart rate is 140.

Heart

The apex of the heart is between the fourth and fifth intercostal space, lateral to the left sternal border.

Abdomen

Juan's abdomen shows a palpable liver, 2–3 cm below the right costal margin; kidneys are palpable 1–2 cm above the umbilicus. The umbilical cord is bluish-white at birth with two arteries and one vein (note: it is important to inspect the cord). Femoral pulses are equal bilaterally and the abdomen is cylindrical in shape.

Genitourinary

His urethral opening is midline at the tip of the glans penis. Scrotum is edematous, covered with rugae with testes palpable. Urinary stream is at midline. His back and rectum show that his spine is intact, no openings, no tufts of hair, and no masses or prominent curves. The anal opening is patent.

Musculo/Skeletal-Neuro

The trunk incurvation and anal reflexes are present. Baby's extremities show full range of motion. There are ten fingers and toes; his nail beds are pink. There is symmetry of the extremities with equal muscle tone bilaterally, and there are equal bilateral brachial pulses. The sole of baby's foot is flat with creases on the anterior two-thirds of the sole. Holding the baby up, we observe equal gluteal folds and leg folds. The baby's extremities are in flexion, with hands loosely fisted. There is no single transverse palmar crease. The baby can turn his head from side to side when prone and is able to hold his head in a horizontal line when held in the prone position; there is head lag while pulling the baby up to sitting and a momentary ability to hold his head erect. There is no arching of the back, and no tremors or twitches.

Neuro Reflexes

Neurologically, the following reflexes are present in baby Juan: sucking reflex, rooting reflex, palmer grasp, stepping, Moro, Babinski, and plantar grasp. Juan's muscle tone is normal. He has symmetrical extremity movements. During the exam the health care practitioner observes how the parents recognize and respond to the baby's needs. Juan responds to his mother's voice and touch. She is comfortable holding and feeding him. His father expresses concern over whether he will be able to care for the baby. It is important to place Juan in his father's arms, helping him to feel comfortable holding the baby, and to be sure that he will have a class on giving the baby bath and changing Juan's diaper before being discharged. The health care professional should observe or ask the parents about their support networks.

- **What guidance is appropriate to give Mr. and Mrs. Hernandez concerning washing their new baby?**

During the examination the health professional should talk to Mr. and Mrs. Hernandez about the importance of washing the baby's scalp and demonstrate how to wash it gently over the fontanels. The scalp should be washed every day to prevent cradle cap—a crush of yellow scales on the head common in babies. Bathing is usually a daily routine parents do with their baby. Many new parents are scared to wash their tiny infant. The provider can suggest that an experienced person be there the first time to help the family and relieve any anxiety. The nurse demonstrates bathing at the bedside while the umbilical cord stub is still present.

Once the cord falls off (usually in about 10–14 days), the baby will be ready for a baby bath. For bathing newborns, use fragrance-free soaps and lotions. For areas of dry skin and creases, moisturizing lotions are recommended. Powders are not recommended because they may be inhaled, causing respiratory problems. To prevent diaper rash, the health care provider advises Mrs. Hernandez to clean the baby after wet diapers or stools, and change them frequently. Diaper creams or ointments will be helpful, but it is important to clean the area well and dry the area before putting on the cream and diaper. While the cord is intact, keep the diaper folded below the umbilicus and air-dry the cord, keeping it free of urine and feces. The use of alcohol is not recommended, nor are belly bands on the umbilicus. It is important for the provider to tell the parents to always wash their hands with warm soap and water before touching the baby. All visitors to the household including family should do this.

Now is also the time to discuss whether Juan will have a circumcision in the hospital before going home. The decision should be based on Juan's family and their cultural needs. The health provider should discuss the pros and cons of circumcisions with the parents in an informative, unbiased manner.

Screenings that are done on baby Juan before leaving the hospital or birthing center include glucose screening, bilirubin screen, hearing, and PKU (see box "Major Developmental Characteristics of Hearing") (DeMichele and Ruth 2010; Fouzas et al. 2009; Porter and Dennis 2002; Wagner et al. 2013; Wolf et al. 2007).

Major Developmental Characteristics of Hearing

Birth

Responds to loud noise by startle, or Moro reflex

Responds to sound of human voice more readily than to any other sound

Quieting effect from low-pitched sounds, such as lullaby, metronome, or heartbeat

8–12 Weeks

Turns head to side when sound is made at the level of ear

12–16 Weeks

Locates sound by turning head to side and looking in same direction

16–24 Weeks

Locates sound by turning head to side and then looking up or down

24–32 Weeks

Locates sounds by turning head in a curving arc

Responds to own name

32–40 Weeks

Localizes sounds by turning head diagonally and directly toward sound

40–52 Weeks

Knows several words and their meaning, such as "no," and names of family members

Learns to control and adjust own response to sound, such as listening for the sound to occur again

Source: *Harlor, A.D. and Bower, C. and The Committee on Practice and Ambulatory Medicine, The Section on Otolaryngology-Head and Neck Surgery. (2009). Clinical report—Hearing assessment in infants and children: Recommendations beyond neonatal screening.* Pediatrics, *124(4), 1252–1263.*

- **What kind of anticipatory guidance would you give for the newborn and his family?**

Getting Family Support: The health care provider should speak with the parents about the importance of having people they can turn to for help and support them physically and emotionally, and be able to ask questions of. Explain to the parents that people want to help but often don't know what the parents exactly want them to do. Parents need to give these helpers specific instructions on what they can do to help, such as "could you get some items at the store for me when you go shopping?", "could you watch the baby for an hour while I have my check-up?", or "could you be with me while I bath the baby?"

Feeling good: Remind Mr. and Mrs. Hernandez that all parents get upset at least some times while they are caring for their babies. They may not understand why their baby is crying or they may have just changed the baby from head to toe and the baby soils its diaper and you need to begin again and you are running out of undershirts (onesies) and need to do the laundry. Ask, "So what do you do when you get upset?" Explain that when you have upset feelings it helps to have someone to call or ask for help. Suggest the parent put the baby down in a safe place like a crib. It is important to never hit, yell at, or shake your baby. Suggest the parents identify activities that are difficult for them to do now that they are a new mom, such as laundry, grocery shopping, vacuuming, washing the dishes, and preparing meals. It is important for Mrs. Hernandez to get the rest and sleep she needs and to spend some time on herself along and with her partner. One way is to sleep whenever the baby is sleeping. This time spent is important for Mrs. Hernandez and for her family to be able to care for her baby. It will help her to stay happy, feel nurtured, and be healthy. If she is feeling tired, sad, or overwhelmed, she might feel the "baby blues." This is common in the first few weeks with a new baby. If these feelings continue for more than a few days, Mrs. Hernandez will need to let her health care provider and Mr. Hernandez know, so that they can get the right resources to help his wife. The provider may administer the Beck Depression Scale and seek appropriate counseling for Mrs. Hernandez. She may find a parent support group helpful as well (Hockenberry and Wilson 2011; Burns 2009; Hefner 2010).

Building a relationship between parent and child: Even from the start, Juan will enjoy watching his parent's face and will soon start reacting to their expressions and sounds with vocalizations and smiles by around 6 weeks. This is a good time to begin telling your child that you love them and also expressing this emotion by giving baby Juan hugs and kisses. He will also enjoy looking at and listening to mobiles and also hearing the words from books that are read to him, even at this young age. It is important to remember that babies need play time apart from feeding. From early infancy relationships are being built by the interactions of parent/caregiver and child as they respond to each other in a kind of "serve and return" dance (National Scientific Council on the Developing Child 2009). The infant coos, the parent responds by cooing and saying "you're so cute"; the infant smiles and the parent smiles back and may say, "look, you are smiling at me." This is play in infancy: it fosters the architecture of the developing brain, which grows to 85% of its adult capacity during the first 3 years of life (National Scientific Council on the Developing Child 2007). But also remind Mr. and Mrs. Hernandez that newborns do sleep and eat most of the time; as they grow, more time will be spent in play.

Advice for first week home: Health care providers should review with the parents the contents of the *Bright Futures Parent Handout* (American Academy of Pediatrics 2010a) for the first week. It contains bulleted sections on parents' well-being, baby's nutrition and feeding, baby care, getting used to baby, newborn to 1-month suggestions on routines and behavior, safety suggestions, and a general list of topics for the first-month visit. The handout can be accessed at American Academy of Pediatrics (2010). *Bright Futures Parent Handout 2–5 Day (First Week) Visit.* Elk Gove, IL: American Academy of Pediatrics. Viewed online: May 27, 2014 at http://brightfutures.aap.org/pdfs/Visit%20Forms%20by%20Age%20110/Newborn,%202-5%20 Day/A.Inf.PH.2-5day.pdf.

- **What do you do when you suspect there will be problems or that the parents are at high risk for problems when they take baby Juan home?**

A high-risk parent is someone who needs to be supported with emotional and physical help and resources. They are potentially abusive or neglectful if not supported. Parents at high risk for problems when they take their babies home should be referred to a social worker for follow-up home visits. Indicators for high risk include

- Adolescent pregnancy
- Lack of prenatal care
- Thinking about adoption
- Unwanted pregnancy
- Insufficient support from those at home
- Physical limitations of parent
- Inadequate housing/food resources/finances
- Domestic violence
- Positive toxicology
- Incarcerated parent
- Emotional disorders
- Parent with mental retardation

Other families at risk include those with babies who have special health care needs and those with multiple small children in the household. Parents can also be concerned about how their other children will react to the new baby in the family. Spending individual time every day with the other children and doing things they like to do, such as having a special project, going to the library, singing favorite songs, and reading a book, help children know they are still wanted and loved. Older children being asked to help care for the baby with something that is within their capability to do also helps them feel wanted and loved in adjusting to the new baby. It is important not to leave the baby alone or unsupervised with their young siblings.

- **What kinds of infant behaviors should Mr. and Mrs. Hernandez anticipate when they take baby Juan home?**

The health provider should explain to Mr. and Mrs. Hernandez that Juan may have different cries and fuss at different times of the day. It is normal for babies to fuss or cry an hour or two each day in the first few months, especially in the early evening. Mr. and Mrs. Hernandez should make sure that they have taken care of Juan's needs. Holding and caressing Juan, carrying him and rocking him, and touching him are all important in caring for him. Physical contact helps keep Juan feeling safe and makes him understand he is loved and cared for. Also, Juan should be talked to as Mr. and Mrs. Hernandez go about their daily routines with Juan, communicating love, warmth, laughter, and making eye contact, and smiling. He will respond to his parents' voices and will be calmed by them and by 6–8 weeks Juan will start smiling back (Dixon and Stein 2006).

- **What health and safety precautions should the parents take in their home?**

Whenever the parents are going to handle Juan, they should first wash their hands. Also, all visitors to the house should wash their hands with soap and warm water for at least 30 s upon entering and before they touch the baby. Also when going out, the parents should not take the baby into crowds of people and not allow anyone to touch him without washing hands. Explain to Mr. and Mrs. Hernandez that the reason for these cautions is that babies don't have a mature immune system yet. The immunity Juan receives is passive immunity from the antibodies in his mother's breast milk and will lack his own immune system for the first 3 months of life (see box "Advantages of Human Milk").

When putting Juan to sleep it is important to put him on his back, to prevent sudden infant death syndrome (SIDS). Cigarette smoking in the household also increases the risk for SIDS. Juan should not sleep in the bed with his parents. If Mrs. Hernandez is feeding Juan in bed, it is important to put him back in his crib after he is finished and burped, when he is ready to go back to sleep. There should be no loose or soft bedding, or soft toys in the baby's crib. Babies like to be swaddled in thin blankets and placed on their back in the crib, with the sides of the crib raised.

Fall prevention is also important. Mr. and Mrs. Hernandez should never leave Juan unattended on a changing table, bed, or any raised surface. They should also be careful not to leave any objects around that Juan could accidentally ingest, such as plastic pieces, holders, deflated balloons, small buttons, and coins. As babies grow, putting things in their mouths is the way they explore the world and we need to keep it safe for them right from the beginning.

Pacifier use: Since Mrs. Hernandez is breastfeeding, we would not recommend that she use a pacifier until Juan is over a month old. There is evidence that a pacifier given to an infant while sleeping on his back reduces the incidence of SIDS (American Academy of Pediatrics, Taskforce on Sudden Infant Death Syndrome 2011). Make sure that the pacifier used is one piece.

Temperature: Room temperature for babies should be comfortable—not too hot or too cold while the baby is sleeping. If Mrs. Hernandez is comfortable, baby Juan will be.

Composition of Human Milk

Human milk contains the following elements that are beneficial for human babies:

- Correct amount of protein
- Higher amount of lactalbumin (which produces easily digested curds) than casein (which produces large, hard curds)
- Lactose, which stimulates the growth of friendly microorganisms in the intestine, synthesizes B vitamins and reduces the growth of harmful bacteria
- Monounsaturated fatty acids, which enhance absorption of fat and calcium
- Readily absorbable iron and zinc
- More favorable ratio of minerals that are bioavailable except fluoride
- Adequate amounts of vitamins A, B complex, and E
- Vitamin C content depends on maternal intake of vitamin C
- Low but more absorbable levels of vitamin D
- Immunologic benefits, including immunoglobulin A, macrophages, granulocytes, T- and B-cell lymphocytes, and other substances that inhibit bacterial growth
- Has laxative effect
- Is readily available and affordable
- Fosters a close bond between infant and mother during feeding

Sources:

American Academy of Pediatrics, Committee on Nutrition. (2009). Pediatric nutrition handbook, 6th ed. *Elk Grove Village, IL: American Academy of Pediatrics*

Ballard, O. and Morrow, A.L. (2012). Human milk composition: Nutrients and bioactive factors. Pediatric Clinics of North America, 60, *49–74.*

Burns, C.E., et al. *Pediatric Primary Care: A Handbook for Nurse Practitioners*, 4th ed. Philadelphia, PA: W.B. Saunders, 2009.

Schanler, R.J., Krebs, N.F., Mass, S.B. (Eds.). (2014). Breastfeeding handbook for physicians, 2nd ed. *Elk Grove Village, IL & Washington, D.C.: American Academy of Pediatrics & American College of Obstetricians and Gynecologists.*

Schanler, R.J., Krebs, N.F., Mass, S.B. (Eds.). (2014). Composition of human milk. In: American College of Obstetricians and Gynecologists & American Academy of Pediatrics. Breastfeeding handbook for physicians, 2nd ed, Chapter 3. *Elk Grove Village, IL & Washington, D.C.: American Academy of Pediatrics & American College of Obstetricians and Gynecologists.*

- **What supports can you offer to Mrs. Hernandez to sustain breastfeeding?**

Mrs. Hernandez has chosen to breastfeed, which is good for all newborns. She can expect Juan to nurse about every 1–2 h for the first week to make up for the weight he loses right after birth and this also helps while the milk supply is coming in for the mother to produce enough milk. Subsequently the baby will nurse every couple of hours for the first month or two, with hopefully a longer period at night.

Some babies initially get nights and days mixed up and may need to be woken to feed more often during the day to have the longer sleep at night. Babies will nurse between 8 and 12 times in 24 h (Feldman 2011).

The health care provider should talk to Mrs. Hernandez about the common concerns new mothers have about breastfeeding in the first days and weeks after birth. These concerns will usually center around difficulty with the infant feeding at the breast, breastfeeding pain, and milk quantity. These risks for the mother stopping to breastfeed can be overcome with appropriate support to Mrs. Hernandez. Teach Mrs. Hernandez different positions to ease breast pain, enable better latching on, and toughening the nipples between feedings. Tell her to take warm showers before nursing and use a light ointment, like HPA (pure) lanolin, to lubricate and prevent cracked nipples. A local lactation consultant or La Leche League leader can help with these challenges (Burns et al. 2009; American Academy of Pediatrics 2014; American Academy of Pediatrics, Committee on Nutrition 2009; American Academy of Obstetrics and Gynecology 2014; Ballard et al. 1991).

- **What advice would you give if the baby had been bottle-fed?**

If she had chosen to formula feed, Mrs. Hernandez would prepare two ounces of the infant formula every 2–3 h, increasing the amount of formula needed at each feed, based on the baby's appetite. Use only commercially prepared, iron-fortified formulas.

One food to avoid for babies is honey. Infants in the first year of life are not allowed to have honey because it contains botulism that cause neurotoxicity in infants. Honey should not be put in the bottle, only formula. Neurotoxicity affects baby's nerves and muscles. Infant botulism is very serious and occurs worldwide (Koepke et al. 2008; Centers for Disease Control and Prevention 2010; Centers for Disease Control and Prevention 2011; American Academy of Pediatrics, Committee on Infectious Diseases 2014).

Formula hints (Zickler 2011; Burns et al. 2009; American Academy of Pediatrics 2010; Hagan 2008):

1. Only commercially prepared, iron-fortified formulas should be used: powder, concentrate, ready-to-feed. Do not dilute ready-to-feed; do not reuse if it has been more than 4 h since opened.
2. Mix formulas with bottled water for first month; continue if on well or unsure of water quality. Store in refrigerator if open no longer than 24 h.
3. Specialized formulas have similar preparation directions. Goat's milk, whole cow's milk, and rice milk have inadequate amounts of vitamins and minerals.
4. Serve formula at room temperature. Do not microwave to heat. Do not let formula sit out at room temperature to warm for more than 15–20 min.
5. Clean off formula cans with soap and water before opening. Use hot soapy water and bottlebrush to clean nipples and bottles or clean in dishwasher.
6. Hold during feedings; burp every 1–2 oz.
7. Hold in upright, semireclined position for feedings. No bottle propping.
8. Newborn will drink 0.5–1 oz of formula/feeding every 2–3 h for first 24 h (60–100 mL/kg/day). There may be days when the baby takes more or less, depending on sleep patterns. Baby should take in 90% of feeding in the first 20 min.

- **What patterns of elimination can you expect in the newborn infant?**

For newborns, feedings generally start with 5 min on each breast, with burping or diaper change in between. As Juan gains weight, he will nurse longer at each breast up to 20 min on each breast. Juan should have 6–8 diapers in 24 h and he may have one stool per feeding or may go a number of days without a stool. Stools of breastfed children will be loose; this is normal. During the first 48 h, the stools will be dark olive green, tar-like substance, called meconium—the transition stool from what the infant injected during utero. After 2–3 days of breast or bottle-feeding, the stool will change to yellow pasty consistency. Infants can have 1–6 stools a day depending on whether they are bottle-fed (fewer) or breastfed (more). Karo syrup should not be used with infants who may be constipated.

Mrs. Hernandez should continue taking her prenatal vitamins to make sure that she is getting vitamin B-12.

- **What safety tips for car and home can you give to the parents before they take baby Juan home?**

Car seat safety: A rear-facing car seat should be used for transportation. Check with the manufacturer what the safety warrantee is if using a used seat. During all times of traveling, babies must be in a rear-facing car seat for infants and not in the first row of seats—the back seat is the safest place. Parents can borrow new car seats from the local AAA office without charge if they can't invest in one themselves or don't have a car. Some seat models come with adaptable strollers for travel.

Home Safety Tip

Working smoke detector should be on each floor of the household.

No smoking around baby or wearing clothes that have smoke on them. Research has demonstrated increased otitis media when babies are exposed to people who smoke (American Academy of Pediatrics 1997).

- **When can Juan be taken outside?**

He can go outside, but not be near crowds of people or exposed to direct sunlight. Keep him well bundled up and away from others, for example in a baby carrier or sturdy stroller. Explain to the parents that this advice is due to the baby's immature immune system. Babies should also not go outside in extremes of temperature days. Give the parents a handout of information to take home with them about their baby's care during the first week of life, such as *Bright Futures Parent Handout 2 to 5 Day (First Week) Visit* (American Academy of Pediatrics 2010a).

- **What are the immunization needs of the baby?**

Provider should generally explain to parents about immunization needs based on *Recommended Immunization Schedule for Persona Aged 0 through 6 Years—United States 2010*. Centers for Disease Control and Prevention web site http://www.cdc.gov/vaccines/recs/acip. Accessed June 2, 2011.

For immunizations at this age, consult the CDC, ACIP, or AAP web sites for the current immunization schedule recommendations:

(a) CEC National Immunization Program (NIP): http://www.cdc.gov/vaccines

Title: Tips for Successful Bottle Feeding (American Academy of Pediatrics 2009)

Hold baby in semireclining position.

Try burping every 1–2 oz.

Formula should be fed to baby at room temperature.

Do not microwave to heat as it may become too hot for baby.

Warm formula bottle in bowl of hot water for a few minutes.

Formula should not sit out to warm for more than 15–20 min.

Use the clean technique to mix formula. Sterile technique is not necessary.

1. Always clean off cans with soap and water before opening.
2. Use hot soapy water and bottlebrush to clean nipples and bottles.
3. Bottles can also be cleaned in dishwasher.

Avoid propping the bottle.

Pacifiers can be used for non-nutritive sucking. Breastfeeding should be well established before starting infant on a pacifier, but babies who suck pacifiers are at decreased incidence of sudden infant death.

No smoking or drinking hot beverages while holding baby.

Guidelines for Breastfeeding

Advantages and Duration of Breastfeeding

- Best source of nutrition for the first year of life
- Recommend exclusive breastfeeding for first 6 months
- Supplemental foods added after 6 months with continued breastfeeding beyond the first year
- Protects against many diseases and infections
- Stimulates contractions of uterus for new mother

How Breastfeeding Works

- Lactation is governed by the interplay of three mechanisms to produce the milk supply:
  - Release of the hormones oxytocin and prolactin.
  - Frequent breast emptying.
  - Sufficient sucking of the child on the breast.
- Composition of human milk changes over time:
  - Colostrum is the first milk that women excrete beginning in pregnancy.

Colostrum provides maternal antibodies, fats, proteins, carbohydrates, and other substances that human babies need.
It is thick, yellow, and is often called "liquid gold."
It has three times the amount of protein as the mature milk.
- The "mature milk" appears 48–72 h after giving birth.
It appears less thick and creamy and can be thin looking at times.
It contains foremilk and hind milk.
Foremilk (milk excreted when baby starts a feeding) contains water and nutrients.
Hind milk contains fat and calories.
Babies need both types of milk to thrive.

When Not to Breastfeed

- Infants have galactosemia.
- Maternal HIV.
- Active tuberculosis being treated with chemotherapy.
- Herpetic lesions on the mother's nipple or areola.
- Drug abuse by the mother.
- Mother taking specific medicines that may be harmful to the baby:
  - Each one will need to be checked about its likelihood to pass through the breast milk barrier.
  - For further information on medications and breastfeeding, see LactMed section of TOXNET (http://toxnet.nlm.nih.gov).

Maternal Preparation

- Discuss with pregnant and new mother how to maintain a healthy breastfeeding diet.
- Situations that may require a lactation consultant include
  - Breast or nipple surgery or thoracic surgery
  - Presence of inverted or flat nipples
  - Previous negative breastfeeding experiences
  - Current medications and/or medical treatments

Infant Challenges

Situations that may require consultation with a lactation consultant and/or specialists may include

- Congenital illness
- Early gestational age
- Infant receiving medications or procedures
- Oral or facial malformation
- Tongue or lip ties

Breastfeeding in the First Days

- Encourage breastfeeding with skin-to-skin contact immediately after birth.
- Feed when the infant is quiet and alert.
- Discourage use of any supplements.
- Encourage exclusive breastfeeding without the use of bottles or pacifiers.
- Teach the correct method for latching on to the breast.
- Explain infant feeding cues to look for, such as rooting, increased alertness, putting fists in mouth, and crying.
- If waking baby to feed, the best time is during REM sleep.

Proper Latch Techniques and Positions

- Preparation:
  - Mother should wash her hands with warm soapy water before beginning each breastfeeding session.
  - The mother should be in a comfortable position, supported by pillows (sitting or reclining).
  - If sitting up, pillows should be put under the mother's arms so the baby is sufficiently supported while being held by mother.
  - Other positions the mother might choose for breastfeeding are the side-lying position, cradle position, and football hold.
- Holding the infant:
  - The mother should hold the baby with the opposite arm from the breast being used.
  - Support the head by placing the thumb by one ear and the rest of the fingers by the other palm on shoulder blades of the baby.
  - Baby's tummy should be facing mother's tummy with the legs through mother's arm.
  - Line baby's nose up to nipple, help baby flex head up and wait for a wide open mouth, and bring the baby in from the shoulder blades so the head is in flexed-up position, chin and cheeks close as possible with the nose clear.
  - With the hand on the same side of the breast, sandwich the breast tissue using a "c" hold being sure that your fingers are not too close to the areola so they do not end up in the baby's mouth.
  - Stroking the baby's cheek may help get baby to open its mouth.
  - If the latch is done properly, the infant's lips will be around the areola with the chin and cheek touching the breast and the infant's tongue will be over the gum ridge and cup the areola.

- Removing baby from beast:
  - If the baby continues to suck and the mother wants to switch sides, the mother can insert her finger to break the suction.
  - If the latch is not complete, use this method to break the suction and begin again.
- Signs for good latch and sufficient feeding:
  - The mother should feel a gentle tugging sensation when baby is suckling.
  - There should not be nipple pain.
  - Mother's breast should become softened after feeding, and nipple should remain the same shape as before the feeding.
  - Mother will feel her uterus contract during the first days and increased lochia flow.
  - Opposite breast may leak.
  - The baby will make audible swallowing sounds of suck and swallow pattern with occasional pauses.

    In the early days there may be more sucks per swallow.

    Once the milk comes in there should be consistent one-to-one suck swallow breathe pattern sustained for at least 3–5 min with intermittent pausing to be sure that it's a good feeding.
  - Babies should be eating at least eight feedings a day and have 6–8 wet diapers and 2–4 bowel movements a day.
  - A baby will look relaxed and sleepy after a good feeding with hands open and relaxed.
  - Baby will appear satisfied and appear to be gaining weight.
- Spacing between feedings:
  - First 3 months:

    If the infant falls asleep during feeding or does not wake for feedings after more than 3 h during the day, unwrap her or rub her feet to wake her up.

    Mother should empty one breast before going on to the next one because the fat content is higher at the end of the feeding.

    The first few days after birth the amount of colostrum is very small, but sufficient to nourish the baby.

    If the baby does not wake or is unable to create a good seal or latch on the breast, then the baby still needs to be fed ideally with mother's pumped milk.
  - Infant over 3 months:

    As baby grows, the interval between feedings usually lengthens between 2 and 4 h, with often a longer stretch at night.

    As baby grows the baby will need increased production of breast milk to meet their nutritional needs. The baby will want to nurse more often to increase the supply of milk to meet their needs.

- Breastfeeding the infant when they want without supplementing is best to meet the changing nutritional needs of the baby.

Red Flags When Breastfeeding

- Don't see swallowing and hear sucking sounds within a few minutes of starting the feeding.
- Lack of frequent wet diapers—at least six per day, and fewer than two stools a day.
- Baby not gaining weight.
- Blood in the stool:
  - Most often an indication of allergy, does not mean to stop breastfeeding but maternal diet may need to change, often starting with elimination of dairy and soy.
  - Referral to a specialist.
- Malodorous stools most often allergy—referral to a specialist

When Mother and Infant are Separated

- Mothers should be encouraged to express milk when they will be away from their infant and to store the milk in the freezer.
- Mother can build up a stored milk supply by expressing milk from each breast after a feeding. This milk can be stored in the freezer for emergencies.
- Expressing milk can be done using a pump or by hand.
- The mothers' breasts should be emptied a minimum of eight times a day to maintain a milk supply while separated from the baby.
- According to federal law, all places of work need to provide mothers with private space where she can collect her milk and a refrigerator to store it in.
- An insulated bag with an ice pack should be used for transporting milk.
- The breast milk should be labeled with date and then frozen unless it is going to be used within 24 h.

Sources:

American Academy of Pediatrics, Committee on Nutrition. (2009). Pediatric nutrition handbook, 6th ed. *Elk Grove Village, IL: American Academy of Pediatrics*

Burns, C.E., et al. *Pediatric Primary Care: A Handbook for Nurse Practitioners*, 4th ed. Philadelphia, PA: W.B. Saunders, 2009.

Feldman, A.L. (2011). Guidelines for Breastfeeding, Chapter 5, pp. 35-56. In Richardson, B.E., Ed. Pediatric Primary Care: Practice Guidelines for Nurses. *Sudbury, MA: Jones & Bartlett Publishers.*

Kramer, Shoshana R. RN, BSN, IBCLC. Lactation Consultant, Queens, New York.

Schanler, R.J., Krebs, N.F., Mass, S.B. (Eds.). (2014). Breastfeeding handbook for physicians, 2nd ed. *Elk Grove Village, IL & Washington, D.C.: American Academy of Pediatrics & American College of Obstetricians and Gynecologists.*

United States Department of Labor. Employment protections for workers who are pregnant or nursing. *Accessed August 17, 2015 at: http://www.dol.gov/wb/maps/.*

United States. Office of Personnel Management. (2013). Guide for establishing nursing mother's program. *Washington, DC: U.S. Office of Personnel Management. Accessed August 17, 2015 at: https://www.opm.gov/policy-data-oversight/worklife/reference-materials/nursing-mother-guide.pdf*

(b) American Academy of Pediatrics *Red Book*: http://www.aapredbook.org

Checklist:

References

American Academy of Obstetrics and Gynecology, American Academy of Pediatrics (2014a) Breastfeeding handbook for physicians, 2nd edn. American Academy of Pediatrics, Elk Grove Village, IL

American Academy of Pediatrics, Committee on Nutrition (2009) Pediatric nutrition handbook, 6th edn. American Academy of Pediatrics, Elk Grove Village, IL

American Academy of Pediatrics (2009) Committee on Nutrition: Pediatric nutrition handbook, 6th edn. American Academy of Pediatrics, Elk Grove Village, IL

American Academy of Pediatrics (2010a) Bright Futures parent handout 2-5 day (first week) visit. American Academy of Pediatrics, Elk Gove, IL. http://brightfutures.aap.org/pdfs/Visit%20Forms%20by%20Age%20110/Newborn,%202-5%20Day/A.Inf.PH.2-5day.pdf. Accessed 27 May 2014

American Academy of Pediatrics (2010b) Car safety seats: a guide for families 2010. Healthy Children website. http://www.healthyc. (hildren.org/English/safety-prevention/on-th-go/pages/Car-Safety-Seats-Information-for-Families-2010.aspx. Accessed 2 June 2011

American Academy of Pediatrics (undated) Infant-food and feeding. http://www.aap.org/en-us/advocacy-and-policy/aap-health-initiatives/HALF-Implementation-Guide/Age-Specific-Content/Pages/Infant-Food-and-Feeding.aspx. Accessed 18 June 2014

American Academy of Pediatrics. Committee on Environmental Health (1997) Environmental tobacco smoke: a hazard to children. Pediatrics 99:639–642

American Academy of Pediatrics. Committee on Infectious Diseases (2014) Recommended childhood and adolescent immunization schedule—United States, 2014. Pediatrics 133(2):357–363

American Academy of Pediatrics, Taskforce on Sudden Infant Death Syndrome (2011) SIDS and other sleep-related infant deaths: expansion of recommendations for a safe infant sleeping environment, technical report. Pediatrics 128(5):e1341–e1367

Ballard JL, Khoury JC, Wedeg K et al (1991) New Ballard Score expanded to include extremely premature infants. Pediatrics 119:417–423

Burns CE et al (2009) Pediatric primary care: a handbook for nurse practitioners, 4th edn. W.B. Saunders, Philadelphia, PA

Centers for Disease Control and Prevention (2010) Recommended immunization schedule for persons aged 0 through 6 years—United States 2010. http://www.cdc.gov/vaccines/recs/acip. Accessed 2 June 2011

Centers for Disease Control and Prevention (2011) Recommendations and guidelines: childhood and adolescent immunization schedules. http://www.cdc.gov/vaccines/schedules/index.html. Accessed 11 Dec 2014

DeMichele AM, Ruth RA (2010) Newborn hearing screening. Medscape reference. http://emedicine.medscape.com/article/836646. Accessed 2 June 2011

Dixon SD, Stein MT (2006) Encounters with children: pediatric behavior and development, 4th edn. Mosby, St. Louis, MO

Feldman AL (2011a) Guidelines for breastfeeding. In: Richardson B (ed) Pediatric primary care: practice guidelines for nurses. Jones & Bartlett Learning, Burlington, MA, pp 35–56; Chapter 5

Feldman AL (2011b) Guidelines for breastfeeding. In: Richardson BE (ed) Pediatric primary care: practice guidelines for nurses. Jones & Bartlett Publishers, Sudbury, MA, pp 35–56; Chapter 5

Fouzas S, Mantagou L, Skylogianni SM et al (2009) Transcutaneous bilirubin levels for the first 120 post-natal hours in healthy neonates. Pediatrics 125(1):e52–e57

Hagan JF, Shaw JS, Duncan P (eds) (2008) Bright futures: guidelines for health supervision of infants, children, and adolescents, 3rd edn. American Academy of Pediatrics, Elk Grove Village, IL

Hefner AM (2010) The well infant. In: Burns CE, Richardson B, Brady MA (eds) Pediatric primary care case studies. Jones & Bartlett Publishers, Sudbury, MA, pp 75–84

Hockenberry MJ, Wilson DW (2011) Wong's nursing care of infants and children, 9th edn. Elsevier/Mosby, New York, NY

Hurley DS (2000) Developing fine and gross motor skills: birth to three. PRO-ED, Inc, Austin, TX. www.proedinc.com. Retrieved 11 Dec 2014

Koepke R, Sobel J, Arnon SS (2008) Global occurrence of infant botulism, 1976-2006. Pediatrics 122:e73–e82

LactMed (n.d.). http://toxnet.nlm.nih.gov

Marcdante KJ, Kliegman RM, Jenson HB et al (eds) (2011) Nelson essentials of pediatrics, 6th edn. Saunders, Philadelphia, PA

McInerny TK, Adam HM, Campbell DE et al (eds) (2009) Textbook of pediatric care. American Academy of Pediatrics, Elk Grove Village, IL

National Institute of Health. Osteoporosis and Related Bone Diseases National Resource Center (2012) Calcium and vitamin D: important at every age. http://www.niams.nih.gov/Health_Info/Bone/Bone_Health/Nutrition/. Accessed 23 Dec 2014

National Scientific Council on the Developing Child (2007) The timing and quality of early experiences combine to shape brain architecture (working paper no. 5). Harvard Center for the Developing Child, Boston, MA. http://developingchild.harvard.edu/index.php/resources/reports_and_working_papers/working_papers/wp5/. Accessed 18 Nov 2014

National Scientific Council on the Developing Child (2009) Young children develop in an environment of relationships (working paper no. 1). Harvard University Center on the Developing Child, Cambridge, MA

Porter ML, Dennis BL (2002) Hyperbilirubinemia in the term newborn. Am Fam Phys 65(4):599–607. American Academy of Family Physicians website. http://www.aafp.org/afp.org/afp/2002/0215/p599.html. Accessed 2 June 2011

Potts NL, Mandleco BL (eds) (2012) Pediatric nursing: caring for children and their families, 3rd edn. Delmar Cengage Learning, Clifton Park, NY

Samour PQ, King K (2005) Handbook of pediatric nutrition, 3rd edn. Jones and Bartlett Publishers, Sudbury, MA

Taylor M (2001) Imaginary companions and the children who create them. Oxford University Press, New York, NY

Thureen PJ, Hall D, Deacon J et al (2005) Obstetric considerations in the management of the well newborn. In: Assessment and care of the well newborn, 2nd edn. W.B. Saunders, Philadelphia, pp 3–20

Wagner EA, Chantry CJ, Dewey KG et al (2013) Breastfeeding concerns at 3 and 7 days postpartum and feeding status at 2 months. Pediatrics 132:e865

Wolf A, Hubbard E, Stellwagen LM (2007) The late preterm infant: a little baby with big needs. Contemp Pediatr 24(11):51–59

Zickler CF (2011) Making newborn rounds. In: Richardson B (ed) Pediatric primary care: practice guidelines for nurses. Jones & Bartlett Learning, Burlington, MA, pp 26–33; Chapter 4

8 Two-Week Visit

Abeba is brought by her mother, Mrs. Owusu, and her grandmother, Mrs. Jalloh, to the clinic for her 2-week visit while Abeba's father is at work. The grandparents live with the family. Abeba's birth weight was 2.95 kg (6.5 lb). Upon discharge at 72 h after birth, Abeba weighed 2.7 kg. Her current weight is 2.97 kg. Her length is 46.25 cm (18.5 in.). Her head circumference is 32.2 cm (12.8 in.). Abeba is being breastfed. The grandparents immigrated from Ethiopia; the mother was born in the United States. Abeba is their first child. Mrs. Owusu appears very tired and quiet. The grandmother holds the baby and undresses the child for weighing and the physical exam.

Upon questioning, Mrs. Owusu states that she breastfeeds Abeba about every 3 h, six times a day, and Abeba sleeps 4 h during the night at one time and has five wet diapers daily with a soft, yellow pasty stool every other day. Abeba also cries every evening from 5 to 7 p.m. The provider asks what happens when the baby is crying in the evening. Mrs. Owusu states that she lets the baby cry because she is afraid of spoiling her but Mrs. Jalloh, the grandmother, picks up Abeba and swaddles and rocks her. Mrs. Owusu states that she is having trouble sleeping and goes from periods of happiness to sadness. She is greatly concerned that she will have a spoiled child. Mrs. Owusu says that her nipples are irritated but not cracked. Abeba's umbilical cord stub has fallen off. Abeba continues to have head lag and she sleeps on her back as instructed by the nurse at the hospital. The parents do not do any tummy time play with the baby. Abeba startles at the sound of a cart banging in the hallway outside. The grandmother rushes over to sooth her and the mother starts to weep.

Questions:

- **Are Abeba's height and weight appropriate for her?**

Yes. It is normal for newborns to lose 5–8% of their birth weight and regain their weight within 10–14 days.

- **Identify Abeba's current stage of psychosocial development and assess how Mrs. Owusu can help her master this stage.**

According to Erikson, Abeba is in the trust versus mistrust stage of development which is concerned with gaining a sense of trust and overcoming mistrust. This lasts

D. Kramer, *Primary Well-Being: Case Studies for the Growing Child*,
DOI 10.1007/978-3-319-56708-2_8

from birth to 1 year. Infants need consistent care at this age; by picking up the child when they cry, mother is helping Abeba develop trust. There is no concern about spoiling an infant for the first 6 months. Delayed gratification during this time period leads to mistrust on the part of the baby. When we respond quickly, we are sending a message and showing the baby that the world is a warm, trusting place.

- **Assess the psychosexual development of a 2-week-old child.**

  According to Freud, Abeba is in the oral stage of development, in which she gains gratification from sucking. The oral stage lasts for the first year. It is important to provide sucking opportunities for the infant, on the breast, on a pacifier if bottle-fed, on hands, and later on toys, to meet their sucking gratification needs. Rooting and sucking reflexes are especially important, since the infant derives pleasure through oral gratification, such as sucking and tasting. Another way baby Abeba develops a sense of trust is through having her oral needs met. Also, babies need physical contact with their caregivers. They need to be held securely, touched, and stroked. They need to hear human voices and see our smiling faces looking at them. No baby is too young to talk to, coo with, and laugh with. All these interactions promote a healthy relationship and build Abeba's ability to form relationships with other people as she grows (Hagan et al. 2006; Brazelton 1974; Evans and Porter 2009).

- **Assess the cognitive development of a 2-week-old child.**

  According to Piaget, a child's cognitive development is in the sensory motor phase from birth to 1 month, in which they repeat a pattern of reflexes. The infant is learning about their environment through their reflexes. Sucking, swallowing, rooting, grasping, crying, tasting, putting fists in mouth, kicking their feet, flailing their arms, and moving their head, all are examples of this phase.

- **The nurse asks Mrs. Owusu if Abeba has different cries.**

  The nurse is trying to assess the emotional state of the mother and see if there is attachment developing. It the mother identifies different cries, that is a positive sign that bonding is occurring. If the mother seems sad or not knowledgeable about her child, she may be experiencing postpartum depression. This should not be neglected. It is important to assess the mother for depression using a few questions (Hagan et al. 2006) such as the following:

- *What is it like for you taking care of the baby?*
- *Do you have time to take care of yourself?*
- *Sometimes people feel sad or blue or may have periods of crying after a new baby comes into the family; is this true for you?*
- *Are you interested in doing things?*
- *Are you getting pleasure from doing things with your baby?*

The primary care provider should listen without judgment to the mother's words and assess the interaction between the mother and her child. Reassure the mother that there is support available and that she is not alone. There are standardized screening tools that can be used to assess mother's depression symptoms. The Edinburg Post-Partum Depression Scale or the Beck Depression Inventory and the Parenting Stress Index are commonly used. If any of these symptoms are present—feeling down, having no energy, inappropriate guilt, excessive worrying about baby's health, and any thoughts of death or psychoses present—assess whether to take the mother to the emergency room immediately, give her treatment, or guide her through the referral process to obtain treatment (Tanski et al. 2010; Beck 2001; Brazelton and Sparrow 2006; Culbert and Olness 2010; Evans and Porter 2009; McGrath et al. 2008; Medoff-Cooper 1993; Wilson et al. 2000).

- **What milestones of gross and fine motor development could Abeba expected to display?**

  Abeba's symmetrical primary reflexes are present. Also present are doll's eyes reflex, and dance reflex. Tonic neck reflex will be evident when supine. Abeba's grasp reflex is strong. Abeba responds to sounds by Moro reflex. She looks at faces and follows a person with her eyes. She responds to her mother and father's face and eyes. When on her stomach, Abeba lifts her head. She can stay awake for an hour or longer, and can sleep for 3–4 h.

- **Assess the social behaviors that Abeba may exhibit at this age.**

  Abeba may communicate distress signals such as crying, arching her back, and gagging. She will be responsive to talking, singing, facial expressions, and tone of voice of those caring for her. Abeba will enjoy being held, rocked, soothed, and touched.

- **Identify the characteristics of play at this age and suggest appropriate playthings and activities to encourage Abeba's development.**

  Play is an integral part of human social behavior, but in our society, as children grow, we have been giving less and less time to allowing natural play in early childhood programs and at home (Entin 2011). Here is what play looks like in an infant: Looking at the infant at close range, hanging bright toys 8–10 in. from baby's face; speaking, cooing, or singing softly, playing soft music; holding, caressing, and cuddling; swaddling the infant with hand and face wrapped securely; rocking the infant; and taking them for a walk in a stroller or carriage or in an appropriate baby carrier for this age that are safe and approved for a 2-week-old infant.

- **Assess visual and hearing development to the parents.**

  Newborns are able to see objects at 8–12 in. Acuity and accommodation improve in the first 4 months. Abeba's eyes are sensitive to light. She will prefer bright colors and edges. She will be able to distinguish her mother's voice from others. Hearing soft-pitch lullabies and heart sounds will decrease activity in infants. Abeba will readjust her body to the language pattern around her (American Academy of Pediatrics, Bright Futures 2014; Burns et al. 2009; Duderstadt 2006; Hagan et al. 2006; Hockenberry and Wilson 2011; McInerny et al. 2009; Richardson 2011; Zickler 2011a; Zickler 2011b).

Now is a good time to start introducing books to the baby. Explain to Mrs. Owusu that it is not too early for a baby to be read to. Abeba will enjoy the sound of her mother's voice or others in the household and begin to absorb their speaking patterns. Recent research and a policy statement by the American Academy of Pediatrics emphasizes that in addition to early literacy and language skills, early reading at least once a day helps develop nurturing, interactive relationships between parent and child that promote early brain development and lead to school readiness (American Academy of Pediatrics 2014).

- **Assess immunization needs for this age.**

For immunizations at this age, consult the CDC, ACIP, or AAP web sites for the current immunization schedule recommendations (U.S. Centers for Disease Control 2012):

– CEC National Immunization Program (NIP): http://www.cdc.gov/vaccines
– American Academy of Pediatrics *Red Book*: http://www.aapredbook.org

- **What information can be given about nutrition for mother and baby and breastfeeding at this age?**

At this point, Abeba should be breastfeeding about 15 min from each breast. She will be sleeping about 16 h a day but have wakeful periods of up to 1 h. She should be nursing 8–12 times a day. At 2 weeks, Abeba is having a growth spurt—meaning she will nurse more frequently to increase the milk production. To prevent nipple confusion, the health care provider would usually not recommend the use of a pacifier between feeds at age 2 weeks.

Remind Mrs. Owusu that it is normal for newborns to feed every 2 or 3 h. When Abeba is hungry, she will make sucking motions, move her lips, and be restless. Mrs. Owusu should feed for about 10 min on one breast and then switch to the other side until it is soft and empty. Ask if Mrs. Owusu feels a tingling sensation in the breast at the beginning of the feeding. This will be the "let-down" reflex working to push the milk out at the beginning of the feeding when the milk usually comes out spraying and she will hear Abeba swallowing quickly. Advise Mrs. Owusu to keep a feeding log till the next visit to have an idea of the frequency and length of the feedings and when Abeba sleeps. Suggest to Mrs. Owusu that she seek out an accredited breastfeeding group such as La Leche League (see http://www.llli.org/ to find local groups in your area) for breastfeeding and new parent support. La Leche League also runs a 24-h hot line for questions related to breastfeeding usually manned by local group leaders.

No other food is necessary for the baby (American Academy of Pediatrics 2009), but Mrs. Owusu needs to be sure that she herself is well hydrated and is eating a healthy diet. Nursing mothers should continue to take their prenatal vitamin, and may need an extra 400–500 calories a day to keep up her energy. She should opt to use nutrient-rich foods such as whole grains, fresh fruit and vegetables, and iron-rich foods, in combination with vitamin C to enhance absorption, proteins, and foods rich in calcium such as dairy products and supplement with vitamin

D. Regarding fish, it is a good source of protein and omega 3 fatty acids, but excessive amounts of mercury passed through the breast milk should be avoided. It is advised to limit fish to 6 oz a week while breastfeeding. Low-mercury fish includes canned light tuna, salmon, shrimp, and catfish. Fish in mercury like swordfish, mackerel, tilefish, and shark should be avoided while Mrs. Owusu is nursing. Some foods the mother eats can cause possible allergic reactions in the baby such as cow's milk, tree nuts, wheat, soy, eggs, and fish. Also foods that cause excessive gas may upset the baby, like garlic, broccoli, and cabbage. Symptoms would be blood in the stool, increased fussiness, a rash, or diarrhea after nursing. Parents should eliminate foods to see what is causing the situation. It is not recommended for breastfeeding mothers to drink alcohol, and they should limit caffeinated drinks to two cups a day (American Academy of Obstetrics and Gynecology, American Academy of Pediatrics 2014; American Academy of Pediatrics Committee on Nutrition 2009; American Academy of Pediatrics 2010; American Academy of Pediatrics undated).

- **Mrs. Owusu says that she is concerned because Abeba is picked up by the grandmother when she begins to cry. Discuss this with them.**

Mrs. Owusu is concerned that her daughter will be spoiled which is not the case; she is crying because she has a need at this age to be held. By being picked up and cuddled right away, Abeba is developing trust in her surroundings and the people who care for her and that her needs will be met.

- **Identify the anticipatory guidance that would be helpful for Mrs. Owusu and the grandmother.**

Immune system: Babies at 2 weeks of age do not have their own immune system and it is preferable not to take baby out yet to crowded places.

Adjustment to baby: Ask Mrs. Owusu how her family is adjusting to the new baby. This is a time of transitions. Reassure Mrs. Owusu that she is getting to know Abeba and initial uncertainty will give way to assurance as she gets more comfortable with Abeba. Advise Mrs. Owusu to rest when Abeba sleeps to help her feel calm and good. Mrs. Owusu can let the grandmother do some of the routines. For now, grandma is holding, bathing, changing, and dressing Abeba, as well as calming Abeba when she is crying.

Sleep: Explain about changing sleep-wake patterns; how Abeba may sometimes have days and night confused and wake up frequently at night while sleeping longer during the day. Mrs. Owusu can help her baby to develop sleep and feeding routines. Reassure Mrs. Owusu that she can offer to nurse Abeba at least every 3 h during the day. Eventually, Abeba will sleep for longer periods at night.

Abeba should be put to sleep in the same place each time. This should be a crib with a firm, flat mattress and with slats no more than 2 and 3/8 in. apart. Nothing else should be in the crib and the top rails of the crib should be in a raised position while the baby is in it. The drop side of the crib should require two distinct actions to prevent accidental release by the child.

Routines: It is important to start setting routines at this age for feeding, bathing, and sleep. Babies like to be read to even at this early age and hear parents' voices.

Reading can be done from a magazine or book. Include talking to the baby in all the routines, as simple as just describing what you are doing with the baby. The routine for feeding could include diapering the baby first to get her fully awake for nursing, or diapering in between breast sides so if she falls asleep, she is ready to be put down in her crib. As much as possible, parents and other caregivers of Abeba should talk to her, sing softly, read, and communicate their love and concerns to her as they go about their daily routines.

When to call the doctor: Mrs. Owusu should call the doctor if Abeba has any fever over 100.4 °F.

Car safety: She should obtain a rear-facing car seat for Abeba that meets the guidelines of the federal regulations: see http://www.ghsa.org/html/stateinfo/laws/childsafety_laws.html for guidance for each age (American Academy of Pediatrics 2010).

References

American Academy of Obstetrics and Gynecology, American Academy of Pediatrics (2014) Breastfeeding handbook for physicians, 2nd edn. American Academy of Pediatrics, Elk Grove Village, IL

American Academy of Pediatrics (2010) Car safety seats: a guide for families 2010. American Academy of Pediatrics Healthy Children website. http://www.healthychildren.org/English/safety-prevention/on-th-go/pages/Car-Safety-Seats-Information-for-Families-2010.aspx. Accessed 2 June 2011

American Academy of Pediatrics (2009) Committee on Nutrition: Pediatric nutrition handbook, 6th edn. American Academy of Pediatrics, Elk Grove Village, IL

American Academy of Pediatrics (2012) Breastfeeding and the use of human milk. Pediatrics 129(3):e827–e841

American Academy of Pediatrics, Bright Futures (2014) Recommendations for preventive pediatric health care. http://www.aap.org/en-us/professional-resources/practice-support/Periodicity/Periodicity%20Schedule_FINAL.pdf. Accessed 24 July 2014

American Academy of Pediatrics. Committee on Environmental health (1997) Environmental tobacco smoke: a hazard to children. Pediatrics 99:639–642

American Academy of Pediatrics. Task Force on Sudden Infant Death Syndrome (2011) SIDS and other sleep-related infant deaths: Expansion of recommendations for a safe infant sleeping environment. Pediatrics 128:1030–1039

Beck CI (2001) Predictors of postpartum depression, an update. Nurs Res 50(5):275–285

Brazelton TB (1974) Mother-infant reciprocity. In: Klaus MH, Leger T, Trause MA (eds) Maternal attachment and mothering disorders. Sausalito, CA, Johnson & Johnson Baby Products

Brazelton TB, Sparrow JD (2006) Touchpoints-birth to three, 2nd edn. Da Capo Press, Cambridge, MA

Burns CE et al (2009) Pediatric primary care: a handbook for nurse practitioners, 4th edn. W.B. Saunders, Philadelphia, PA

Culbert TP, Olness K (eds) (2010) Integrative pediatrics. Oxford University Press, New York, NY

Duderstadt K (2006) Pediatric physical examination. Elsevier, St. Louis, MO

Entin E (2011) All work and no play: Why your kids are more anxious, depressed. The Atlantic, Oct 12.

Evans CA, Porter CI (2009) The emergence of mother-infant co-regulation during the first year: links to infant developmental status and attachment. Infant Behav Dev 32(2):137–238

Hagan JF, Shaw JS, Duncan P (eds) (2006) Bright futures: guidelines for health supervision of infants, children, and adolescents, 3rd edn. American Academy of Pediatrics, Elk Grove Village, IL

Hockenberry MJ, Wilson DW (2011) Wong's nursing care of infants and children, 9th edn. Elsevier/Mosby, New York, NY

Klingler B, Scott E (2009) A pediatric perspective on nutritional therapeutics. In: Culbert TP, Olness K (eds) Integrative pediatrics. Oxford University Press, New York, NY, pp 314–339; Chapter 9

McGrath JM, Records K, Rice M (2008) Maternal depression and infant temperament characteristics. Infant Behav Dev 31(1):71–80

McInerny TK, Adam HM, Campbell DE, Kamat DM, Kelleher KJ (eds) (2009) Textbook of pediatric care. American Academy of Pediatrics, Elk Grove Village, IL

Medoff-Cooper (1993) the early infant temperament questionnaire. J Dev Behav Pediatr 14(4):230–231

Potts NL, Mandleco BL (eds) (2012) Pediatric nursing: caring for children and their families, 3rd edn. Delmar Cengage Learning, Clifton Park, NY

Prymula R, Siegrist CA, Chlibek R et al (2009) Effect of prophylactic paracetamol administration at time of vaccination on febrile reactions and antibody responses in children: two open-label, randomized controlled trials. Lancet 374(9698):1339–1350

Richardson B (ed) (2011) Pediatric primary care: practice guidelines for nurses. Jones & Bartlett Learning, Burlington, MA

Tanski S, Garfunkel LC, Duncan PM, Weitzman M (eds) (2010). Performing preventive services. A Bright Futures handbook. Elk Grove, IL: American Academy of Pediatrics. Retrieved June 12, 2014 from: http://brightfutures.aap.org/pdfs/Preventive%20Services%20PDFs/Forward%20and%20Introduction.pdf

U.S. Centers for Disease Control (2012) Talking with parents about vaccines for infants: strategies for health care professionals. http://www.cdc.gov/vaccines/hcp/patient-ed/conversations/downloads/talk-infants-bw-office.pdf. Accessed 20 Nov 2014

Wilson ME, White MA, Cobb B et al (2000) Family dynamics, parent-fetal attachment and infant temperament. J Adv Nurs 32(1):204–210

Zickler CF (2011a) One-month visit. In: Richardson B (ed) Pediatric primary care: practice guidelines for nurses. Jones & Bartlett Learning, Burlington, MA, pp 63–73; Chapter 7

Zickler CF (2011b) Two-week visit. In: Richardson B (ed) Pediatric primary care: practice guidelines for nurses. Jones & Bartlett Learning, Burlington, MA, pp 57–62; Chapter 6

Two-Month Visit

9

Harry is brought into the pediatrician's office by his mother and father, Mr. and Mrs. Smith. Harry weighed 3.6 kg (7 lb 9 oz) at birth and was 51 cm (20.4 in.). His head circumference was 36 cm (14.4 in.), putting him in the 50th percentile for weight, length, and head circumference at birth. Upon discharge at 72 h after birth, Harry weighed 3.24 kg. His current weight is 5.4 kg (11.8 lb); current length is 58 cm (23.2 in.) and his current head circumference is 48 cm (inches) (19.2 in.), still in the 50th percentile. Harry is being breastfed. His mother is excited that Harry is smiling and cooing and in general responding to her when she talks to him. Harry's father is wondering when he will sleep through the night. Harry sleeps in his own crib and likes to look at a mobile when he is awake. Mother has been breastfeeding Harry every 2–3 h and the baby is sleeping most of the day. Mrs. Smith is concerned that Harry is sleeping too much and has short frequent waking periods during the day. Mrs. Smith's sister-in-law keeps telling her that she should be giving the baby a pacifier between feeds. Harry has four yellow pasty stools a day and seven wet diapers. Mrs. Smith wants to know when Harry will start getting shots for immunization.

- **Are Harry's height and weight appropriate for him?**

Harry's height and weight are appropriate for his age. His height, weight, and head circumference are at the 50th percentile for a 2-month-old. He has maintained his growth curb since birth. Infants gain 0.05–0.075 oz per day (about 2 lb/month for the first 4–5 months). Infants double their weight by 4–6 months and triple their weight by the end of the first year. Infants grow 2.5 cm a month in length for the first 6 months and their head circumference increases 0.5 cm a month for the first year. Upon physical exam, the posterior fontanel should be closed.

- **Identify Harry's current stage of psychosocial development and assess how Mrs. Smith can help him master this stage.**

Infants have certain psychosocial tasks they need to accomplish in the first year of life. Trust is the first and basic foundation of these tasks. Harry is at Erikson's stage of trust versus mistrust. Parents can nurture trust by meeting the child's needs through feeding, comfort, and stimulation. Feeding is the most important activity

D. Kramer, *Primary Well-Being: Case Studies for the Growing Child*,
DOI 10.1007/978-3-319-56708-2_9

the infant engages in. Comfort means being held, having diapers changed, and being soothed. Providing appropriate stimulation, such as a smiling face, tactile and visual stimulation such as mobiles over the crib, and tummy time also contribute to the infant having a positive perception of his caregiver.

Trust is also nurtured by developing routines for the baby, including playtime-face to face, and tummy, and lap play such as reading, and playing with bright safe objects, and mirrors. Routines also include nap time, feeding time, and diapering/bathing time. It is important for parents to talk to their infants as they care for them throughout the day. It is also important to remind parents that they cannot spoil a child of this age by picking them up. Rather the parents are establishing trust in their baby that the world is a good/positive place every time they meet their baby's needs.

Harry will have a social smile with his parents. He will turn to sounds. These activities to build trust also contribute to attachment—the child forming a bond with one or more of the people caring for him. Attachment is a part of an infant's social development and human physical contact is extremely important in developing this bond. Play and stimulation and socializing are the cornerstones of attachment that parents engage in with their baby in a normal, healthy family.

- **Assess the cognitive development of a 2-month-old child.**

According to Piaget, Harry is in the Sensory Motor Development Stage II: Primary Circular Reactions. In this stage babies will replace what were merely reflexes at birth with learned activity. Just like the newborn starts making faces or coos in response to us and then later they learn to make faces or coo deliberately to get us to react. Now, at 2 months, more learned responses are occurring, such as finding out that sucking one's fingers is pleasurable. At around age 3 months Harry will grab toys that are put near him, such as a musical rattle, and learn to initiate the sound. Parents should continue to provide stimulation such as using bright objects to look at, safe toys, singing and talking, and tummy time. Babies may also like to be in a swing; how much time in the swing will depend on the baby.

- **The nurse asks Mrs. Smith if Harry has different cries and what kind of baby he is, e.g., active and calm, in other words his temperament.**

Temperament. All babies are born with their own personalities and temperament—how babies react to the world. Some are more relaxed, and some more high strung. As a health care provider, you want to be able to assess the infant's temperament and the parents' comfort level with it. It is also an opportunity, if there are older siblings present, to get a glimpse into the parents' reaction to all the children's temperaments and the mix of temperaments in the family and how to treat them as individuals. It is important for the health care provider to help the parents understand the infant's temperament and how to relate to it.

For parents, it is easier to relate to a baby that likes to cuddle versus one that arches his back or stiffens up when touched. As a health care provider you want to teach parents how to tune in to these babies. Suggestions include massaging the infant's back and helping assess the infant for any neurological issues, such as sensory motor integration, hypotonia or hypertonia, or cerebral palsy. Dr. T. Berry

Brazelton has done extensive work on infant temperaments and how to understand baby's different temperaments (Brazelton and Sparrow 2006) (see "Red Flags for the Health Care Provider" box on page 8). Infants with more difficult temperaments for mothers to relate to may contribute to maternal depression. These mothers need to be screened for depression (Beck 2001; McGrath et al. 2008).

Resources for assessing temperament include the Revised Temperament Questionnaire and the Early Infant Temperament Questionnaire. These surveys can be given to parents to help them better understand their infant's temperament and how to best care for their child (Medoff-Cooper 1993).

Distinguishing cries and sounds. Crying is a form of communication. At this age—2 months—parents should be able to differentiate among their baby's cries. Babies also at this age coo and will vocalize to a familiar voice. Harry should already have a social smile. Encourage Harry's parents to talk back to their infants in response to his coos and respond to Harry when he cries. Mr. and Mrs. Smith should also smile to Harry and he will respond to his parents' smile. When parents meet the child's needs, the crying should cease. If the child has difficulty calming down, that is a red flag to check for possible underlying conditions (see "Red Flag" box). While discussing the child's temperament, it is important to listen if there are any frustrations on the part of the parent or a potential for abuse and/or neglect. These may be signs of an attachment disorder (Wilson et al. 2000; Zeanah and Fox 2004).

Fussy periods. It is normal for babies to have a fussy time, often in the evening for about an hour or two, especially around 2–3 months of age. Then it usually decreases. This might require extra comforting and nurturing efforts such as sitting with the baby in a rocking chair or walking around and singing or talking to the baby. If Mr. or Mrs. Smith aren't available, another caring person can take over at these times. It is also helpful to encourage Mrs. Smith to sleep while Harry is sleeping and to do activities that nurture and calm her, such as a warm bath, or a walk, or whatever relaxes her. T. Berry Brazelton has identified different behaviors in infants and divided them into quiet baby, average baby, and active baby categories (Brazelton 1983).

- **What milestones of gross and fine motor development could Harry be expected to display?**

At 2 months, baby's hands are often open rather than clenched. The crawling reflex and doll's eye reflex have disappeared and grasp reflex is fading. There is less head lag when pulled to a sitting position. Harry should be developing head control. When Harry is prone, he can lift his head to a 45° angle off a flat surface. When held in a sitting position, Harry bends forward and can be held up. The asymmetrical tonic neck reflex is intermittent at this age rather than all the time. Harry follows an object from side to midpoint beyond midline and turns his head to the side where the sound is. Infants at this age have peripheral vision up to 180°. Labyrinth righting (Harry being able to raise his head) appears at 2 months (see box "Red Flags" below on page 8 for signs of developmental delays). Mr. and Mrs. Smith can foster Harry's development by doing physical exercise with him. See box "Helping Your Child's

Physical Development—2–4 Months." (American Academy of Pediatrics, Council on Early Childhood 2014; Bright Futures 2005; American Academy of Pediatrics Bright Futures 2014; Brazelton 1974, Burns 2009; Culbert and Olness 2010; Duderstadt 2006; Evans and Porter 2009; Richardson 2011; Zickler 2011)

Helping Your Child's Physical Development: 2–4 Months

1. *Rolling: Side Lying to a Supine Position*: Place your baby on his back in front of you while you are sitting on the floor. Gently roll him to one side and then onto his back, and then onto the other side and back to his back.
2. *Grabbing*: Encourage child to grab for toys. Place toys—such as small rattles that make sounds or toys with different textures—on the floor within baby's reach.
3. *Reaching Upward*: Dangle a toy over the baby's chest after diapering or dressing so they can grab it.
4. *Hands to Midline*: Play clapping games with your baby such as pat-a-cake and clapping to music. When playing on the floor, place a childproof mirror and toy in front of the baby.

Source: *Hurley, D.S. (2000).* Developing fine and gross motor skills: Birth to three. *Austin, TX: PRO-ED, Inc.*

- **Identify the characteristics of play at this age and suggest appropriate playthings and activities to encourage Harry's development.**

At 2 months Harry needs visual, auditory, tactile, and kinetic stimulation. He will enjoy bright objects, being talked to, being caressed while bathing or diaper change, and being in an infant swing. Make his room bright using pictures or mirrors. Mrs. Smith should take him from room to room as she moves about the home and place Harry in an infant seat so he can see what is going on from a safe surface. Include Harry in family get-togethers and trips outside the home. Offer rattles, and use wind chimes and musical mobiles. Give him a massage and comb his hair with a soft brush. Take him for rides in the car. Move Harry's arms and legs in a swimming motion for exercise. Be sure to give him tummy time and not keep him strapped in a seat for any length of time. See box "Toys for Babies 2- to 6 Months."

- **Assess visual and hearing development**

Harry reacts to loud noises by startle and responds to human sound. He is soothed by low-pitched sounds, such as a lullaby, soft music, or heartbeat. He has good visual acuity (20/100 to 20/400) and able to focus on a moving object within 45° in close range—about 8–10 in. away. His eye and head movements are not well integrated and doll's eye reflex is still present. This reflex should disappear between 6 and 12 weeks. If not, there may be a neurologic problem (Hockenberry and Wilson 2011).

- **Is Harry getting enough to eat? Can Mrs. Smith tell by his wet diapers and stool?**

Harry's weight gain has maintained him on the 50th percentile. Currently he is being breastfeed every 2–3 h during the day. He has seven wet diapers a day and four pasty stools, which indicates that Harry is getting enough to eat. Since Harry is breastfeeding and getting enough to eat, at 2 months the health provider could recommend a pacifier between feeds if Harry is fussy.

The health care provider can help parents understand the importance of good food choices for their developing child. The standard recommendation is that mothers breastfeed for a year with the first 6 months being only breast milk and then introduce solid foods. Research supports that breastfeeding is the best choice for babies. Reassure Mrs. Smith that breastfeeding leads to reduced risk for asthma, atopic dermatitis, food allergies, and respiratory allergies (Klingler and Scott 2010).

- **Discuss immunization for babies with Mr. and Mrs. Smith.**

Baby Harry has gotten the appropriate dose of hepatitis B vaccine soon after birth in the hospital. Health care providers need to review the risks, side effects, and benefits of Harry receiving immunizations with Mr. and Mrs. Smith and have them sign a consent form to have vaccines administered. Best practice is to get immunizations completed by the first 2 years of life following the schedule that has been developed by the US Centers for Disease Control (CDC). Combination vaccines are often used to decrease the number of injections given to a child. Depending on the situation, providers can spread the injections out over a longer period of time. For standard immunizations at this age, consult the CDC, ACIP, or AAP web sites for the current immunization schedule recommendations:

- CEC National Immunization Program (NIP): http://www.cdc.gov/vaccines
- American Academy of Pediatrics *Red Book:* http://www.aapredbook.org

Use of pain medication in infants: There is controversy as to whether to administer acetaminophen prophylactically after immunization because of possible effects on the liver (Prymula et al. 2009), as well as decreasing the immunity.

Vaccine refusal: Some parents refuse to accept immunizations (US Centers for Disease Control 2012). If parents refuse immunization for their child the health care provider should document the refusal and have the parents' state that they have been provided with the opportunity to read a statement about each vaccine from the CDC, and the opportunity to discuss the recommendation and refused to accept the vaccination. The CDC has materials for providers and parents to help discuss vaccines as well as a form for parents to sign when they reject them. See http://www.cdc.gov/vaccines/hcp/patient-ed/conversations/index.html for helpful resources.

- **Mrs. Smith says that she is concerned because Harry sleeps a lot. Discuss this with them.**

Infants at this age sleep on average 16 h a day, which is needed for them to develop and grow.

- **What information can be given concerning breastfeeding?**

The health care provider should continue to encourage Mrs. Smith to breastfeed. The American Academy of Pediatrics recommendation is for 6 months of exclusive breastfeeding and with supplementation up to a year or more and encourages health care providers to be knowledgeable about the benefits of breastfeeding to mother and child as well as the economic and business case for breastfeeding (American Academy of Pediatrics 2012). (See breastfeeding guidelines under newborn.) Remind Mrs. Smith about common growth periods when Harry will be nursing more frequently to build up the milk supply to keep pace with his growing body. These increased nursing periods usually occur at 3 months, 6 months, and 9 months.

No solids should be offered to Harry before 6 months of age while he is breastfeeding or until he doubles his weight.

- **Anticipatory guidance**

At 2 months the health care provider can talk to Mr. and Mrs. Smith about safety practices with Harry, their baby's vulnerable immune system, being careful about taking baby out, activities to stimulate growth and development, next stages of development to expect, and red flags to be aware of (Tanski et al. 2010). Harry will be seen for a regular appointment again at 4 months. Between 2 and 4 months he will acquire many new skills—babbling, cooing, trying to roll over, and more (see boxes "Skills Developed Between 3 and 4 Months of Age," and "Appropriate Toys for Infancy"). Harry's parents can encourage him in learning these skills by the following activities (Hurley 2000). Share with the parents the following box containing activities to stimulate the next stages of development.

Activities to Stimulate Next Stages in Development: 3–4 Months

- Rolling baby from side to side
  - Place the child on his back in front of you while you are sitting on the floor.
  - Gently roll your child to one side and then onto his back, and then onto the other side and back to his back.
- Encouraging the child to grab for toys
  - Place toys, such as small rattles that make sounds or toys with different textures, on the floor within the child's reach.
- Reaching upward:
  - Dangle a toy over your child's chest after diapering or dressing so the baby can grab it.
- Hands to midline
  - Play clapping games with your child such as pat-a-cake and clapping to music.
  - When playing on the floor, place a childproof mirror and toy in front of the baby.

Skills Developed Between 3 and 4 Months of Age

Note: If any of these skills are not present by 4 months of age, this is a red flag and the child should receive a full developmental assessment.

- Around 3 months of age, child will hold a rattle.
- At around 4 months he will start grabbing the rattle and other items.
- At around 4 months child will start rolling over.
- Child's hand naturally will be held in a loosely open position at 3 months.
- Child's grab reflex will disappear at 3 months.
- Child will start to pull on his clothes or blanket at 3 months.
- At 3 months, the child will be able to hold his head erect when sitting, but it will still bob forward; he will have less head lag when pulled to a sitting position and he will be able to raise his head and shoulders from a prone position to 45–90° angle from the table and support himself on his forearms.
- The child will start to look at his hands at 3 months.
- The child will coo, babble, and squeal with pleasure at 3 months. And "talk" when spoken to.
- The child will start to recognize parents and will stop crying when the parent enters the room.

Toys for Babies 2–6 Months

Babies at this age like bright objects, soft items, rattles that make sound, safe mirrors, balls, and items with different textures. There are many resources with suggestions for obtaining free or low-cost playthings for babies on the Internet.

One that links development to interactive activities for the birth to 3 years is ***Recipes to Play, A community PLAYbook for fun and learning,*** created by a group of interdisciplinary professionals who work with infants and toddler. It is available to download free for the parents at http://nyztt.org/pdf_DOCSrecipesPlaybook_4-2-%202013.pdf

Appropriate toys for this age include

- Plastic rattles
- Keys
- Unbreakable mirror attached to a crib or playpen
- Soft balls—some can make sounds—textured toys that make sounds
- Toys with finger holds
- Musical toys that make bell sounds (no loose parts)
- See-through rattles that show the parts making the noise
- Old magazines with bright pictures
- Baby books with hard cardboard, cloth, or vinyl pages

Red Flags for the Health Care Provider

Note: These red flags mean that the provider should follow up with immediate attention to the child. This may involve specialists, hospital admission, and in-depth study.

- Breathing difficulties
- Seizures
- Any fever
- Irritability most of the time
- Poor feeding, difficulty feeding and sucking, feedings take longer than 45 min of sucking if breastfeeding, baby wakes up every hour for feeding
- Fast or slow breathing or sweating while feeding (tachypnea, bradycardia, or diaphoresis)
- Vomiting
- No urine output in 12 h
- Black or decreased bowel movements
- Child not smiling or cooing
- Slow weight gain—less than 1 lb a month
- Head circumference not increasing or growing too quickly: >2 standard deviations on head chart
- No regulation of sleep/wake cycle
- Asymmetrical movements versus symmetrical (at same time for both sides of body)
- Hypotonia and/or hypertonia (loose muscle tone and/or tight muscle tone)
- No attempt to raise head when placed on stomach
- Hands fisted with oppositional thumb
- Baby doesn't turn to sound
- Baby doesn't look and follow people or items

Anticipatory Guidance

Sleep: The safe position is sleeping on the back for Harry (American Academy of Pediatrics 2011). He should always be on a firm sleep surface, without bumpers, soft objects, or any loose bedding. Harry can be in the same room as his parents but not in their bed. Wedges and positioners should be avoided. Harry's room should not be too hot or too cold. The ideal room temperature is between 65° and 74° (American Academy of Pediatrics 2011). Avoid overheated rooms.

Bathing: Harry should be bathed in warm water in a warm room, but never hot or cold, as babies loose body heat quickly. Never leave Harry unattended in the bathtub, even for half a minute. Mr. and Mrs. Smith should take everything they need with them into the bathroom before giving Harry his bath. At this age, baby Harry should be placed in an infant bath tub.

Preventing falls: Remind Mr. and Mrs. Smith to always keep a hand on baby Harry when changing him on tables or other raised surfaces, when on the sofa or other surfaces off the floor to avoid risk of falling.

Car safety: Harry should be placed in a car seat that is Federal Motor Vehicle Safety tested and approved. It should be installed properly in the backseat, facing backward in the car. Car seats can be rented or borrowed from local hospitals, fire departments, or March of Dimes chapters.

Smoking: Avoid anyone smoking around baby Harry or in the house. Smoking, including secondary smoke, increases the risk of SIDS, ear infections, and respiratory problems such as asthma in children (Hagan et al. 2008). Advise family members who smoke outside the house to change their clothes after they smoke. The family housing should also have a working smoke detector on each floor and batteries should be replaced annually. A fire evacuation plan and occasional drills are also recommended to be prepared. A carbon monoxide detector is also a good idea.

Sun exposure: Babies should be limited in exposure to the sun to about 20 min a day. If sunscreen is used, it should have an SPF rating of at least 15 but baby should still be limited in exposure to the sun. Protect Harry by using hats and long-sleeved shirts and pants.

References

American Academy of Pediatrics (2012) Breastfeeding and the use of human milk Pediatrics, 129(3):e827–e841

American Academy of Pediatrics, Council on Early Childhood (2014) Literacy promotion: an essential component of primary care pediatric practice. Pediatrics 124(2):404–409

American Academy of Pediatrics, Task Force on Sudden Infant Death Syndrome (2011) SIDS and other sleep-related infant deaths: Expansion of recommendations for a safe Infant sleeping environment Pediatrics, 135(4):E1105

Bright Futures (2005) Developmental milestones check list. http://www.tnaap.org/Files/EPSDT/DevelopmentalMilestonesChecklist.pdf. Accessed 1 June 2015

American Academy of Pediatrics, Bright Futures (2014) Recommendations for preventive pediatric health care. http://www.aap.org/en-us/professional-resources/practice-support/Periodicity/Periodicity%20Schedule_FINAL.pdf. Accessed 24 July 2014

Beck CI (2001) Predictors of postpartum depression: an update. Nurs Res 50(5):275–285

Brazelton TB (1974) Mother-infant reciprocity. In: Klaus MH, Leger T, Trause MA (eds) Maternal attachment and mothering disorders. Sausalito, CA, Johnson & Johnson Baby Products

Brazelton TB (1983) Infants and mothers: differences in development. Dell, New York, NY

Brazelton TB, Sparrow J (2006) Touchpoints: birth to three, 2nd edn. Da Capo Press, The Perseus Books Group, Boston, MA

Burns CE et al (2009) Pediatric primary care: a handbook for nurse practitioners, 4th edn. W.B. Saunders, Philadelphia, PA

Culbert TP, Olness K (eds) (2010) Integrative pediatrics. Oxford University Press, New York, NY

Duderstadt K (2006) Pediatric physical examination. Elsevier, St. Louis, MO

Evans CA, Porter CI (2009) The emergence of mother-infant co-regulation during the first year: links to infant developmental status and attachment. Infant Behav Dev 32(2):137–238

Hagan JF, Shaw JS, Duncan P (eds) (2006) Bright Futures: guidelines for health supervision of infants, children, and adolescents, 3rd edn. American Academy of Pediatrics, Elk Grove Village, IL

Hockenberry MJ, Wilson DW (2011) Wong's nursing care of infants and children, 9th edn. Elsevier/Mosby, New York, NY

Hurley DS (2000) Developing fine and gross motor skills: Birth to three Austin, TX: PRO-ED, Inc

Klingler B, Scott E (2010) A pediatric perspective on nutritional therapeutics. In Culbert TP, Olness K (Eds) Integrative pediatric. New York: Oxford University Press Chapter 9

Medoff-Cooper B (1993) The early infant temperament questionnaire. J Dev Behav Pediatr 14(4):230–231

McGrath JM, Records K, Rice M (2008) Maternal depression and infant temperament characteristics. Infant Behav Dev 31(1):71–80

Prymula R, Siegrist CA, Chlibek R et al (2009) Effect of prophylactic paracetamol adeministration at time of vaccination on febrile reactions and antibody responses in children: Two open-label, randomized controlled trials Lancet 374(9698):1339–1350

Richardson B (ed) (2011) Pediatric primary care: practice guidelines for nurses. Jones & Bartlett Learning, Burlington, MA

Tanski S, Garfunkel LC, Duncan PM, Weitzman M (eds) (2010) Performing preventive services. A Bright Futures handbook. American Academy of Pediatrics, Elk Grove, IL. http://brightfutures.aap.org/pdfs/Preventive%20Services%20PDFs/Forward%20and%20Introduction.pdf. Accessed 12 June 2014

U.S. Centers for Disease Control 2012 Talking with parents about vaccines for infants: Strategies for health care professionals (Information for health care professionals)

Wilson ME, White MA, Cobb B et al (2000) Family dynamics, parent-fetal attachment and infant temperament. J Adv Nurs 32(1):204–210

Zeanah CH, Fox NA (2004) Temperament and attachment disorders. J Clin Child Adolesc Psychol 33(1):82–87

Zickler CF (2011) One-month visit. In: Richardson B (ed) Pediatric primary care: practice guidelines for nurses. Jones & Bartlett Learning, Burlington, MA, pp 63–73. Chapter 7

Four-Month Visit

10

Maria Gonzales is brought to the pediatric clinic by her single mother, Evelyn Gonzales, age 24. Ms. Gonzales lives in a subsidized housing project in a one-bedroom apartment. Maria weighed 3.5 kg (almost 7.5 lb) at birth in the 25th percentile and was 47 cm (18.8 in.) in length (25th percentile). Her head circumference was 33.4 cm (13.36 in.). Her current weight is 5.5 kg (12.1 lb). Her current length is 59 cm (23.6 in.). Her current head circumference is 40 cm (16 in.)—at the 25th percentile. Maria is being bottle-fed. She has not yet doubled her weight. Maria's mother is concerned because she notices that Maria no longer startles when there is a loud noise. When Maria hears her mother's voice she turns to her. Maria holds a rattle in her hand and brings it to her mouth. Maria drinks 5 oz six times a day usually every 3 h with a longer stretch at night. She has seven wet diapers a day and semiformed stools once daily.

Maria sleeps four times a day for about 1.5 h each time and Ms. Gonzales does tummy time at each diaper change for 7 min. Maria has a longer sleep period at night but not the whole night. A mobile hangs over her crib. Maria coos and squeals when her mother plays with her. Ms. Gonzales is looking for day care for her child while she job hunts. Now that Maria is 4 months old, Ms. Gonzales asks if she can use regular cow's milk instead of formula. Ms. Gonzales is looking forward to getting out and seeing people again.

Questions:

- **Are Maria's height and weight appropriate for her?**

Yes. Maria is consistently on the 25th percentile. Infants should gain 0.5–1 oz/day or about 2 lb/month and double their birth weight between 4 and 6 months. Maria should grow in length on average 1 in./month, and her head circumference should increase by 0.5 cm/month.

- **Is her physical development appropriate for 4-month-old girl? What milestones of gross and fine motor development could Maria be expected to display?**

At this age, Maria will be able to grasp objects, beginning with raking motion. She can bring her hands together and follow objects with eyes to 180°. Maria has good

D. Kramer, *Primary Well-Being: Case Studies for the Growing Child*,
DOI 10.1007/978-3-319-56708-2_10

head control. Maria should have no head lag when she is pulled to a sitting position and can balance her head. She can lift her head and chest when prone. She bears weight on legs, but cannot stand on her own. She can roll from front to back and from her back to her side. Maria will show increased drooling, which indicates functional salivary glands, not teething (Brazelton 1983; Hurley 2000; Porter and Kaplan 2011).

- **What reflexes do you expect her to have?**

Ms. Gonzales says that she is concerned because Maria is no longer startled by a loud noise. This is good news—it means she has outgrown her primitive reflexes. Reassure Ms. Gonzales that it is normal for startle reflexes such as Moro to fade in a 4-month-old. Rooting and palmar grasp also disappear. Babinski is still present, but tonic neck is no longer as prominent, and may disappear by 4 months.

It is a good sign that Maria's startle reflex is fading and she is developing normally. Give the mother lots of encouragement—the fact that she noticed it is gone shows good observation of her child. If the primitive reflexes were still evident, it would be a sign for further consultation with the pediatrician.

It is important to praise Mrs. Gonzales for placing Maria on her stomach and doing tummy time. She should continue to strengthen Maria's trunk, head, and neck muscles by having Maria's arms extended forward, and hold a toy in front of Maria so the baby will hold her head up and look at her mother. Once her head is lifted, Maria will start pushing up her arms and lifting her chest by arching her back. This helps develop strength in Maria's upper body so that she can eventually turn, sit, and stand.

It is good that Maria is bringing things to her mouth. Appropriate toys for this age include plastic rattles, keys, unbreakable mirror attached to a crib or playpen, soft balls—some can make sounds—textured toys that make sounds, toys with finger holds, musical toys such as bells, maracas, tambourines (no loose parts), see-through rattles that show the parts making the noise, old magazine with bright pictures to show her, baby books with hard cardboard, cloth, or vinyl pages. During tummy time, Ms. Gonzales can offer these toys to Maria. Now that Maria is grabbing items, it is time to remove the mobile from her crib.

- **Identify Maria's current stage of psychosocial development and assess how Ms. Gonzales can help her master this stage.**

According to Erikson, Maria is in the trust versus mistrust stage of development. Infants need consistent care to gain trust, such as picking up a child when they cry; delayed gratification leads to mistrust. It is important to be consistent in meeting Maria's needs and responding to her different cries. Maria needs conditions that foster trust, and positive psychosocial feelings as she develop. She has learned to trust her mother who is responsive to her infant's needs and cues. This reinforces trust and does not result in spoiling (Dixon and Stein 2006).

- **Assess the cognitive development of a 4-month-old child.**

Maria is in Piaget's sensory motor stage of development. At this age, Ms. Gonzales will observe that Maria is noticing the way her mother talks and the individual sounds she makes. Maria will continue to learn and build on Piaget's stage of primary circular reactions and start to begin secondary circular reactions. Beforehand Maria was repeating reflexive reactions and recognizing causality—that when she would press the button on the toy it would make a sound. Now Maria will do intentional activity to cause a desired outcome.

Maria is beginning to link an event with action such as quieting when put in a feeding position or upon seeing the bottle. Her ability to wait is beginning to develop as she learns to anticipate a response from her mother.

Maria is cooing, laughing, and squealing. She vocalizes in a variety of ways to initiate and sustain interaction and is beginning to listen when others speak.

- **Assess the social behaviors that Maria may exhibit at this age. Is baby smiling, more responsive, and making a variety of different sounds? Is baby responding to sound by looking at the caregiver, becoming quiet?**

At 4 months, Maria anticipates her feeding when she sees the bottle. She squeals with excitement using her whole body. She begins to make laughter out loud. She starts making consonant sounds: ba, ga, pa, kana. She begins to have eye-hand coordination. Maria inspects and plays with her hands. She can pull a blanket over her face and play. She will try to reach for objects and her toys—and may overshoot them. Maria can play with a rattle placed in her hand, but if it drops she can't pick it up yet. Maria begins to drool in preparation for teething.

Maria is building up relationships. She recognizes her primary caregiver. She has a variety of facial expressions such as smiling, surprise, and fear. She enjoys being cuddled. Her smiles are purposeful.

- **Identify the characteristics of play at this age and suggest appropriate playthings and activities to encourage Maria's development.**

Babies of Maria's age like bright objects, soft items, rattles that make sound, safe mirrors, balls, and items with different textures. Maria likes to be cuddled; she smiles a lot. Encourage the mother to laugh when Maria laughs. Tell Ms. Gonzales to call Maria by her name, place a rattle in her hand, and have squeeze toys with different textures that Maria can easily grasp. Maria enjoys splashing in the bathtub at this age. She shows interest in what is happening around her. See box "Helping Your Child's Physical Development—4–6 Months" for ideas on how Maria's family can help her development.

- **The nurse asks Ms. Gonzales if Maria has different cries?**

Mother is able to recognize Maria's cries for when she is hungry, when she wants to be changed, and when she wants company. Praise Ms. Gonzales for having developed a warm loving relationship with her child.

- **Describe visual and hearing development to the mother.**

Maria can focus on a block that is about ½ in. She can accommodate near objects. She makes many different sounds and makes sounds when prompted by a verbal

Helping Your Child's Physical Development: 4–6 Months

1. *Prone on Forearms*: Place baby on their belly and prop them up on forearms after diapering or dressing for a few seconds and longer as baby tolerates it.
2. *Prone with Arms Extended*: Turn baby onto stomach and prop them on their straightened arms for a few seconds after diapering or dressing.
3. *Sitting with Support*: While baby is sitting on your lap, use one hand to support their back and one to support their chest. As baby gets stronger, decrease the support.
4. *Supine: Feet to Hands or Mouth*: After diapering or dressing your baby, hold baby's feet together and slowly bring them up toward their chest and back down.
5. *Rolling Prone to Side Lying*: Encourage your baby to play on their side by offering toys or a childproof mirror and a pillow along their back for support. When baby is playing on tummy, shake a rattle or toy to try to get them to push themselves onto their side. Lie on your side with baby on their side facing you and gently rock them from their side to their belly and back to their side.
6. *Rolling Prone to Supine*: Roll baby from their back to their belly and then return them to their backside after you diaper or dress them.
7. *Rolling Supine to Prone*: Slowly roll the baby from their back to their tummy while sitting on the floor. Place baby on their back and dangle a toy in front of them so they reach towards it. Slowly move the toy to their side so they turn onto their tummy.

Source: Hurley, D.S. (2000). Developing fine and gross motor skills: Birth to three. *Austin, TX: PRO-ED, Inc.*

cue—when others speak to her. She is able to turn to sounds. Infants at this age have peripheral vision up to 180°.

- **Describe immunization at this age.**

  For immunizations at this age, consult the CDC, ACIP, or AAP web sites for the current immunization schedule recommendations (U.S. Centers for Disease Control and Prevention 2011):

– CEC National Immunization Program (NIP): http://www.cdc.gov/vaccines
– American Academy of Pediatrics *Red Book:* http://www.aapredbook.org

- **What information can be given concerning bottle-feeding and nutrition and starting solid foods and cow's milk?**

Maria's caloric needs are 98–108 kcal/kg/day. She gets this from her bottles and is not yet ready for solid food. Cow's milk can irritate the lining of an infant's stomach and intestines, causing bleeding into the stools. It also contains high concentrations of proteins and minerals and lacks the correct amount of iron, vitamin C, and other vitamins as well as having a form of fat—butter fat—that is hard for babies to digest and not the best for their growth. Infant formulas are iron fortified, which helps prevent iron-deficiency anemia, especially at this age. In addition, most formulas also contain docosahexaenoic acid (DHA) and also arachidonic acid (ARA) which help brain and eye development. Infant formula also contains vitamin D. Some infant formulas contain probiotics, which may prevent infectious diarrhea and atopic dermatitis and may reduce the symptoms of infant colic (American Academy of Pediatrics 2009).

Signs that Maria is ready for solids include that she opens her mouth for the spoon, has good head and neck control, can sit in a supported position, and shows an interest in the food her mother is eating. Also, between 4 and 6 months is usually when an infant doubles their weight, which is an indicator that they can start solid foods. At this age, Maria has lost the reflex to push her tongue against anything inserted in her month and will accept an infant spoon to eat from. Although Maria has not doubled her weight, her iron stores are being depleted and she should have iron supplements of 1 mg/kg/day, especially if Ms. Gonzales is not starting solid foods yet.

Eating foods should be enjoyable (Burns et al. 2009; Clinton 2011a; Clinton 2011b; Hockenberry and Wilson 2011; Marcdante et al. 2011; McInerny et al. 2009; Ontario Society of Nutrition Professionals in Public Health 2014; Potts and Mandleco 2012; samour and King 2005). Maria should be sitting upright to prevent choking. If she is not interested in eating, advise Ms. Gonzales to not force her, and try again in a week. It is not recommended to put food in the baby's bottle unless the child has gastrointestinal reflux.

Traditionally, a single grain iron-fortified cereal is the first food fed in America to babies. Then vegetables are slowly added, and then fruits. Advise Ms. Gonzales to wait at least 3 days between introducing each new food to make sure that there is no adverse reaction, such as diarrhea, rash, or vomiting.

- **Identify the anticipatory guidance that would be helpful for a 4-month-old.**

At 4 months of age, Maria is becoming more mobile. Now is the time to take more safety precautions by babyproofing the home and anticipating Maria's increasing ability to turn over, move around, put things in her mouth, pull at things, and get injured.

Safety for mobile infants: Ms. Gonzales should be advised to begin babyproofing her home to keep Maria safe, and also to be careful when visiting other places to watch for danger. Ms. Gonzales should keep an eye on Maria as she becomes mobile; don't leave her alone in a room without being in a crib or safe play yard. Don't leave Maria alone in tub or on dressing table or on the bed. Mrs. Gonzales should make sure to always have her hand on the baby when the baby is not on the floor. Avoid putting Maria in a walker—they are not a safe toy for babies because they can tip over and also fall down stairs even where there is a gate (see box "Baby Proofing Suggestions").

Baby Proofing Suggestions

Start when the baby is beginning to turn over to babyproof the home.

Clear out bottom cabinets of dangerous items, such as household cleaners, medications, and sharp objects.

Take breakables off low tables.

Put changing table or cabinet in a corner.

Put furniture against walls.

Lock up pills and medicines.

Remove small objects baby could swallow—anything that fits inside your thumb and forefinger rounded together.

Cover outlets.

Install door and drawer safety latches.

Install safety gates, especially at tops of stairs.

Remove cords, wires, and strings.

Remove plastic bags from baby's environment.

Keep houseplants out of reach and remove poisonous plants.

Sleep patterns: Babies at 4 months sleep about four times during the day, ranging from 1 to 2 h.

Personality development: At 5 months Maria will start smiling at her mirror image. She will start patting the bottle. She will start discriminating strangers from family. Advice Ms. Gonzales to use a variety of toys or household objects to stimulate Maria. Introduce Maria to different textures in toys and objects. Continue to talk, read, and sing to Maria.

Fine and gross motor development: At 5 months Maria will pursue a dropped object. She will put an object directly in her mouth. She will grasp an object voluntarily. She will play with her toes. Maria will be able to turn from her abdomen to her back and her birth weight will double. Ms. Gonzales should avoid use of a walker for Maria. They limit development of the baby's core muscles. Encourage floor "tummy" time so Maria can begin to explore her surroundings.

General safety: The health care provider should stress at every visit some essentials of general safety and hygiene for baby and family (see box on "General Safety and Hygiene").

Feeding: Advise Ms. Gonzales to allow Maria to self-regulate the amount she eats. Mother should watch for cues that Maria is finished eating, such as Maria turning her head away to say she is done. Secure Maria in a high chair for eating foods. Never leave her alone in the high chair.

General Safety and Hygiene

General: Parents need to be worried as their babies become mobile about the increased risk for injury, poisoning, burns, drowning, choking and suffocation, falls, and other preventable injuries. If the home was babyproofed at a younger age, the family should look at their babyproofing again in light of new development stages.

Illness Prevention:

- Stress the importance of hand washing by all caregivers including family members.
- Children should wash hands upon entering the home, coming in from the outdoors, and before eating.
- Mouth should be covered when coughing.
- Wash hands after blowing the nose.
- Avoid honey and corn syrup (Karo) for the first year of life to prevent infant botulism.

Injury Prevention:

- Use gates at steps and in entranceway to kitchen that has no door and at the tops and bottom of stairways.
- Use window guards for all windows above the ground floor and have screens on all windows.
- Keep doors locked to the outside and public hallways.
- Use covers on all electric outlets and sockets.
- Use door and drawer safety latches.
- Remove strings, plastic bags, cords, and electric wires to a safety box.
- Remove sharp objects that could injure baby.
- Always use an age-appropriate car seat when traveling in an automobile.
- Children under 20 lb should be placed in a car seat that faces backwards.
- When a child is over 20 lb and over 1 year of age, the car seat can face forward.
- As children enter toddlerhood and begin sports activities, always use appropriate sports safety gear, i.e., helmets, mouth guards, eye protection, and knee pads.
- Never leave a child alone in a car.
- Never leave a child alone in a high chair.
- Keep all guns under lock and key and store ammunition separately in a locked cabinet.

(continued)

Burn Prevention:

- Keep babies under 6 months out of direct sun exposure. Dress them in long, loose, lightweight garments.
- If unable to prevent exposure to the sun, use a minimal amount of sun screen to small areas for young babies.
- Use sunscreen of at least SPF 15+ and avoid prolonged sun exposure for babies over 6 months and children.
- Maintain a smoke-free environment.
- Have working smoke detector on each floor of the household as well as a carbon monoxide detector.
- Keep matches out of reach.
- Keep hot oil from splattering while cooking by using the back burner and also turning pot handles inward.
- Always check that bathwater temperature is not too warm.

Heat Stress:

- Check the back seats of a vehicle to ensure that no children are left inside.

Drowning Prevention:

- Keep the bathroom door closed.
- Keep the toilet lid down.
- Remove buckets of water.
- Never leave a child alone in a bathtub.
- Children should have swim lessons with qualified instructors and not be near water unless there is an adult next to them.
- Child should always be in sight and no more than arms-length if the child is near water.

Choking Prevention:

- Keep floor and low tables empty of small items baby could ingest.
- Avoid the following dangerous food items that can cause choking until child is over age 3; however caution should continue to be taken with children through the preschool and early school-age years: hard candies and jellybeans, whole grapes (cut them into halves or quarters), nuts and seeds, hot dogs (slice lengthwise even for older children), hard candies, popcorn, peanut butter (add jelly when on bread and avoid eating by spoonful), chunks of raw vegetables (such as carrot sticks), chewing gum, and chunks of meat (mince in small pieces).

- Remove items that can be choking hazards, including coins, buttons, toys with small parts, marbles, balloons, button batteries, small magnets, plastic tags from clothing, plastic garbage bags and bag pieces, and band aides.
- Teach children not to run with a lollypop or other hard item in their mouths.

Poisoning Prevention:

- Keep the poison control phone number and other emergency numbers on the refrigerator and next to the telephone.
- Keep medicines and other nonfood items locked up and in a high cabinet well off the floor.
- Always keep poisons/nonfood items (such as laundry and dishwasher cakes) in original container and store in locked cabinet.
- Remove poisonous plants.
- Keep plants out of reach.

Suffocation Prevention:

- Keep stuffed animals, bumpers, and pillows out of cribs.
- Remove all plastic bags.
- Remove toys with small pieces.

Abduction Prevention:

- Avoid wearing personalized clothing in public places.
- Teach the child not to go anywhere with strangers.
- Teach the child about safe touch.
- Never leave children alone in a car, at home, or in public.

After Maria finishes eating or at least once a day (such as at bath time), cleanse her gums with a soft cloth or gauze when she starts eating solid foods (American Academy of Pediatrics 2009). Once she has a tooth, her teeth should be brushed twice a day with a small amount of fluoride toothpaste (American Academy of Pediatrics 2009).

Limit setting and discipline: Begin exploring parental ideas about discipline with Ms. Gonzales. As Maria grows and explores her environment, Ms. Gonzales may feel the need to discipline her. Ms. Gonzales should teach Maria gently to avoid touching dangerous items in other people's homes where it may not be babyproofed. The Primary Health Provider should talk about corporal and physical punishment with Ms. Gonzalez and stress that these are not appropriate methods for any child.

Discipline at this age is about change of tone to express disapproval. Spanking teaches that violence is acceptable and it may potentially harm the child not only physically over time but psychologically and emotionally as well. If the only reason a child is not misbehaving is because of fear of corporal punishment when a parent is around, they may misbehave more when the parent is absent (Cain 2008; Larzele 2008).

Ms. Gonzales should give positive reinforcement for good behaviors and set realistic goals for acceptable behaviors. Positive reinforcement includes offering praise, smiling, and patting. She should call attention to unacceptable behavior as it is happening, use distraction to change behavior such as offering a different toy when one is grabbed from another child's hands, or exchanging a loud toy for a quiet toy if the child is making too much noise (Larzele 2008; Cain 2008).

The health care provider should review with Ms. Gonzales the guidelines for when to call the healthcare provider and worrying illness concerns (i.e., fever, vomiting, diarrhea) (see box "When to Call Your Health Care Provider").

When to Call Your Health Care Provider

- Breathing difficulties
- Behavior changes or irritability
- No urine output in 12 h
- Dehydration signs: irritability, sunken fontanel, sleepiness, decrease in tears, low urine output, sunken eyes
- Fever of 101 °F (38.3 °C) or higher
- Rash
- Infant having tremors
- Continued primitive reflexes: Moro, rooting, tonic neck beyond 4 months
- Concerns

References

American Academy of Pediatrics (2009) Committee on nutrition: pediatric nutrition handbook, 6th edn. American Academy of Pediatrics, Elk Grove Village, IL

Brazelton TB (1983) Infants and mothers: differences in development. Dell, New York

Burns CE et al (2009) Pediatric primary care: a handbook for nurse practitioners, 4th edn. W.B. Saunders, Philadelphia, PA

Cain DS (2008) Parenting online and lay literature on infant spanking: information readily available to parents. Soc Work Health Care 47(2):174–184

Centers for Disease Control and Prevention (2011) Recommendations and guidelines: childhood and adolescent immunization schedules. http://www.cdc.gov/vaccines/schedules/index.html. Accessed 11 Dec 2014

Clinton P (2011a) Four-month visit. In: Richardson B (ed) Pediatric primary care: practice guidelines for nurses. Jones & Bartlett Learning, Burlington, MA, pp 75–80. Chapter 9

Clinton P (2011b) Six-month visit. In: Richardson B (ed) Pediatric primary care: practice guidelines for nurses. Burlington, MA, Jones & Bartlett Learning, pp 81–84. Chapter 10

Dixon SD, Stein MT (2006) Encounters with children: pediatric behavior and development, 4th edn. Mosby, St. Louis, MO

Hagan JF, Shaw JS, Duncan P (eds) (2008) Bright futures: guidelines for health supervision of infants, children, and adolescents, 3rd edn. American Academy of Pediatrics, Elk Grove Village, IL

Hockenberry MJ, Wilson DW (2011) Wong's nursing care of infants and children, 9th edn. Elsevier/Mosby, New York, NY

Hurley DS (2000) Developing fine and gross motor skills: Birth to three. PRO-ED, Inc, Austin, TX. www.proedinc.com

Larzele RE (2008) Disciplinary spanking: The scientific evidence. J Dev Behav Pediatr 29(4):334–335

Marcdante KJ, Kliegman RM, Jenson HB et al (eds) (2011) Nelson essentials of pediatrics, 6th edn. Saunders, Philadelphia, PA

McInerny TK, Adam HM, Campbell DE, Kamat DM, Kelleher KJ (eds) (2009) Textbook of pediatric care. American Academy of Pediatrics, Elk Grove Village, IL

Mindell JA, Owens JA (2009) A clinical guide to pediatric sleep: diagnosis and management of sleep problems, 2nd edn. Lippincott Williams & Wilkins, Philadelphia, PA

Ontario Society of Nutrition Professionals in Public Health (2014) Pediatric nutrition guidelines (birth to six years) for health professionals. Ontario, Canada. http://www.healthunit.org/professionals/nutrition/Pediatric%20Nutrition%20Guidelines%20for%20Primary%20Health%20Care%20Providers.pdf. Accessed 28 Aug 2015

Porter, RS, Kaplan, JL (2011) The Merck manual online. http://www.merck.com/mmpe/index.html. Accessed 11 Dec 2014

Potts NL, Mandleco BL (eds) (2012) Pediatric nursing: caring for children and their families, 3rd edn. Delmar Cengage Learning, Clifton Park, NY

Samour PQ, King K (2005) Handbook of pediatric nutrition, 3rd edn. Jones and Bartlett Publishers, Sudbury, MA

Six-Month Visit

11

Mrs. McDoungh brings her son Jimmy into the pediatric clinic for his 6-month checkup. Jimmy's weight is 8.5 kg (18.7 lb) (75th percentile), his length is 68 cm (27.2 in.) (75th percentile), and his head circumference is 43.4 cm (17.36 in.) (75th percentile). Jimmy's anterior fontanel is still open, with no overriding sutures palpated. He has doubled his birth weight (at birth 3.8 kg–8.36 lb) and is exclusively breastfed. The mother is concerned about starting solid foods. She has a friend whose baby has allergies and the mother thinks she should only breastfeed to prevent Jimmy from getting allergies. He is turning over from back to front and front to back and likes rolling. He plays with rattles, shaking them in his hands and putting them in his mouth. Mrs. McDoungh notices that Jimmy sometimes rolls under the table. Jimmy has eight wet diapers a day and soft stools twice a day. He is down to two naps daily and makes sounds such as ba and da. When playing with objects, he shakes and bangs them. Mrs. McDoungh is starting to play peekaboo with Jimmy. She wonders if she uses a walker with him whether he will begin to walk sooner. Jimmy also likes to be read picture books that rhyme.

- **Are Jimmy's height and weight appropriate for him?**

Yes, Jimmy remains in the 75th percentile. Children of this age need 95–105 kcal/kg/day. His head circumference should be increasing about 1 cm (0.5 in.) each month and length about 1 cm (0.5 in.) a month. He has doubled his birth weight between 5 and 6 months. His length has increased 0.5 in./month. Growth may occur in spurts; and should always be plotted. Jimmy's infant stores of iron have been used up and Mrs. McDoungh should be advised to introduce solid foods that have been fortified with iron at this time.

- **Identify Jimmy's current stage of psychosocial development and assess how Mrs. McDoungh can help him master this stage.**

Jimmy is an active, social 6-month-old infant with his family. It is normal for Jimmy at this age to develop stranger anxiety. It shows that he is able to differentiate his caregivers from others. (Clinton 2011; Burns et al. 2009; Dixon and Stein 2006; Hagan et al. 2008; Hockenberry and Wilson 2011; Marcdante et al. 2011; McInerny et al. 2009; Potts and Mandleco 2012). His parents are comfortable in their role and look forward to their infant's new achievements.

D. Kramer, *Primary Well-Being: Case Studies for the Growing Child*,
DOI 10.1007/978-3-319-56708-2_11

- **Assess the cognitive development of a 6-month-old child.**

According to Piaget, Jimmy is in the sensory motor stage of cognitive development. Jimmy is starting to look for dropped objects, a sign of cognitive development. Separation anxiety is another sign. At 6 months of age, many pediatrician's offices start distributing books at the well-baby visit to encourage parents to read to their babies. One such national program is Reach Out and Read, but there are many others. Babies at this age can begin to understand words and parents can point to pictures and say the names of objects. Books are a vehicle for parents to interact with their babies that promotes literacy and language development as well as building a warm, nurturing relationship (High et al. 2014). Jimmy has begun to imitate sounds, doing one syllable utterances, such as ho, mo, da, and he. Jimmy likes hearing his own sounds, which reinforces his utterances. He likes looking at his mirror image and pictures of other babies.

- **What milestones of gross and fine motor development could Jimmy be expected to display?**

When Jimmy is prone he can lift his chest and upper abdomen off the surface and bear weight on his hands. He lifts his head when pulled to a sitting position. He can sit with his back straight in a high chair. And he now rolls from his back to his abdomen.

Jimmy bears almost all his weight when he is held in a standing position. He rakes objects and grasps them with his hands. He also transfers objects between hands and drops, shakes, and bangs them. Jimmy can pick up a dropped object. If his mother gives him one toy he drops the other he is holding. He can manipulate and grasp small objects. He holds the breast when breastfeeding, and he grasps his feet and pulls them to his mouth when he is lying on his back. See box **Helping Your Child's Physical Development—Six to Nine Months (page 122)**.

- **What reflexes do you expect him to have?**

Jimmy's Moro and tonic neck reflexes have completely disappeared, as well as grasp and rooting reflexes.

- **Assess the social behaviors that Jimmy may exhibit at this age.**

Jimmy recognizes and enjoys interacting with parents. He likes to be picked up.

Jimmy expects that his needs will be met and expresses frustration when they are not. He exhibits frequent mood swings, from one moment to the next. When his face is hidden in a towel, he enjoys the game of hiding and revealing—peekaboo. Separation anxiety is emerging. He begins to differentiate angry or friendly tone of others and responds accordingly. He uses gestures to gain attention such as pointing and reaching.

- **Discuss what you would say to Mrs. McDoungh about using a walker for Jimmy.**

Mrs. McDoungh is asking about using a walker to help Jimmy walk earlier. Walkers actually reduce development of the baby's core and do not promote walking. They are not recommended for use and can be dangerous—Jimmy could fall down the stairs or tip over in the walker and be seriously hurt (American Academy of Pediatrics 2001).

Explain to Mrs. McDoungh that in a pediatric advisory, the American Academy of Pediatrics recommends walkers not in compliance with new voluntary safety standards not be sold in the USA (American Academy of Pediatrics 2001. It has high risks for injury and no clear benefits. Thousands of young children are treated in the emergency room every year for fractures, and head injuries related to use of walkers. Most have a parent at home during the time of injury.

Muscles used to move a walker are different from ones needed for walking. In fact, using a walker delays learning to walk as it encourages walking on tiptoe, making it harder for the child to balance. A stationary play center without wheels is safer than a walker to entertain and stimulate Jimmy.

- **Identify the characteristics of play at this age and suggest appropriate playthings and activities to encourage Jimmy's development and safety.**

Mr. and Mrs. McDoungh can foster normal development through play, by encouraging a variety of physical activities such as creeping activities, weight-bearing activities, using objects, and playing various games (Hurley 2000). Jimmy's ability to explore his environment will improve his cognitive ability as well (Hurley 2000). See box **Helping Your Child's Physical Development—Six to Nine Months** for ideas on how to stimulate Jimmy's development and give Mrs. McDoungh a copy to take home. Also see box **Toys for Babies Two to Six Months** on page 107.

Helping Your Child's Physical Development: Six to Nine Months

1. Place your baby on the floor on their tummy. Put your child's favorite toy about 6 in. away in front of them to encourage them to move towards the toy. If they are not yet able to move, place the toys a little closer and gradually move them farther and farther away.
2. To practice weight bearing, stand your child up by holding them around their chest after diapering or dressing them. Count to 5 or 10 and then return them to a sitting position.
3. Your child will begin to bang objects together at this age. Give them two objects at a time.
4. When feeding them in the high chair, use a plastic-coated safety baby spoon to bang against the tray. You can say "bang, bang" while banging objects together to promote language development.
5. You can encourage your child to transfer toys hand to hand around seventh month of age, by showing them how to do it.
6. Encourage use of the pincer grasp by providing 4–6 cheerios on the high-chair tray at a time, provided that there are no allergy contraindications, so baby can pick them up one at a time.

7. When diapering your baby, encourage the child to play with a rattle or toy held in their hand.
8. Reaching: prone on forearms—When baby is on their tummy, propped up on their forearms, they will shift their weight onto one forearm while reaching with the other arm. Your baby assume the prone on forearm position while on the floor and offer a toy so that they must reach for it with one hand. Place a few toys on baby's left side so they will reach with their left hand to get them and repeat on the right side.
9. Bridging—After diapering or dressing your baby, lay them on their back. Bend their knees, hold their feet to the ground, and gently raise and lower their buttocks.
10. Help stand with support—After dressing or diapering your baby, stand the baby up with support and count or sing a song.
11. Sitting balance—After dressing or diapering the baby, place them in a sitting position. While holding their hands, play a game like pat-a-cake or sing a song to encourage trunk control.
12. Transition: Prone to and from sitting—Help your baby raise themselves onto a hands and knees position from lying on their belly by lifting their belly off the floor.
13. Transition: supine to and from sitting—Place your baby on their side. While gently holding down their hips and legs, help them push themselves up by using their arms and hands.
14. Transition: supine to and from hands and knees—Roll baby from their back to tummy and onto back again. Then, roll them from back to tummy and lift up their chest and tummy so that they are in hands and knees position.
15. Crawling—Place baby in the hands and knees position and help them move their arms and legs in an alternating way, such as right arm, left leg, left arm, and right leg.
16. Pulls up to tall kneeling—Sit on the floor with your baby in the hands and knees position. Place a favorite toy on your thigh to encourage baby to place their hands on your thighs so that they are tall kneeling. Bend your knees if baby needs to be more upright.

Source: Hurley, D.S. (Hurley 2000). *Developing fine and gross motor skills: Birth to thre*e. Austin, TX: PRO-ED, Inc.

- **Describe visual and hearing development to the mother.**

Vision: At 6 months, infants are better at spotting small objects and at tracking moving objects. Jimmy can see all the colors of the rainbow and see them more brightly. Visual acuity has increased and he has approximately 20 × 25 vision. He has better eye-hand coordination so he can pick something up and put it in his mouth. Prior to 6 months, Jimmy's eyes were not always coordinated but by 6 months they should be. If his eyes were not coordinated by this time, he should see a pediatric ophthalmologist.

Hearing: Jimmy should be able to follow sounds with his eyes and respond to changes in voice and tone. He will pay attention to music and notice that some toys make sounds. He should be babbling in a speechlike way and use different sounds, including *pa, ba,* and *ma*. He should laugh and babble when excited and make gurgling sounds when playing (National Institute of Health, National Institute on Deafness and Other Communication Disorders 2010). If any of these behaviors are not present, Jimmy should be referred for a hearing test.

- **Assess nutrition and dental needs.**

Dental: Jimmy should be starting to teethe at this age. He will be mouthing objects, drooling, and waking up in pain from throbbing gums. His first teeth to emerge will be two lower center incisors. Baby Jimmy may chew and bite on objects as well as occasionally during breastfeeding.

Breastfeeding should be encouraged to continue, but firmly remove him when he bites and say "Mommy is not for biting."

Nutrition: A child who is 6 months old will start to use their fingers to eat food. Now is a good time to introduce solid foods if not before, but encourage Mrs. McDonough to continue breastfeeding at least until Jimmy's first birthday.

According to the American Academy of Pediatrics, Jimmy's first food should be iron-fortified rice cereal, mixed with some breast milk as he is still breastfed. Then gradually Mrs. McDonough can introduce pureed vegetables and then strained or pureed fruits. Some experts suggest starting vegetables before fruits although there is no evidence to suggest that children won't eat vegetables because they are not as sweet as fruit (American Academy of Pediatrics 2009). Give Jimmy new foods one at a time and start with 1–2 teaspoons.

Offer a new food only after 3 days to check for any allergic reaction. Some experts suggest starting with pureed meat for babies, especially those who were breastfed, because they have a more easily digestible form of iron and zinc. Meat also contains more nutrients than cereals. Mrs. McDoungh should be made aware that it is better to use commercial baby vegetables in the first year, particularly spinach, beets, squash, and carrots, as they pick up nitrates from the soil and too much could cause anemia in babies. Baby food manufacturers test for this (American Academy of Pediatrics 2008). Eventually baby crackers like Zwieback or other foods that can be softened in the mouth can be offered, like small pieces of banana, cheerios, or wafers.

Mrs. McDoungh should offer solid foods to Jimmy 2–3 times/day so that Jimmy will become accustomed to new textures and tastes. Mrs. McDoungh should introduce solids with a spoon. She should never put cereal in a bottle, unless Jimmy is experiencing reflux.

If Mrs. McDoungh is worried about there being a reaction, besides waiting a few days between each food introduced, she should also check that Jimmy is not having diarrhea, a rash, or vomiting, or even a mood change. These all can be signs of an allergy to the food introduced. Mrs. McDoungh should stop using the new food and consultant with me as her health care provider for Jimmy. If Jimmy has a severe allergic reaction such as hives, swelling, or trouble breathing, take him immediately to the emergency room. If this does occur, Mrs. McDoungh will be told to carry an EPI pen (auto injectors) with her to give immediately when this reaction occurs.

Because Jimmy is being breastfed, now is a good time to add vitamin D (400 IU) and iron supplements (1 mg/kg/day) (8 mg for Jimmy who weighs 8 kg).

As food is added to Jimmy's diet, his stools will change. Mrs. McDoungh may see pieces of food, and changes in color and odor, and in texture. Foods that generate more allergic reactions are eggs, fish, nuts, and chocolate—these are started usually after the first year of life. Soy, wheat, and milk may also be allergens. Honey is also delayed until over 1 year due to botulism contamination. Infants with strong family history of allergies should avoid foods with high allergy potential (strawberries, eggs, etc.) until end of first year (Samour and King 2005).

- **Describe immunization needs at this age.**

  For immunizations at this age, consult the CDC, ACIP, or AAP web sites for the current immunization schedule recommendations (U.S. Centers for Disease Control 2001):

- CEC National Immunization Program (NIP): http://www.cdc.gov/vaccines
- American Academy of Pediatrics *Red Book*: http://www.aapredbook.org

- **Mrs. McDoungh says that she is concerned because Jimmy is rolling under the furniture. What guidance would you offer?**

  It is normal for babies to roll from side to side at this age. It is a baby's way of getting around and mastering their environment. Now is the time to make sure that everything is babyproofed. Mrs. McDoungh should make sure that no tablecloths are hanging down, no small objects are near the floor, and dangerous items are locked away. Babyproof the environment with outlet covers, door and drawer latches, and safety gates. She should remove cords, wires, string, and plastic bags from the baby's environment. Also, do not put heavy or hot objects on tables that have tablecloths and could be pulled down.

- **Identify the anticipatory guidance that would be helpful for a six-month-old.**

  Teething: In the coming months, Jimmy may have teeth erupt, starting with two lower central incisors, and he will start chewing and may bite. These later skills lay the foundation for mastering more advanced skills, such as eating whole foods, growing toward independence, and self-regulation.

  Mrs. McDonough can rub Jimmy's gums with a cold teething ring when he is in pain. The mother should make sure that the teething ring is large and made from one piece so no separation can take place. The same rules apply to pacifiers, which may be used at this age.

  Over-the-counter preparations like Baby Orajel or Anbesol should not be given because they can numb the whole mouth, suppressing the gag reflex. Treat teething discomfort with oral massage, frozen wet washcloths, other cold hard objects for chewing, as well as acetaminophen or ibuprofen if necessary. Talk to Mrs. McDonough about the fluoride source in their community, e.g., water supply, and suggest supplementation if needed.

Physical Growth and Development: Jimmy will start sitting up and leaning forward on his hands and he will lift his head off a table spontaneously. He will be able to bear weight on one hand when he is on his stomach prone. He will be able to sit erect for a moment and bear full weight on his feet. His parachute reflex (putting his arms up) will appear.

By 7 months Jimmy will bounce actively when held in a standing position. He will transfer objects from one hand to the other, display a unidextrous (one-handed) approach, and grasp for objects. He will be able to hold two objects of about the same size and weight more than momentarily and bang objects on the table. He will rake at a small object. By 8 months Jimmy will begin to show regular patterns in bladder and bowel elimination. He will sit steadily without support, bear weight on his legs when supported, and may stand holding on to furniture. He will also be able to adjust his posture to reach an object.

By 8 months, Jimmy will begin using the pincer grasp—using his index, fourth, and fifth fingers against the lower part of his thumb. He will be releasing objects at will, ringing a bell purposely, and holding two objects while looking at a third object. He will be able to obtain an object by pulling on a string and he will stretch persistently for toys beyond his reach.

Jimmy's growth rate will begin to slow down at around 6 months, going to 90–150 g weekly for the rest of the first year (3–5 oz). Jimmy will continue to grow about 0.5 in. (1.25 cm) each month. The health care provider can share with Mrs. McDoungh the box **Helping Your Child's Physical Development: Six to Nine Months.**

Social and Cognitive Development: Socially, at 7 months, Jimmy will show increasing fear of strangers and be distressed when his parent disappears; he will imitate simple acts and noises and try to attract attention by coughing or snorting. He will enjoy playing games such as peekaboo. The health care provider should encourage Mrs. McDonough to do reading activities with Jimmy, using picture books and infant board books.

Jimmy may exhibit oral aggressiveness by biting and mouthing objects and people. He will show expectation after repeated exposure to the same stimuli, such as when seeing food taken from the refrigerator he will expect to be fed.

Jimmy will be able to focus on very small objects, respond to his own name, figure out where sound is coming from by turning his head in an arc, and develop an awareness of depth and space. He will start producing vowel sounds and "chained syllables" like baba, dada, and kaka. By 7 months he will have four distinct vowel sounds and "talk" when others are talking.

He will make the consonant sounds *t, d,* and *w* and listen selectively to familiar words. His vocalizations will contain emphasis and emotion. While he will combine syllables, he will not yet know their meaning, such as *mama.* Jimmy will exhibit increasing anxiety when a parent, especially mother, leaves. Stranger fear is also elevated. Jimmy may dislike dressing and changing his diaper and will respond to the word "no."

For general safety, food, and hygiene reminders for Mrs. McDoungh, see box General Safety and Hygiene (page 115). Also review with Mrs. McDoungh when to call the health care provider (see box When to Call Your Health Care Provider on page 117). The health care provider should also see the Red Flags For the Health Care Provider box (page 107) for further follow-up.

References

American Academy of Pediatrics, Committee on Injury and Poison Prevention (2001) Injuries associated with infant walkers. Pediatrics, 108(3), 790–792. http://pediatrics.aappublications.org/content/108/3/790.full. (Reaffirmed in 2005) Accessed 11 Dec 2014

American Academy of Pediatrics (2008) Starting solid foods. Updated May 28, 2013. www.healthychildren.org/. Accessed 25 Mar 2014

American Academy of Pediatrics, Committee on Nutrition (2009) Pediatric nutrition handbook, 6th edn. American Academy of Pediatrics, Elk Grove Village, IL

Burns CE et al (2009) Pediatric primary care: a handbook for nurse practitioners, 4th edn. W.B. Saunders, Philadelphia, PA

Centers for Disease Control and Prevention (2011) Recommendations and guidelines: childhood and adolescent immunization schedules. http://www.cdc.gov/vaccines/schedules/index.html. Accessed 11 Dec 2014

Clinton P (2011) Six-month visit. In: Richardson B (ed) Pediatric primary care: practice guidelines for nurses. Jones & Bartlett Learning, Burlington, MA, p 81. Chapter 10

Dixon SD, Stein MT (2006) Encounters with children: pediatric behavior and development, 4th edn. Mosby, St. Louis, MO

Hagan JF, Shaw JS, Duncan P (eds) (2008) Bright futures: guidelines for health supervision of infants, children, and adolescents, 3rd edn. American Academy of Pediatrics, Elk Grove Village, IL

High PC et al (2014) Literacy promotion: an essential component of primary care pediatric practice. American Academy of Pediatrics. http://pediatrics.aappublications.org/cgi/doi/10.1542/peds.2014-1384. Accessed 2 June 2015

Hockenberry MJ, Wilson DW (2011) Wong's nursing care of infants and children, 9th edn. Elsevier/Mosby, New York, NY

Hurley DS (2000) Developing fine and gross motor skills: birth to three. PRO-ED, Inc, Austin, TX. www.proedinc.com. Accessed 11 Dec 2014

Marcdante KJ, Kliegman RM, Jenson HB et al (eds) (2011) Nelson essentials of pediatrics, 6th edn. Saunders, Philadelphia, PA

McInerny TK, Adam HM, Campbell DE, Kamat DM, Kelleher KJ (eds) (2009) Textbook of pediatric care. American Academy of Pediatrics, Elk Grove Village, IL

National Institute of Health, National Institute on Deafness and Other Communication Disorders (2010) Your baby's hearing and communicative development check list. http://www.nidcd.nih.gov/health/hearing/pages/silence.aspx. Accessed 17 June 2014

Potts NL, Mandleco BL (eds) (2012) Pediatric nursing: caring for children and their families, 3rd edn. Delmar Cengage Learning, Clifton Park, NY

Samour PQ, King K (2005) Handbook of pediatric nutrition, 3rd edn. Jones and Bartlett Publishers, Sudbury, MA

Nine-Month Visit 12

Li-Ling is a round-faced 9-month-old brought to the pediatric clinic by her grandmother, Mrs. Chang, for her monthly checkup. Her birth weight was 2.5 kg (5.5 lb) and birth length was 45 cm (18 in.), putting her in the third percentile at birth; her head circumference at birth was 32 cm (12.8 in.), also third percentile. Li-Ling now weighs 6.8 kg (14.7 lb), her height is 64.8 cm (25.9 in.), and her head circumference is 41.6 cm (16.2 in.). Grandma is concerned about Li-Ling's weight when she is told that the child is in the third percentile. Li-Ling is still breastfed at night but takes a bottle during the day while her mother works. Mrs. Chang describes how Li-Ling crawls all over the place, pulling herself up to stand. She pulls down items on low tables and grabs at tablecloths. Li-Ling has difficulty separating from her mother and cries when her mother goes to work. Her mother gives her a set of toy keys when she leaves each day. Li-Ling also has a favorite stuffed bear. Li-Ling also expresses fear when new people talk to her. She is eating finger foods like rice cakes, tofu, beans, cereals like oat cheerios, cornflakes, steamed corn, cut-up fruit like bananas, and strawberries, and cooked fruit like apples, pears, peaches, or apricots. Li-Ling still takes two naps but the nap in the afternoon is shorter. The grandmother sings a particular song to Li-Ling before nap and bedtime. Li-Ling is combining sounds, waves bye-bye to visitors, and loves to play peekaboo. She says dada and mama to everyone and responds to her name. She looks for hidden objects. The grandmother is concerned about babyproofing. There are many wires and cords on the floor in the apartment.

- **Are Li-Ling's height and weight appropriate for her?**

There are many factors that influence children's height and weight: family history, heredity, and nutrition. If a child remains consistently on their height and weight curve, they are growing according to their individual trajectory. The health care provider should reassure grandma that Li-Ling is consistently on the third percentile growth curve and is doing fine. At this age, Li-Ling needs between 98 and 100 kcal/kg/day.

- **Assess Li-Ling's current stage of psychosocial development and how her mother and grandmother can help her master this stage.**

According to Erikson, Li-Ling is in the trust versus mistrust stage of development. Infants need consistent care to gain a sense of trust, and should be picked up

D. Kramer, *Primary Well-Being: Case Studies for the Growing Child*,
DOI 10.1007/978-3-319-56708-2_12

when they cry, for example. The health care provider can explain to Li-Ling's grandmother how delayed gratification leads to mistrust and not to fear giving Li-Ling what she needs at this age.

All of the pulling and grabbing behaviors that Li-Ling is showing are normal for this stage of development, such as pulling down the tablecloth and pulling herself up to stand. It is wonderful that the mother and grandmother are developing routines with Li-Ling around eating and naptime, and when the mother leaves for work with singing and special toys like the keys. This stage is full of movement. The need to explore is critical for Li-Ling's cognitive development. She is rapidly gaining new motor and cognitive skills.

This age presents new challenges to parents and caregivers because of the increasing mobility and knowledge of the child. Review with grandma the box General Safety and Hygiene (page 115). Remind grandma and parents to put gates on stairs, and barriers around space heaters or radiators; to keep electric cords out of baby's reach; and use safety outlet covers. Also avoid placing hot foods on the tablecloth where your baby can pull them down. The grandmother and mother should try to consolidate the cords and wires in the apartment so Li-Ling cannot reach them. Li-Ling should always be within sight and not more than an arm length away if she is near water. That includes the bathtub and bathroom. Also, remind parent about removing blind or drapery cords, and hanging objects. Use outlet covers, door and drawer latches, and safety gates. Remove cords, wires, string, small objects, and plastic bags from baby's environment. Keep medicines locked up.

- **Assess the cognitive development of a nine-month-old child.**

Li-Ling is rapidly gaining new motor and cognitive skills daily. She is in Piaget's stage of sensory motor development. She is in Piaget's scale of coordination of secondary schemas and their application to new situations. She is able to remember objects she no longer sees (object permanence), as we see when she looks for a ball that rolls under the coach; she looks for objects and goes after them. She understands the meaning of some words and combines syllable. She imitates speech sounds and expressions. She has learned that she is separate from her mother and is upset when her mother leaves. She combines sounds, waves good bye, and says dada and mamma in response to everyone. Li-Ling responds to her name and turns her head toward sound. She has more depth perception and responds to simple verbal commands. She understands "no." (High 2014).

- **What milestones of gross and fine motor development could Li-Ling be expected to display?**

Li-Ling has good fine motor coordination. Her Pincer grasp is developed (thumb and index finger). Li-Ling has a clear dominant hand; she can grasp a third object and compare two objects by bringing them together. She is able to pick up small objects and is beginning to poke with her index finger. She can drop, bang, and throw objects. She can feed herself finger foods cut into small pieces.

She has good gross motor development. Li-Ling sits up well, is creeping and crawling on hands and knees around the house, and has begun to pull herself up to a standing position and hold on to the furniture. She can bear her weight when pulled to stand. She can sit for sustained periods (about 10 min). Li-Ling recovers her balance when she leans forward but cannot do so when learning sideways. Provide Li-Ling's parents with a copy of the Box **Helping Your Child's Physical Development—Nine to 12 Months,** to help them foster Li-Ling's development (Burns 2009; Clinton 2011; Hagan et al. 2008; Hockenberry and Wilson 2011; Marcdante et al. 2011; McInerny et al. 2009).

Helping Your Child's Physical Development: Nine to 12 Months

1. *Isolated Index Finger Action:* When diapering your baby, have them point to different body parts (nose, mouth, eyes) both on themselves and on you.
2. *Holds Crayon Adaptively:* When baby is sitting in high chair, put some pudding or whip cream on the tray and let them smear it with their fingers. Hold baby on your lap while you are sitting at a table. Put a big, fat crayon or marker in baby's hand and help them scribble on a piece of paper. Repeat with other hand.
3. *Stacking Blocks:* While sitting on floor with baby, show baby how to stack the blocks into a tower. Start with large blocks and gradually decrease the size of the blocks.
4. *Pivots While Sitting:* Place a few favorite toys on either side of your baby on the floor so they must turn to reach them. After diapering or dressing them, lay them on their back and gently rotate their trunk by bending their knees and bringing them to one side, then to the middle, and then to the other side.
5. *Transition: Sitting to and from Hands and Knees:* When your baby is sitting, place their hands on the floor and gently lift their buttocks so they assume the hands and knees position.
6. *Transition: Pulls Up to Stand from Hands and Knees:* While playing on the floor, give the baby opportunities to pull herself up to a standing position. Let them use furniture, pillows, and you for support. Supervise them closely to prevent falls.
7. *Cruising Sideways:* Stand the baby next to couch or coffee table and gently move their legs one at a time so that they move sideways while supporting them at hips.
8. *Standing: Leaning for Support:* Stand the baby in front of a sturdy object such as a sofa or coffee table and place their favorite toys in front of them. Provide support at the trunk or hips and encourage them to play with the toys.
9. *Walking with Support:* Practice walking your baby using both your hands for support. Gradually decrease the support to one hand, and then to no hands. Stay close by in case baby loses their balance. Provide toys that can be pushed around the house, such as push-pull toys and an overturned laundry basket.

Source*:* Hurley, D.S. (2000). Developing fine and gross motor skills: Birth to three. *Austin, TX: PRO-ED, Inc.*

- **What reflexes do you expect Li-Ling to have?**

Primitive reflexes should be absent by 9 months, but the parachute reflex emerges. Babinski reflex (toe fanning) is still evident.

- **Assess the social behaviors that Li-Ling may exhibit at this age.**

Li-Ling waves bye, bye and plays peekaboo. Her mother is increasingly important to Li-ling and gives Li-Ling a transitional object when she leaves for work to soothe the child. Li-Ling shows increasing interest in pleasing her parent but also in expressing wants. She begins to show fears of going to bed and being left alone and also of strangers. Grandma helps Li-Ling by singing a familiar lullaby. Li-Ling will put up her arms in front of her face to avoid it being washed.

- **Identify the characteristics of play at this age and suggest appropriate playthings and activities to encourage Li-Ling's development and safety.**

Children of this age like moving, sitting, and exploring. They like toys that roll and blocks. They like stacking pyramid peg toys. They can start doing simple puzzles with big pieces and knobs. They can put things into a receptacle like a bottle or bucket and they like to play with containers. Encourage floor time for Li-Ling to provide opportunities to explore her environment. Talk with her while engaging in other activities (e.g., grocery shopping, riding in a car, walking in the neighbor in her stroller). Grandma and mother should continue singing and movement activities with Li-Ling. They should play games such as "peekaboo." Grandma and mother should encourage reading activities with picture books and infant board books. They can foster Li-Ling's ability to self-soothe with transitional objects such as blanket, stuffed toy, or keys (Dixon and Stein 2006). (See also Box **Helping Your Child's Physical Development—Six to Nine Months.)**

- **Describe visual and hearing development to the grandmother.**

Li-Ling is able to locate the origin of sounds and look for objects. She has good vision and hearing (National Institute of Health 2010). Normal vision is 20/40 at this age.

- **Assess nutrition, immunization, and dental needs for this age.**

For immunizations at this age, consult the CDC, ACIP, or AAP web sites for the current immunization schedule recommendations (Centers for Disease Control and Prevention 2011):

(a) CEC National Immunization Program (NIP): http://www.cdc.gov/vaccines
(b) American Academy of Pediatrics *Red Book*: http://www.aapredbook.org

Nutrition: Li-Ling is still breastfed at night and gets breast milk in a bottle during the day. At this stage she is obtaining most of her most nutrients from solid foods. The mother should be encouraged to continue breastfeeding through the first year, with 3–5 feedings a day of breast milk. Cow's milk should not be introduced until after 12 months. Grandma should make sure that Li-Ling is getting plenty of iron-rich foods such as cooked, mashed, and strained spinach, and infant cereal with iron mixed with breast milk to thicken. Tender chopped meat can be added at this age for increased iron. Li-Ling should be offered a variety of fruits and vegetables cut up into finger size—no bigger than Li-Ling's thumb, so that Li-Ling can use her fine pincer grasp. Remind the grandma that it can take up to 10–15 tries to get Li-Ling to accept new food.

At this age, Li-Ling should be having solid food 4–6 times a day, with at least two main meals and two snacks (American Academy of Pediatrics 2009). As Li-Ling grows, her stomach empties every 2 h and snacks can be increased as she desires, as long as they are healthy, including finger foods like banana and tofu, crackers made of rice or wheat, peeled cucumber, or ripe avocado. Products like "happy puffs," organic vegetables made into little puffs, are often enjoyed by babies this age. Breast milk can be offered from a cup but advise Mrs. Chang to limit water to 1 oz a day and limit baby juice to 4–6 oz a day. Avoid foods Li-Ling could choke on, such as grapes, raisins, peanuts/peanut butter, popcorn, hard candy, carrots, celery, other hard vegetables and fruits, and hard meats. No honey or corn syrup (Karo) should be given until after the first year.

Grandma Chang and mother should be creating a relaxed, pleasant atmosphere and not worry about Li-Ling creating a mess. Mother and grandma should encourage Li-Ling to self-feed and provide her with a spoon. They can avoid overfeeding by watching for clues that Li-Ling is full such as when she turns her head away from the food offered, throws food over the edge of the high chair, clamps her mouth shut, or starts to cry (American Academy of Pediatrics 2005; American Academy of Pediatrics 2008; American Academy of Pediatrics 2014; Potts and Mandleco 2012; Samour and King 2005).

Dental care: After eating or at least once a day, Mrs. Chang should use a soft toothbrush without toothpaste to clean Li-Ling's teeth. Talk to Mrs. Chang about the fluoride source in their community, e.g., water supply, and suggest supplement if necessary. Advise mother to avoid giving Li-Ling a bottle in bed to prevent dental carries.

- **Assess sleep and bedtime rituals at this age.**

At 9 months, Li-Ling is sleeping less, usually between 10 and 14 h a day. Night awakenings are common, 1–2 times, but she should be able to put herself back to sleep. Grandma has already noticed that Li-Ling sleeps less in the afternoon but she is still taking two naps a day, in the morning and afternoon, sleeping from 1 to 3 h (Hagan et al. 2008). She has well-established bedtime rituals including listening to a story book, listening to her grandmother sing a special song, and cuddling for a few minutes. Li-Ling's room should be dimly lit at bedtime and not overly warm. At night Li-Ling's mother is there to nurse her to sleep. This is also a good age to lower the crib mattress to its lowest position in preparation for Li-Ling standing and trying to climb out of bed (Mindell and Owens 2009).

- **Mrs. Chang says that she is concerned because Li-Ling is pulling tablecloths and other objects off tables. What guidance would you offer?**

Suggest that Mrs. Chang and mother assess the situation. Many of the factors Mrs. Chang is concerned about show that Li-Ling is developing normally. It is better to rearrange the environment to be safer for Li-Ling than trying to tell the baby not to touch things. Mrs. Chang can study where she can use table coverings that don't hang down and move reachable objects to higher levels. She will also want to remove breakable objects or small objects from low levels for the time being, especially while Li-Ling is still putting objects in her mouth as she explores her environment. We want an environment where Li-Ling can explore safely and not be told "No, no" all the time. This is also the time for the family to remove blind and drapery cords, and wires from floors. For a full list of safety guidelines, see the box General Safety and Hygiene (page 115).

- **What information can be given concerning stranger anxiety and separation anxiety?**

  Separation anxiety is normal development. Grandma and mother should remain calm, sing a song, talk about mommy going and coming back, or sing it in a song. Stranger anxiety is also normal as Li-Ling differentiates people in her world. Distraction is also useful for stranger anxiety. Don't have someone new pick up Li-Ling until she is comfortable with them. Having grandmother or mother talk calmly to the stranger will help Li-Ling gradually accept the new person.

- **Identify the anticipatory guidance that would be helpful for a nine-month-old.**

  Safety. Review the box **General Safety and Hygiene** (page 115) and ask what babyproofing measures Mrs. Chang has already taken. She should be praised for taking steps to keep Li-Ling safe and also be reminded of some basic safety issues when caring for Li-Ling. Give grandma the box to take home to review with Li-Ling's mother.

  Mrs. Chang should especially have the poison control number (to be placed by telephone and on the refrigerator). A list of other emergency phone numbers and locations should be pasted on the refrigerator as well.

  Growth and development: Between 9 and 12 months Li-Ling is able to cruise and walk holding on, and by the 12-month visit may be able to walk on her own. Other things change between 9 and 12 months: Li-Ling will continue to like eating finger foods but may decrease food intake when she is about 1 year. Grandma and mother should not be concerned that there is something wrong with the baby when she eats less. By 12 months, most children triple their weight and have grown twice as tall as their birth length. Li-Ling will have 6–9 teeth by the end of her first year of life. The anterior fontanel is almost closed. A lumber curve will develop and lordosis (curvature of the spine) will be evident during walking.

References

American Academy of Pediatrics (2005) Infant-Food and Feeding. http://www.aap.org/en-us/advocacy-and-policy/aap-health-initiatives/HALF-Implementation-Guide/Age-Specific-Content/Pages/Infant-Food-and-Feeding.aspx. Accessed 18 June 2014

American Academy of Pediatrics (2014) Healthy active living for families 2014. healthychildren.org/growinghealthy. Accessed 16 Dec 2016

American Academy of Pediatrics Committee on Injury and Poison Prevention (2001) Injuries associated with infant walkers. Pediatrics 108(3):790–792. http://pediatrics.aappublications.org/content/108/3/790.full. (Reaffirmed in 2005) Accessed 11 Dec 2014

American Academy of Pediatrics (2008) Starting solid foods. Updated May 28, 2013. www.healthychildren.org/. Accessed 25 Mar 2014

American Academy of Pediatrics, Committee on Nutrition (2009) Pediatric nutrition handbook, 6th edn. Elk Grove Village, IL, American Academy of Pediatrics

Burns CE et al (2009) Pediatric primary care: a handbook for nurse practitioners, 4th edn. W.B. Saunders, Philadelphia, PA

Centers for Disease Control and Prevention (2011) Recommendations and guidelines: childhood and adolescent immunization schedules. http://www.cdc.gov/vaccines/schedules/index.html. Accessed 11 Dec 2014

Clinton P (2011) Six-month visit. In: Richardson B (ed) Pediatric primary care: practice guidelines for nurses. Jones & Bartlett Learning, Burlington, MA, p 81. Chapter 10

Dixon SD, Stein MT (2006) Encounters with children: pediatric behavior and development, 4th edn. Mosby, St. Louis, MO

Hagan JF, Shaw JS, Duncan P (eds) (2008) Bright futures: guidelines for health supervision of infants, children, and adolescents, 3rd edn. Elk Grove Village, IL, American Academy of Pediatrics

High PC et al (2014) Literacy promotion: an essential component of primary care pediatric practice. Pediatrics. http://pediatrics.aappublications.org/cgi/doi/10.1542/peds.2014-1384. Policy Statement: American Academy of Pediatrics, released June 24

Hockenberry MJ, Wilson DW (2011) Wong's nursing care of infants and children, 9th edn. Elsevier/Mosby, New York, NY

Hurley DS (2000) Developing fine and gross motor skills: birth to three. PRO-ED, Inc, Austin, TX. www.proedinc.com. Accessed 11 Dec 2014

Marcdante KJ, Kliegman RM, Jenson HB et al (eds) (2011) Nelson essentials of pediatrics, 6th edn. Saunders, Philadelphia, PA

McInerny TK, Adam HM, Campbell DE, Kamat DM, Kelleher KJ (eds) (2009) Textbook of pediatric care. American Academy of Pediatrics, Elk Grove Village, IL

Mindell JA, Owens JA (2009) A clinical guide to pediatric sleep: diagnosis and management of sleep problems, 2nd edn. Lippincott Williams & Wilkins, Philadelphia, PA

National Institute of Health, National Institute on Deafness and Other Communication Disorders (2010) Your baby's hearing and communicative development check list. http://www.nidcd.nih.gov/health/hearing/pages/silence.aspx. Accessed 17 June 2014

Potts NL, Mandleco BL (eds) (2012) Pediatric nursing: caring for children and their families, 3rd edn. Clifton Park, NY, Delmar Cengage Learning

Samour PQ, King K (2005) Handbook of pediatric nutrition. In: 3. Jones and Bartlett Publishers, Sudbury, MA

One-Year Visit

13

Taisha is an active 1-year-old brought to the pediatric clinic by her mother and father, Mr. and Mrs. Jones. Her birth weight was 2.6 kg (5.7 lb) (10th percentile), and is now 8 kg (17.6 lb) (10th percentile) which is three times her birth weight. Taisha's length at birth was 46 cm (18.4 in.) and she is now 66 cm (26.8 in.); and her head circumference at birth was 32.4 cm (12.96 in.) and now it is 42.24 (16.89 in.), also on the 10th percentile. She is eating much less and less frequently and some days she wants more or less—while a month ago she was more consistent. The Jones' are concerned about this. Taisha continues to be breastfed and eats a variety of table foods, enjoys finger foods, and has about three meals and two snacks a day. Mrs. Jones is trying to decide if she should continue breastfeeding and what Taisha should drink if she is not breastfeeding. Should she use a bottle or a cup. Taisha is walking holding on and enjoys it. She can hold a crayon crudely and makes marks on a paper, but still tries to put the crayon in her mouth. The apartment they live in often does not provide sufficient heat and the parents frequently resort to a space heater in the winter. The parents are concerned that Taisha will turn the heater over and get hurt. Taisha doesn't like going to sleep in the evening and wakes up in the middle of the night crying. She naps for a long time in the morning and at about 2 p.m. She says dada and momma specific to her parents. Taisha understands "no" and "hot" but sometimes throws temper tantrums when something is denied to her. Her parents are used to disciplining older children as they each teach sixth grade. They ask about using time out at Taisha's age. When her parents name something in the room, Taisha will look for it. She likes talking and singing games, and naming body parts.

- **Are Taisha's height and weight appropriate for her?**

Taisha's height and weight are appropriate for her individual growth pattern. At 12 months she needs 98–100 kcal/kg/day. She has tripled her birth weight, and at a year, the brain size usually doubles. Taisha's growth rate is decreasing so she is eating less. Toddlers have food fads; one day they will eat one thing; another day they will eat something else. Parents should not be concerned if there is inconsistency. Reassure Mr. and Mrs. Jones that toddlers' eating patterns will vary from meal to meal; they should think in terms of several days when reviewing recommended servings of food. (American Academy of Pediatrics 2014; American

D. Kramer, *Primary Well-Being: Case Studies for the Growing Child*,
DOI 10.1007/978-3-319-56708-2_13

Academy of Pediatrics Undated; American Academy of Pediatrics 2008; American Academy of Pediatrics Committee on Nutrition 2009; Ontario Society of Nutrition Professionals 2014)

- **Identify Taisha's current stage of psychosocial development and assess how her parents can help her master this stage.**

  Taisha has successfully completed Erickson's psychosocial stage of trust versus mistrust. She is now moving to autonomy versus shame and doubt. This is when the toddler wants to do things on her own and learns to say "no." Taisha has now gained trust from having her parents meet her needs and develop routines and show affection and approval. Toddlers have a sense of control over their environment but still want to meet the approval and affection of their primary care providers. This is the time to offer choices to children pointing to the red top or the blue top—to give Taisha a sense of autonomy but making sure that both choices are acceptable to the caregiver. During this stage, Taisha may be upset as Mrs. Jones nudges her to wean from breastfeeding. At other times she may refuse to nurse. Welcome Mr. and Mrs. Jones to the world of the toddler. There is nothing consistent about the toddler.

- **Assess the moral development of a year-old child?**

  Taisha is in stage one of moral development: premoral stage, the preconventional level. This stage remains until 18 months of age. In this stage infants learn how to behave by trying to avoid punishment and seeking to obtain praise from adults and older individuals in their environment, especially their primary caregiver.

- **Assess the cognitive development of a year-old child.**

  Taisha remains in Piaget's sensorimotor stage of coordination of secondary schemas and their application to new situations. This is demonstrated by Taisha's moving away from her parents by exploring new surroundings, working to find a toy that is out of reach, and actively searching for hidden objects. She has a curiosity about her environment and actively observes other's actions and listens to their talk. She continues to touch and mouths objects as a way to explore. With her first birthday, Taisha will be entering the sensory motor stage of tertiary circular reactions. In this stage, Taisha will use her physical skills and curiosity to explore her environment. She will be able to do nesting cups—put smaller objects in larger ones, put objects into a container and take them out, start exploring draws, and open doors. Things are no longer "out of sight out of mind." Taisha is increasingly moving around her environment, practicing her locomotor skills.

  Taisha's language development is increasing. She understands the meaning of words and simple verbal commands and gestures that have meaning like waving bye-bye, signaling to come. Taisha uses 1–2 words together, knows 3–5 words besides "dada" and "mama," and understands others she doesn't speak. Comprehension always comes before verbalization at this age. She knows how to call her parents using "dada" and "mamma." She imitates sounds, especially animal sounds, and responds to simple verbal commands and gestures. She understands "no," and "hot." She can look for objects named by others.

- **What milestones of gross and fine motor development could Taisha be expected to display?**

Taisha is now able to walk while holding on with one hand. She enjoys cruising around the furniture in her apartment and occasionally stands alone for a few seconds or takes a step in preparation for walking. She can sit down from a standing position on her own. Her pincer grasp is well developed. Taisha can put an object in a cup, like a block or ball. She tries to build a block tower but fails after two blocks, but she loves to knock down a tower built by others. She also likes trying to insert a small object into a narrow-necked container. She likes to turn pages in books, usually several at a time, and likes to make marks on a paper, holding a crayon or pencil. See box "Helping Your Child's Physical Development—12 to 18 months." If Taisha were not walking holding on, not standing when supported, doesn't say at least one word, doesn't point to things, or doesn't gesture, these would be red flags for further developmental assessment.

Helping Your Child's Physical Development: 12 to 18 Months

1. *Crawling Up and Down Stairs*: Parents can place a gate on the second or third step of a flight of stairs and sit behind their child as they crawl up and down one or two stairs. Demonstrate crawling up and down steps.
2. *Placing Objects into Containers*: Have toys for your baby to play with such as shape sorters and wooden puzzles with handles to learn how to place objects in and take them out of containers.
3. *Turning Pages in a Book*: When parents read to their child before naptime or bedtime, let them practice turning the pages.
4. *Self Help: Dressing*: Partially remove your child's clothing while undressing, and encourage them to finish the task, i.e., taking off socks.
5. *Walking Independently*: Extend your arms about 3 ft from your child as they lean against the couch or armchair and encourage them to walk towards their parent.
6. *Seats Self in Chair*: Sit on the floor and encourage your child to walk toward their parent, turn, and sit on their lap.
7. *Rolling a Ball*: Roll a ball back and forth with your child as you sit on the floor across from them with your legs wide apart.

Source: Hurley, D.S. (2000). Developing fine and gross motor skills: Birth to three. *Austin, TX: PRO-ED, Inc. Retrieved Dec. 11, 2014 from www.proed-inc.com.*

- **Assess the social behaviors that Taisha may exhibit at this age.**

Taisha is having temper tantrums that are to be expected at this age when she doesn't want to do something or is frustrated. Consistent rules and appropriate discipline will help reduce tantrums. Advise Mr. and Mrs. Jones that the best approach to managing tantrums is to have consistent and developmentally appropriate expectations. They should praise Taisha when she is cooperative. They can offer Taisha options so that she can continue to feel autonomous. It is important that Mrs. and Jones be flexible in their expectations for Taisha. Having established routines for bedtime, when children typically have difficulty slowing down, or anytime when there is a transition, so that Taisha can prepare herself for the transition, and Mr. and Mrs. actively communicating what is going to be happen, can help prevent tantrums and discipline problems.

- **How can the primary care provider help promote Taisha's emotional development at this age and reduce the occurrence of temper tantrums?**

Advise the parents that it is usually best to ignore the tantrum and give comfort once the child is able to control her emotions. Tell Mr. and Mrs. Jones to not give into what the tantrum was about. See the accompanying box for when tantrums are a concern, such as when the child bangs their head, when they become aggressive, or when they show violent behavior, if they occur frequently in child care or school settings (see "Temper Tantrums" box). Other emotions are emerging such as anger and affection, jealousy, and fear. Taisha may give a hug or kiss on request. She may still be anxious around strangers. She may become attached to a blanket or favorite toy and want to take it wherever she goes. This is also the age to start discussing discipline and what that means with parents (see box "Discipline of the Young Child") (Rains 2011; Potts and Mandleco 2012; McInerny et al. 2009; Marcdante et al. 2011; Hockenberry and Wilson 2011; Hagan et al. 2008; Dixon and Stein 2006; Clinton 2011; Burns 2009; American Academy of Pediatrics 2014).

Discipline of the Young Child

Discipline and limit setting are positive aspects of parenting to help children learn socially acceptable behavior, to have self-control, and to produce constructive activity from uncomfortable feelings like anger, frustration, and fear, and learning that others are there to set limits that will protect them. When the infant is 1 year of age it is a good time to think about the family's attitude to discipline and limit setting and form a plan to grow with their baby. Discipline is a consequence for a behavior that is not acceptable. It is important to focus on the behavior, not on the child. For example: Say to Taisha, "our hands are not for hitting." Or "I am unhappy when I see Mary hit. She is not for hitting." Instead of saying "Taisha is bad for hitting Mary.

To minimize unacceptable behavior:

- Have realistic expectations and prepare the environment for the child.
- Give your child opportunities to feel empowered, such as dressing herself, making a block tower, taking a book off the shelf, bringing an object to a parent, and sending a kiss to grandma.
- Review expected behavior with your child in new environments and situations, e.g., "we are going to grandma's house and we don't touch objects on the table" or "this is what we expect at dinner in the restaurant."

Hopefully grandma will put away her fragile objects and put toys in their place while Taisha visits.

- At this age distraction is the best way to redirect behavior.
- Be aware of the child's temperament and energy level—such as fatigue—which makes the child more vulnerable to misbehavior.
- Offer reasons for delaying a child's request that they can understand but tell them you will do it at a certain time later. At 1 year, a child may not understand the word later—better to say today at and give an activity associated with time, such as after dinner.
- Always keep your word for anything you will tell your child you will do.
- Use 'No" sparingly. Try to redirect the child instead or provide explanations instead.
- Model appropriate behavior, such as not screaming and keeping calm.
- Keep rules few and simple and be consistent. Don't go into long explanations with young children aged 1–3.
- Identify an unacceptable behavior when it occurs and implement discipline immediately.
- Disciplining a child should be done in a way to allow privacy so they will not feel ashamed and embarrassed in front of others.
- Consequences for behaviors should take place in a time-limited fashion. If using time out, it should be 1 min/year of age. No lecturing, or scolding, or criticism about the incident should be made afterwards.
- Praise your child on accomplishments and positive behaviors. For young children a stars chart to record positive behavior is appropriate. For older children, use tokens that can be exchanged for goods and services.
- Avoid physical punishment.

Sources: *Clinton, P. (2011). Twelve-month visit. In: Richardson, B. (Ed.), Pediatric primary care: Practice guidelines for nurses. Burlington, MA: Jones & Bartlett Learning.*

Hockenberry, M.J. and Wilson, D.W. (2011). Wong's Nursing care of infants and children, 9th ed. New York, NY: Elsevier/Mosby.

- **Identify the characteristics of play at this age and suggest appropriate playthings and activities to encourage Taisha's development and safety.**

Taisha likes to wave "bye-bye." She enjoys hand games like "pat-a-cake" and when stories and songs are acted out, like "wheels on the bus," and finger games like "where is thumpkin." One-year-olds like playing at naming things, body parts, and people. Taisha imitates the activity of other children and adults. Toys to introduce at this stage include push-pull toys to practice walking, stacking blocks, nesting cups, and shape sorters. Squeaky animal and doll toys, large puzzles, jack in the box, books with textures and objects on them (like Pat the Bunny), books with rhymes, and rhythmic type songs are also good playthings for this age to encourage fine and gross motor coordination, cognitive development, and imaginary play.

Taisha's parents should continue to talk, sing, and tell stories to her. Mr. and Mrs. Jones should make it a habit to describe what they are doing to Taisha (e.g., "this is how we put on socks"). They can play games such as naming things, body parts, and people. They can encourage reading activities with picture books and infant board books. If television is watched in the home, Mr. and Mrs. Jones should limit viewing for Taisha to 1 h or preferably less per day.

- **What nutrition advice would you offer Taisha's parents?**

  Although breastfeeding is continuing Taisha is getting most of her nutrients from food. If Mrs. Jones wants to decrease the number of times she is breastfeeding per day, she can start offering Taisha whole milk up to 16–24 oz/day from a cup. Three meals a day and two snacks is an appropriate amount of food for a 1-year-old—usually a serving size is one tablespoon per food/year/age. The health care provider should advise the parents that food should be continued to be chopped into small pieces to prevent choking and food such as grapes, raisins, and hotdogs should be cut in half lengthwise. Raw vegetables such as carrots, apples, and celery should be cut in very small pieces. Foods such as peanuts and popcorn should be avoided to help prevent chocking. Peanut butter should be avoided until age 3. Toddlers enjoy finger foods. Since they have little patience to sit, they like feeding themselves, and trying to use a spoon and cup. Taisha will be able to use a cup with a lid and hold it with both hands. Parents should expect Taisha to turn the spoon over before it gets to her month—but she will eventually learn how to do it. Most important is for Mr. and Mrs. Jones to provide a varied nutritious diet and give Taisha time to enjoy eating. Taisha should be drinking milk and water instead of sugar-containing beverages.

- **Describe visual and hearing development to the parents.**

  Taisha can localize sounds and listens for sound to recur (National Institute of Health 2010). It is important for the practitioner to assess for amblyopia at this time (lazy eye). Taisha can recognize some geometric forms, like circle and triangle, and follow a fast-moving object.

- **Assess immunizations for this age to the parents.**

  For immunizations at this age, consult the CDC, ACIP, or AAP web sites for the current immunization schedule recommendations (Centers for Disease Control and Prevention 2011):

– CEC National Immunization Program (NIP): http://www.cdc.gov/vaccines
– American Academy of Pediatrics *Red Book*: http://www.aapredbook.org

- **Assess dental needs for this age.**

  At this age, Taisha continues to be breastfed and eats a variety of foods. She has a cup for liquids. Now is the time for her first dental visit to assess for any caries, and to get her used to going to the dentist. Mr. and Mrs. Jones can use a soft toothbrush, with a small pea-size amount of fluoridated toothpaste. The local fluoride source should be determined and supplemented as necessary (Casamassimo and

Hold 2014; Centers for Disease Control and Prevention 2001). For guidelines on oral health, see *Bright Futures in Practice: Oral Health, pocket guide* by Paul Casamassimo and Katrina Hold, Washington, DC: National Maternal and Child Oral Health Resource Center, Georgetown University, 2014.

- **Assess sleep needs for this age.**

Taisha is having two naps a day. At this stage, she should take an early afternoon nap instead of one in the morning and afternoon. Taisha should be sleeping on average 12–14 h per day with 0–1 night awakening and 1–2 naps a day. She may nap from 1 to 3 h and should continue to sleep in her crib. Mrs. and Mr. Jones should continue established bedtime rituals with Taisha and be consistent about bedtime. Taisha may continue to use transitional objects such as a stuffed animal. At this age bedtime resistance may occur and night waking is not unusual. The parents should avoid letting Taisha nap late in the day, as this will interfere with her nighttime sleep. By now, Taisha's mattress should be in the lowest position to keep her from climbing out of the crib. If that occurs, Mr. and Mrs. Jones should transfer her to a youth bed or regular bed with special safety bars. They should continue to remove all cords, small objects, plastic bags, or latex balloons from the bedroom.

- **Assess toileting needs at this age.**

At 1 year, Taisha is not voiding or evacuating as much as she did. She should show a regular pattern for evacuation, but voiding and evacuation will continue to be involuntary. It is still too early to try toilet training; better to wait until close to 24 months.

- **Mr. and Mrs. Jones say that they are concerned because Taisha is curious about the heaters in the apartment. What guidance would you offer?**

The space heaters need to be gated off to protect Taisha from getting to them and hurting herself. Also the health care provider should get the phone number for lack of heat complaints and call in the complaint as well as give the parents the phone number, so the radiators will be fixed.

- **Identify the anticipatory guidance that would be helpful for a year-old child.**

Review the guidelines for when to call the health care provider listed in the box "When To Call Your Health Care Provider" on page 117.

To foster Taisha's physical development, provide Mr. and Mrs. Jones with a copy of the box Helping Your Child's Physical Development—12 to 18 Months.

References

American Academy of Pediatrics (undated) Infant-food and feeding. http://www.aap.org/en-us/advocacy-and-policy/aap-health-initiatives/HALF-Implementation-Guide/Age-Specific-Content/Pages/Infant-Food-and-Feeding.aspx. Accessed 18 June 2014

American Academy of Pediatrics (2014) Healthy active living for families. healthychildren.org/growinghealthy. Accessed 16 Dec 2014

American Academy of Pediatrics, Committee on Injury and Poison Prevention (2001) Injuries associated with infant walkers. Pediatrics 108(3):790–792. http://pediatrics.aappublications.org/content/108/3/790.full. (Reaffirmed in 2005). Accessed 11 Dec 2014

American Academy of Pediatrics (2008) Starting solid foods. Updated 28 May 2013. www.healthychildren.org/. Accessed 25 Mar 2014

American Academy of Pediatrics, Committee on Nutrition (2009) Pediatric nutrition handbook, 6th edn. American Academy of Pediatrics, Elk Grove Village, IL

Burns CE et al (2009) Pediatric primary care: a handbook for nurse practitioners, 4th edn. W.B. Saunders, Philadelphia, PA

Casamassimo P, Hold K (2014) Bright futures in practice: oral health, pocket guide, 2nd edn. National Maternal and Child Oral Health Resource Center, Georgetown University, Washington, DC. http://www.mchoralhealth.org/pocket.html. Accessed 18 Dec 2014

Centers for Disease Control and Prevention (2011) Recommendations and guidelines: childhood and adolescent immunization schedules. http://www.cdc.gov/vaccines/schedules/index.html. Accessed 11 Dec 2014

Centers for Disease Control and Prevention (2001) Recommendations for using fluoride to prevent and control dental caries in the United States. Morb Mortal Weekly Rep. 50:14

Clinton P (2011) Twelve-month visit. In: Richardson B (ed) Pediatric primary care: Practice guidelines for nurses. Burlington, MA, Jones & Bartlett Learning

Dixon SD, Stein MT (2006) Encounters with children: Pediatric behavior and development, 4th edn. Mosby, St. Louis, MO

Hagan JF, Shaw JS, Duncan P (eds) (2008) Bright futures: guidelines for health supervision of infants, children, and adolescents, 3rd edn. American Academy of Pediatrics, Elk Grove Village, IL

Hockenberry MJ, Wilson DW (2011) Wong's nursing care of infants and children, 9th edn. Elsevier/Mosby, New York, NY

Hurley DS (2000) Developing fine and gross motor skills: birth to three. PRO-ED, Inc., Austin, TX. www.proedinc.com. Accessed 11 Dec 2014

Marcdante KJ, Kliegman RM, Jenson HB et al (eds) (2011) Nelson essentials of pediatrics, 6th edn. Saunders, Philadelphia, PA

McInerny TK, Adam HM, Campbell DE, Kamat DM, Kelleher KJ (eds) (2009) Textbook of pediatric care. American Academy of Pediatrics, Elk Grove Village, IL

Mindell JA, Owens JA (2009) A clinical guide to pediatric sleep: diagnosis and management of sleep problems, 2nd edn. Lippincott Williams & Wilkins, Philadelphia, PA

National Institute of Health, National Institute on Deafness and Other Communication Disorders (2010) Your baby's hearing and communicative development check list. http://www.nidcd.nih.gov/health/hearing/pages/silence.aspx. Accessed 17 June 2014

Ontario Society of Nutrition Professionals in Public Health (2014) Pediatric nutrition guidelines (birth to six years) for health professionals, Ontario, Canada. http://www.healthunit.org/professionals/nutrition/Pediatric%20Nutrition%20Guidelines%20for%20Primary%20Health%20Care%20Providers.pdf. Accessed 28 Aug 2015

Potts NL, Mandleco BL (eds) (2012) Pediatric nursing: caring for children and their families, 3rd edn. Delmar Cengage Learning, Clifton Park, NY

Rains SG (2011) Fifteen- to eighteen-month visit. In: Richardson B (ed) Pediatric primary care: practice guidelines for nurses. Burlington, MA, Jones & Bartlett Learning, pp 97–108. Chapter 13

Samour PQ, King K (2005) Handbook of pediatric nutrition, 3rd edn. Jones and Bartlett Publishers, Sudbury, MA

Eighteen-Month Visit

14

Vladimir is a strappling 18-month-old who comes into the pediatric clinic running ahead of his mother and grandmother, Mrs. Samakov and Mrs. Dovbrinski. Vladimir's weight is 13.6 kg (29.9 lb), which is in the 95th percentile. His height is 87 cm (34.8 in.), in the 97th percentile, and his head circumference is 50 cm (20 in.) in the 97th percentile. His grandmother is concerned that he eats sporadically despite his good weight for his age. At day care they tell Mrs. Samakov that Vladimir eats, but the grandmother doesn't see him eating at home. He was breastfed but now is weaned to a cup. The parents are concerned about his strong will, especially when he has a temper tantrum in reaction to not getting what he wants, for example not sharing his toys with a child in day care. The mother and the grandmother want to talk about toilet training. They have observed that Vladimir stops playing when he is having a bowel movement. His anterior fontanelle is closed and he is a little pot-bellied and bow legged and has 14 teeth. He likes playing with push toys. Vladimir has receptive language and understands most of what is said to him. The family speaks Russian at home but English is spoken in day care. Vladimir says six words in Russian and four words in English. He likes to take off his socks by himself but cannot dress himself. He can point to a body part and uses a spoon and a baby cup. Vladimir can listen to a story being read, look at the pictures, and name the objects. He shows affection. He can walk upstairs with assistance. His daycare director reports that Vladimir engages in parallel play. Boris could be sitting next to Vladimir and each is playing with a separate fire truck and not interacting.

- **Are Vladimir's height and weight appropriate for him?**

Yes. At this age: Vladimir is slowing down in growth as he plows through toddlerhood. He can be expected to gain about 5 lb between 1 and 2 years of age and grow about 3 in. As his energy needs decrease, Vladimir needs less calories and fluids per day—about 102 kcal/kg/day for food, 1.2 g of protein/kg/day, and 115 ml/kg/day of fluids. At this time, he may only grow an average of 4.5 lb/year. At 18

D. Kramer, *Primary Well-Being: Case Studies for the Growing Child*,
DOI 10.1007/978-3-319-56708-2_14

months of age it appears as though the child is becoming anorexic but there are actually decreased growth needs, so it seems as if the child is not eating as much as in earlier stages. This is what accounts for the discrepancy in what the daycare provider sees in school versus the grandmother at home.

- **The mother wants to know what type of milk she should give Vladimir and how much he should drink since he was recently weaned.**

Advise Mrs. Samakov that Vladimir should continue to drink whole milk until he is age 2.

Grandma and mom should see that Vladimir gets 1–2 tablespoons of each food for each year of life, or about 1/4 to 1/3 of adult servings on average over the day or even over the week. Encourage Vladimir's family to offer healthy foods including fruits and vegetables and protein at each meal. Whole milk should be limited to <24 oz/day (three cups). The fat in whole milk enables myelination of the nerves. The calcium and vitamin D in milk are essential for Vladimir's healthy bone development as well as vitamin C. Vladimir needs at least 500 mg/day of calcium and 600 iu/day of vitamin D (American Academy of Pediatrics 2012). Fat should be limited to less than 30% of his diet, protein 15–20%, and carbohydrates less than 55% (including vegetables and fruit). Give Vladimir two to three snacks/day and limit sugar. Since milk is lacking in iron, it is important that Vladimir also eat other sources of iron.

Vladimir and his family should be eating meals together. His family should allow Vladimir to self-feed with hands and utensils and drink from a cup, not a bottle at meals. They should avoid giving him foods he could choke on. They should provide healthy choices, allow experimentation, and not force eating with Vladimir.

Depending on what Vladimir's diet includes, screening for anemia may be appropriate (large amounts of cow's milk/day, especially in a bottle, diet deficient in other iron-rich foods are all indicators for anemia screening) (American Academy of Pediatrics Undated; American Academy of Pediatrics 2012; American Academy of Pediatrics 2014; American Academy of Pediatrics 2008; American Academy of Pediatrics 2009; Samour and King 2005).

- **Identify Vladimir's current stage of psychosocial development and describe how his parents and grandmother can help him master this stage.**

According to Erikson, Vladimir is in the second stage of psychosocial development, which is autonomy versus shame and doubt. Toddlers need to be provided with choices and to do what they can on their own (Dixon and Stein 2006).

- **Assess the cognitive development of an 18-month-old child.**

According to Piaget, Vladimir is still in the sensorimotor stage: intervention of new means through mental combinations. He can point to common objects and know two or three body parts. He can begin to follow directions. He likes to imitate animal sounds and can point to a picture of a specific animal and make the appropriate sound. Vladimir has ten or more words in his vocabulary. He is beginning to be aware of ownership of toys, etc. and differentiate himself from objects. Children of this age can develop dependency on transitional objects such as security blankets. He will look for objects when they are not in view. He understands much of the language spoken to him, but says only a few words. Vladimir will make a large jump in language between 18 months and 2 years of age. He can sit and wait for a short period of time. At this age, Vladimir will start showing a hand preference.

Vladimir is beginning to work on causality at this age. He will show an increase in physical abilities and memory development, like knowing there is an object hidden in the room (object permanence). He is starting to see objects symbolically and is beginning to be imaginative (Rains 2011; Potts and Mandeleco 2012; McInerny et al. 2009; Marcdante et al. 2011; Hockenberry and Wilson 2011; Hagan et al. 2008; Burns et al. 2009).

This is the age to screen for early signs of autism spectrum disorder (ASD), including atypical development in socialization and communication. These symptoms can now be detected by pediatric providers in children as young as 18 months. Consistently, those signs include decreases in frequency of gaze to the examiner's face, reduced social smiles and vocalization to others, preoccupation with the same action/object, for example, repeatedly opening the door or turning the wheels of a toy car, being inconsolable when crying, and not being involved in imaginative play (Hagan et al. 2008). The M-CHAT tool is frequently used to screen for ASD (see m-chat.org) (see box "Red Flags for the Health Care Provider in Assessing Development").

Red Flags for the Health Care Provider in Assessing Development

Eighteen months is a pinnacle age in being able to assess for certain developmental delays, such as autism spectrum disorders. If any of these are behaviors are present, the health care provider should make a developmental assessment referral for the child.

1. Cannot walk up stairs with assistance
2. Does not self-feed with spoon at times
3. Does not mimic actions of others
4. Does not use at least six words
5. Does not point to things they want
6. Is inconsolable when crying

Sources: Hagan, J.F., Shaw, J.S., and Duncan P. (eds.). (2008). *Bright futures: Guidelines for health supervision of infants, children, and adolescents. 3rd ed.* Elk Grove Village, IL: American Academy of Pediatrics.

American Academy of Pediatrics (undated). Achieving bright futures: The eighteen month visit, Implementation of the ACA Pediatric Preventive Services Provision.

Retrieved July 8, 2016 from: https://www.aap.org/en-us/professional-resources/practice-support/Periodicity/11%2018%20Month%20Visit%20F010914.pdffrom.

- **What reflexes do you expect him to have?**

Vladimir has lost all of his primitive reflexes. This is the age when Babinski reflex switches from toes curling in when bottom of food is scrapped to toes fanning out. If toes continue to curl this may be a symptom of central nervous system problem. Also pincer grasp should be refined at this age.

- **What milestones of gross and fine motor development could Vladimir be expected to display?**

Vladimir walks up and down stairs with one hand held. He can walk backwards. He runs clumsily and jumps in place with both feet. Vladimir is able to sit by himself on a chair and to throw a ball overhand. In terms of fine motor coordination, he can turn the pages of a book two or three at a time or in clumps; in drawings he imitates strokes. He can manage a spoon and he can build a tower of three or four cubes. He continues to imitate words and begins using two-word phrases; he pulls a toy along the ground; stacks three blocks; uses a spoon and cup; and listens to a story, looking at pictures and naming objects. He shows affection; kisses; follows simple directions; points to some body parts; and enjoys scribbling. Handedness will begin to be established. Also, see box "Red Flags for Health Care Provider in Assessing Development" (page 144).

Vladimir's family can also be given guidance on some fine and gross motor activities they can do with him to foster his development (Hurley 2000). See box Helping Your Child's Physical Development—18 Months to 2 Years.

Helping Your Child's Physical Development: 18 Months to 2 Years

1. *Building a Cube Tower*: Assist your toddler with stacking 1-in. cubes to make a tower. Demonstrate if needed as you sit next to your toddler.
2. *Imitates Drawing*: Provide your toddler with a large and wide washable crayon or marker. As you sit next to your toddler, hold their hand and help draw lines and circles.
3. *Self-Help: Eating*: Provide spill-proof cups with lids that your toddler can pick up and drink from by themselves. Let your toddler use plastic-coated spoons that they can pick up themselves. Expect mealtime to be messy while your toddler is learning to feed themselves. Provide a wet washcloth to wipe toddler's face and high chair when they finish.
4. *Standing on One Foot*: While dressing your toddler in shorts or pants, have them stand up and hold onto your shoulders and lift one foot at a time.

Source: Staisiunas, D. (2000). Developing Fine and Gross Motor Skills: Birth to Three. *Austin, TX: PRO-ED, Inc. www.proedinc.com*

- **Assess the social behaviors that Vladimir may exhibit at this age.**

At this age Vladimir's growth, development, and socialization are demonstrated in play activities. As he progresses from the sensorimotor play of infancy to parallel play of toddlerhood, he will incorporate fine and gross motor skills and new language skills.

Appropriate toys for Vladimir are swing sets, sandboxes, play kitchens, play tools, musical and "talking" toys (especially interactive ones), riding toys (especially without pedals), push toys, balls, containers, telephones, mirrors, dolls and puppets, large crayons, and books (contact Reach Out and Read for information on setting up a literacy promotion program in clinics and offices: http://www.reachoutandread.org).

Vladimir is utilizing his newly developed locomotion skills to explore and control his environment. He will push and carry large objects; put himself into small spaces such as boxes, cabinets, and under tables; delight in repetitive throwing and retrieving; and scribble on surfaces.

- **What information can be given concerning discipline and breath holding?**

Temper tantrums are common at this age. It is a healthy phenomenon that demonstrates that Vladimir is striving for independence and looking for admiration and positive reinforcement of newly found skills. But Vladimir will still experience dependency. He will walk away, check in, and come back multiple times. Mrs. Samakov and Mrs. Dovbrinski should be encouraged to help Vladimir learn to express emotions such as joy, fear, anger, sadness, weariness, and frustration (also see box "Discipline of the Young Child," page 137).

Vladimir's new mobility and drive for autonomy make discipline a new challenge for the family and caregiver to keep him safe. Appropriate discipline guidelines for Vladimir include offering choices when available, following a "no" with a "yes," keeping rules simple and few, and removing objects about which there is constant disagreement. The parents and grandmother should try to "catch the child being good," and reward positive behaviors with verbal praise and physical affection throughout the day.

When discipline is necessary (such as when Vladimir pushes another child), it is helpful to have Vladimir immediately be isolated from the situation, and be sat down in a place that is quiet without any stimulation, but where he can be observed. Doing this will enable him to associate undesirable behavior with being isolated. This will motivate him not to do the behavior again. It is important for the parent or caregiver to state that they are unhappy with the behavior but not that they are unhappy with the child. Isolation will take several experiences over time to achieve its goal. Spanking or corporal punishment is not an acceptable means of discipline. See box on the WAIST Strategy below for one method of discipline that is evidence based. The health provider should let the family know that they can meet/talk to her if they have further questions about behavior management and discipline.

Using the WAIST Strategy to Discipline the Young Child

Some find the WAIST Strategy helpful for effective time-out. **WAIST** is an acronym to remind the user of the five essential steps in a productive time-out.

- **W is for Warn**—Use one warning only, such as "Rebecca, if you do not stop hitting your sister, you will be in time out."
- **A is for Announce**—Clearly explain why your child is in time-out, such as "Rebecca, because you didn't stop hitting your sister, you are going to time out."
- **I is for Ignore**—Your child will likely try to bargain their way out of time-out. Standing firm makes this strategy more effective.
- **S is for Start**—Start the time-out immediately and tell your child the time-out is not up for discussion.
- **T is for Talk**—After your child has a time-out, you can give them the chance to talk about the behavior. However, time-out must be a clean slate for you as a parent. Do not continue to make a child feel punished after they have already had a time-out.

Sources: *University of Florida. IFAS Extension.* The University of Florida IFAS Extension recommends the WAIST acronym for effective time outs: *http://www.bundoo.com/articles/time-out-tips-behavior-management-that-works/).*

- **Assess visual and hearing development.**

Vision: Vladimir will have binocular vision at 18 months. His visual acuity is 20/40. If his eyes do not seem coordinated, such as lazy eye or strabismus, he should be referred to an eye specialist to prevent amblyopia. Vladimir's depth perception is still developing.

Hearing: At this age it is important to know that Vladimir is hearing well because between 18 and 24 months there is a big language burst. And if Vladimir begins to lose language, the family should be concerned about autism spectrum disorders.

- **Assess immunization needs at this age.**

For immunizations at this age, consult the CDC, ACIP, or AAP web sites for the current immunization schedule recommendations (Centers for Disease Control 2011):

– CEC National Immunization Program (NIP): http://www.cdc.gov/vaccines
– American Academy of Pediatrics *Red Book*: http://www.aapredbook.org

- **Assess dental needs at this age.**

Vladimir has 14 teeth and should have seen the dentist at 1 year of age and go every 6 months for a checkup. His parents or grandmother should have a nightly ritual with him to clean his teeth and also once during the day. They should avoid giving him candy or sweets. For guidelines on oral health, see *Bright Futures in Practice: Oral Health, pocket guide* by Paul Casamassimo and Katrina Hold, Ed., Washington, DC: National Maternal and Child Oral Health Resource Center, Georgetown University (American Academy of Pediatrics 2001; Casamassimo and Hold 2014; Centers for Disease Prevention and Control 2001).

- **Assess sleep needs at this age.**

At 18 months, Vladimir needs about 12–4 h total a day of sleep with at least one nap lasting 1–3 h. He may sleep through the night or have one awakening. He may have difficulty combining morning and afternoon naps. He may have difficulty with sleep, especially going to sleep and falling asleep. Vladimir's parents should continue with the sleep strategies they have been using, including a consistent bedtime, quiet activity such as reading or singing, giving him a transitional object such as a toy or blanket, putting him in bed awake, and comforting him in place as appropriate (Mindell and Owens 2009).

- **Vladimir's mother and grandmother want to talk about toilet training. What advice would you give them?**

Ask Vladimir's parent what she have already done about toilet training and what her goals are. It is not a good idea in general to try to toilet train a child under 24 months of age. The average age to be trained is 30 months. Vladimir's parents should be encouraged to watch Vladimir for signs of readiness. One indicator of sufficient myelination of the nerves for toileting is the ability to peddle a tricycle and to be able to follow two consecutive commands, i.e., "please pick up the block and put it on the table." He will be walking and helping to undress himself.

Other readiness signs include being dry at least 2 h at a time during the day and being dry after naps; bowel movements that are regular and predictable; and facial expressions, posture, or words Vladimir uses indicating that he is about to urinate or have a bowel movement. This is one of the most crucial signs—to be able to tell *prior to the incident*, not just after the event, which is an earlier skill. Vladimir should know the difference between wet and dry, and be able to pull his pants up and down. He may also ask to wear grown-up underwear, or use the potty chair or toilet. He will be uncomfortable with soiled diapers and want to be changed.

Vladimir's parents can read books with him about using the potty and take him into the bathroom with the parent of the same sex or other children to observe the routine of using the toilet. They can obtain a potty chair and allow Vladimir to sit on it clothed and help flush the toilet. He may enjoy a special trip to pick out "big kid" underwear when he is ready to stop using diapers during the day. Vladimir should be praised for sitting on the potty with his clothes on.

Stressful situations will impede toilet training and parents should not pressure their child in any way to train at these times or be surprised if they regress. Stress factors include new sibling arriving, moving, or a family crisis such as death or major illness.

Vladimir's family should use proper names for body parts and for products of elimination. They should pick a potty chair that offers foot support either in the chair itself or because it is low to the floor. They should try to make pottying routine. Everyone generally goes first thing in the morning, before bed, before bath, and after meals. Try at these times for a few minutes with Vladimir when he is ready, but don't fight about it or it will deter the process. Parents and grandma should compliment Vladimir on how well he is trying and be sensitive to his readiness and pace of learning.

- **Identify the anticipatory guidance that would be helpful for an 18-month-old child.**

At this age children can start to turn lids and will ingest nonfood items. Soon they will also be able to open doors. They are very mobile and can do things very quickly. Besides babyproofing the home environment, parents should take a number of safety precautions to prevent injuries, poisoning, and drowning (American Academy of Pediatrics 2001). See box "General Safety and Hygiene" (page 115), for specific suggestions.

References

American Academy of Pediatrics (undated) Infant-food and feeding. http://www.aap.org/en-us/advocacy-and-policy/aap-health-initiatives/HALF-Implementation-Guide/Age-Specific-Content/Pages/Infant-Food-and-Feeding.aspx. Accessed 18 June 2014

American Academy of Pediatrics (2012) Kids and vitamin D deficiency. http://www.aap.org/en-us/about-the-aap/aap-press-room/Pages/Kids-and-Vitamin-D-Deficiency.aspx. Accessed 22 Dec 2014

American Academy of Pediatrics (2014) Healthy active living for families. healthychildren.org/growinghealthy. Accessed 16 Dec 2014

American Academy of Pediatrics, Committee on Injury and Poison Prevention (2001) Injuries associated with infant walkers. Pediatrics 108(3):790–792. http://pediatrics.aappublications.org/content/108/3/790.full. (Reaffirmed in 2005). Accessed 11 Dec 2014

American Academy of Pediatrics (2008) Starting solid foods. Updated 28 May 2013. www.healthychildren.org/. Accessed 25 March 2014

American Academy of Pediatrics, Committee on Nutrition (2009) Pediatric nutrition handbook, 6th edn. American Academy of Pediatrics, Elk Grove Village, IL

Burns CE et al (2009) Pediatric primary care: a handbook for nurse practitioners, 4th edn. W.B. Saunders, Philadelphia, PA

Casamassimo P, Hold K (2014) Bright futures in practice: oral health, pocket guide, 2nd edn. National Maternal and Child Oral Health Resource Center, Georgetown University, Washington, DC. http://www.mchoralhealth.org/pocket.html. Accessed 18 Dec 2014

Centers for Disease Control and Prevention (2011) Recommendations and guidelines: childhood and adolescent immunization schedules. http://www.cdc.gov/vaccines/schedules/index.html. Accessed 11 Dec 2014

Centers for Disease Control and Prevention (2001) Recommendations for using fluoride to prevent and control dental caries in the United States. Morb Mortal Weekly Rep 50:RR-14

Dixon SD, Stein MT (2006) Encounters with children: pediatric behavior and development, 4th edn. Mosby, St. Louis, MO

Hagan JF, Shaw JS, Duncan P (eds) (2008) Bright futures: guidelines for health supervision of infants, children, and adolescents, 3rd edn. American Academy of Pediatrics, Elk Grove Village, IL
Hockenberry MJ, Wilson DW (2011) Wong's nursing care of infants and children, 9th edn. Elsevier/Mosby, New York, NY
Hurley DS (2000) Developing fine and gross motor skills: birth to three. PRO-ED, Inc, Austin, TX. www.proedinc.com. Accessed 11 Dec 2014
Marcdante KJ, Kliegman RM, Jenson HB et al (eds) (2011) Nelson essentials of pediatrics, 6th edn. Saunders, Philadelphia, PA
McInerny TK, Adam HM, Campbell DE, Kamat DM, Kelleher KJ (eds) (2009) Textbook of pediatric care. American Academy of Pediatrics, Elk Grove Village, IL
Mindell JA, Owens JA (2009) A Clinical guide to pediatric sleep: diagnosis and management of sleep problems, 2nd edn. Lippincott Williams & Wilkins, Philadelphia, PA
National Institute of Health, National Institute on Deafness and Other Communication Disorders (2010) Your baby's hearing and communicative development check list. http://www.nidcd.nih.gov/health/hearing/pages/silence.aspx. Accessed 17 June 2014
Ontario Society of Nutrition Professionals in Public Health (2014) Pediatric nutrition guidelines (birth to six years) for health professionals, Ontario, Canada. http://www.healthunit.org/professionals/nutrition/Pediatric%20Nutrition%20Guidelines%20for%20Primary%20Health%20Care%20Providers.pdf. Accessed 28 Aug 2015
Potts NL, Mandleco BL (eds) (2012) Pediatric nursing: Caring for children and their families, 3rd edn. Delmar Cengage Learning, Clifton Park, NY
Rains SG (2011) Fifteen- to eighteen-month visit. In: Richardson B (ed) Pediatric primary care: practice guidelines for nurses. Burlington, MA, Jones & Bartlett Learning, pp 97–108. Chapter 13
Samour PQ, King K (2005) Handbook of pediatric nutrition, 3rd edn. Jones and Bartlett Publishers, Sudbury, MA

Two-Year Visit

15

Teddy is a 2-year-old boy who lives on a farm where his parents work. The mother works in the kitchen and the father works in the fields. Teddy's current weight is 12.6 kg (27.7 lb); his length is 88 cm (35.2 in.), putting him in the 50th percentile for both. His head circumference is 48.5 cm (19.4 in.), putting him in the 60th percentile for head size. The family's income is near the federal poverty level and Teddy has few toys and books. Teddy eats finger foods at meals and has about six small meals each day with about two foods at each meal. His parents are concerned he doesn't sit down to eat but wants to run around during meals. His mother cuts up fruit and provides finger foods for him to eat while at the babysitter. Teddy has a daily bowel movement and urinates about 4–5 times a day. He has not expressed any interest in toilet training but his parents do read books to him on the topic. He takes one nap a day. Teddy runs without falling. He walks up and down stairs unassisted one step at a time and enjoys climbing and exploring. Teddy has temper tantrums when he doesn't get what he wants. His parents discipline him with time-out, but first try to distract him and give words to his feelings. Teddy often needs parental reassurance and engages in play that imitates his parents' behavior. He likes to pretend to sweep the floor and feed the chickens. Teddy enjoys jumping, kicking balls and throwing overhand, and running in the yard. He is able to put on a t-shirt, his socks, and Velcro sneakers, He talks in two- to three-word sentences. Teddy's parents are using good discipline techniques such as distraction, patience, ignoring temper tantrums, and using time-out appropriately.

- **Are Teddy's height and weight appropriate for him?**

Yes. Teddy is growing on the 50% growth curve and is an active boy. His usual weight gain is 1.8–2.7 kg/year. His height at 2 years doubled will be approximately

D. Kramer, *Primary Well-Being: Case Studies for the Growing Child*,
DOI 10.1007/978-3-319-56708-2_15

his adult height. He needs about 102 kcal/kg/day, 1.2 g of protein/kg/day, and fluids to 115 mL/kg/day. He may show signs of being ready to toilet train in the daytime.

- **Identify Teddy's current stage of psychosocial development and assess how his parents can help him master this stage.**

According to Erikson, Teddy is in the autonomy versus shame and doubt stage. Teddy should be provided with choices and be allowed to do what he can on his own. For example, offer two sets of socks that are acceptable to the parent or two food choices so Teddy has the opportunity to choose.

- **Assess the cognitive development of a 2-year-old child.**

According to Piaget, Teddy is in the preoperational stage of cognitive development.

Teddy's vocabulary has a minimum of 50 words. He uses two- or three-word phrases and pronouns such as I, me, and you. He can ask his parents to read a book to him. He understands directional commands and can look for hidden objects. He uses words like "up, down, come, and go" with meaning. He can name a picture that is read to him. He can complete sentences and rhymes in familiar books. If reading a book, he can point to an object or animal if asked "where is __." He can follow two-step commands.

Teddy refers to himself by his first name. He verbalizes his need for toileting, food, or drink and talks incessantly. Teddy is still in parallel play but has a sustained attention span. He can ask people to show him something and displays increased independence from his mother. He can dress himself in simple clothes.

Teddy shows increased pretend play, such as food preparation, caring for baby, and sweeping the floor. He imitates adult behavior like feeding the chickens. He is aware of object permanence and will search for objects. His imitations are becoming increasingly symbolic, such as words and sounds of animals. He has a beginning sense of time in relation to the activities he is doing. For example, he may sit and wait for meals at a table for a short time; he may use the word now and understand "just a minute."

Teddy likes his routines and rituals and is self-centered in thought and behavior; he uses the word "mine" for his toys.

- **What milestones of gross and fine motor development could Teddy be expected to display?**

Gross motor: Teddy goes up and down steps with two feet on each step. He can pick up objects without falling and kick a ball forward.

Fine motor: Teddy can stack 5–6 blocks, make or imitates horizontal strokes and circular strokes with a crayon, and can turn pages one at a time. He is starting to turn doorknobs and unscrew lids. He can align two or more cubes for a train.

See box "Helping Your Child's Physical Development—2–3 Years," for ideas on how Teddy's family can help foster his development (Hurley 2000).

Helping Your Child's Physical Development: 2–3 Years

1. *Playing with Puzzles*: Play with your toddler by handing them puzzle pieces with knobs, and shape sorter pieces. Allow child to turn the pieces around to fit the shapes.
2. *Feeding Self*: Once your child is able to drink from a spill-proof cup give them small amounts of liquid in a regular cup. Play games to foster use of drinking and eating such as house, and restaurant. Ask your child for a pretend breakfast together—when eating the scrabbled egg, pretend to eat it modeling use of utensils.
3. *Kicking a Ball*: Hold your toddler's hand and show them how to kick a nonmoving ball and encourage them to kick the ball.
4. *Stair Climbing*: Let your toddler practice shifting their weight and balancing on one leg by placing thin objects such as a jump rope or rolled-up dish towel on the floor and have your toddler step over them.
5. *Self-Dressing*: Buy cloths that are easy to put on without buttons, etc.; encourage your child to sit on the floor when they slip on their clothes.
6. *Jumping*: Jump up and down with your child holding hands.
7. *Playing ball*: Sit on the floor and roll the ball to each other.
8. *Throwing*: Throw balls and beanbags, into a laundry basket, starting close to the basket and moving farther away as child improves.

Source: Hurley, D.S. (2000). Developing fine and gross motor skills: Birth to three. *Austin, TX: PRO-ED, Inc.*

- **Assess the social behaviors that Teddy may exhibit at this age.**

Teddy plays alongside other children but is not yet skilled at interacting with them. He cannot yet sit in a circle for story time or listen to a long story. He does like to imitate his parents by doing household chores. Teddy will engage in repetitive explorations to satisfy his curiosity such as splashing water outside the tub to see what will happen, making objects fall down the stairs to see how far they will go, or playing with mud to understand what it feels like. He will assert his independence and then hide in back of his parent when other adults appear. He will develop fears of things he can't control, for example of loud sounds like thunder, animals, large moving things, and particular events, such as going to sleep, or going down the drain with the bath water. Giving Teddy support and reassurance will gradually help give him confidence to overcome these fears. At the health office, give Teddy choices such as which ear to examine first, and narrate to him what you are doing during the exam. Teddy may want to remain on his mother's lap for the exam and that is fine.

Teddy should continue to get lots of praise and choices at this age. He can learn simple rules for safety but will take time to internalize them. The temper tantrums will diminish as long as Teddy's parents don't react strongly to them or use them to give negative attention.

During the visit, the health care provider should take note of how Teddy and his parents communicate, what is the tone of their interactions, and the feelings they express. Does the parent teach Teddy the name of the provider or an object in the room? Does Teddy seem free to explore and do his parents set appropriate limits, if needed? Are the parents positive when speaking about Teddy?

- **Identify the characteristics of play at this age and suggest appropriate playthings and activities to encourage Teddy's development and safety.**

Teddy plays next to other children but not yet with them. He likes to imitate housekeeping activities of adults in his life, such as cooking and taking care of the animals on the farm. He plays with blocks and wooden puzzles, and looks at picture books. Shape sorters are good to introduce at this age. Teach Teddy's parents how to make simple toys, like play dough, use a container as a pail and an old spoon as a shovel, and make finger paints. Tell Teddy's parents that there are recipes for homemade, edible play dough (http://www.pinterest.com/explore/edible-play-dough/), finger paints (http://theimaginationtree.com/2011/03/homemade-edible-finger-paint-recipe.html), and other play materials on the Internet or they can ask at the local library.

- **Assess visual and hearing development.**

Teddy is able to discriminate sounds at this age (National Institute of Health 2010). His vision and accommodation are well developed.

- **Describe immunization needs for this age.**

For immunizations at this age, consult the CDC, ACIP, or AAP web sites for the current immunization schedule recommendations (Centers for Disease Control 2011):

- CEC National Immunization Program (NIP): http://www.cdc.gov/vaccines
- American Academy of Pediatrics *Red Book*: http://www.aapredbook.org

- **Assess dental needs at this age?**

Teddy should be brushing his teeth at least two times daily with help from his parents and seeing the dentist every 6 months (Casamassimo and Hold 2014; Centers for Disease Control and Prevention 2001). For guidelines on oral health, see *Bright Futures in Practice: Oral Health, pocket guide* by Paul Casamassimo and Katrina Hold, Ed., Washington, DC: National Maternal and Child Oral Health Resource Center, Georgetown University.

- **Assess sleep needs at this age.**

Sleep needs continue to be 12–14 h in a 24-h period. Teddy is now down to one nap usually lasting about 1–2 h (Mindell and Owens 2009).

- **The parents are concerned about Teddy's sporadic eating and constant activity. What advice would you offer?**

This is normal for a child this age. Finger foods are recommended. Planned snacks can substitute for a meal and should include protein, fruit, and vegetables

(American Academy of Pediatrics Undated; American Academy of Pediatrics 2012; American of Pediatrics 2014; Hagan et al. 2008; Hockenberry and Wilson 2012; Ontario Society of Nutrition Professionals in Public Health 2014; Samour and King 2005).

- **What information can be given concerning toilet training?**

  Teddy's readiness for toilet training should first be assessed. Offer him rewards for sitting on the potty. Read him books on toileting for children. Remember it is a gradual process and can go backwards and forwards, regress and advance, depending on the child's mood, health, family circumstances, and sudden changes in the environment such as a new sibling or illness of a parent or grandparent caregiver (Burns et al. 2009; Dixon and Stein 2006; Hagan et al. 2008; Hockenberry and Wilson 2011; Marcdante et al. 2011; McInerny et al. 2009; Porcher 2011).

- **Assess the anticipatory guidance that would be helpful for a 2-year-old child.**

  This is an extremely mobile time when Teddy is striving for his own independence from adults. Safety precautions are very important and parents or other caregivers should keep a good eye on his location and activities at all times (American Academy of Pediatrics 2011). Also see box on General Safety and Hygiene (page 115).

References

American Academy of Pediatrics (undated) Infant-food and feeding. http://www.aap.org/en-us/advocacy-and-policy/aap-health-initiatives/HALF-Implementation-Guide/Age-Specific-Content/Pages/Infant-Food-and-Feeding.aspx. Accessed 18 June 2014

American Academy of Pediatrics (2011) Task Force on Sudden Infant Death Syndrome. SIDS and other sleep-related infant deaths: Expansion of recommendations for a safe infant sleeping environment. Pediatrics, 128, 1030–1039

American Academy of Pediatrics (2012) Kids and vitamin D deficiency. http://www.aap.org/en-us/about-the-aap/aap-press-room/Pages/Kids-and-Vitamin-D-Deficiency.aspx. Accessed 22 Dec 2014

American Academy of Pediatrics (2014) Healthy active living for families. healthychildren.org/growinghealthy. Accessed 16 Dec 2014

American Academy of Pediatrics, Committee on Injury and Poison Prevention (2001) Injuries associated with infant walkers. Pediatrics 108(3):790–792. http://pediatrics.aappublications.org/content/108/3/790.full. (Reaffirmed in 2005). Accessed 11 Dec 2014

American Academy of Pediatrics (2008) Starting solid foods. Updated 28 May 2013. www.healthychildren.org/. Accessed 25 Mar 2014

American Academy of Pediatrics, Committee on Nutrition (2009) Pediatric nutrition handbook, 6th edn. American Academy of Pediatrics, Elk Grove Village, IL

Burns CE et al (2009) Pediatric primary care: a handbook for nurse practitioners, 4th edn. W.B. Saunders, Philadelphia, PA

Casamassimo P, Hold K (2014) Bright futures in practice: oral health, pocket guide, 2nd edn. National Maternal and Child Oral Health Resource Center, Georgetown University, Washington, DC. http://www.mchoralhealth.org/pocket.html. Accessed 18 Dec 2014

Centers for Disease Control and Prevention (2011) Recommendations and guidelines: childhood and adolescent immunization schedules. http://www.cdc.gov/vaccines/schedules/index.html. Accessed 11 Dec 2014

Centers for Disease Control and Prevention (2001) Recommendations for using fluoride to prevent and control dental caries in the United States. Morb Mortal Weekly Rep 50:RR-14

Dixon SD, Stein MT (2006) Encounters with children: pediatric behavior and development, 4th edn. Mosby, St. Louis, MO

Hagan JF, Shaw JS, Duncan P (eds) (2008) Bright futures: guidelines for health supervision of infants, children, and adolescents, 3rd edn. American Academy of Pediatrics, Elk Grove Village, IL

Hockenberry MJ, Wilson DW (2011) Wong's nursing care of infants and children, 9th edn. Elsevier/Mosby, New York, NY

Hurley DS (2000) Developing fine and gross motor skills: birth to three. PRO-ED, Inc, Austin, TX. www.proedinc.com. Accessed 11 Dec 2014

Marcdante KJ, Kliegman RM, Jenson HB et al (eds) (2011) Nelson essentials of pediatrics, 6th edn. Saunders, Philadelphia, PA

McInerny TK, Adam HM, Campbell DE et al (eds) (2009) Textbook of pediatric care. American Academy of Pediatrics, Elk Grove Village, IL

Mindell JA, Owens JA (2009) A clinical guide to pediatric sleep: diagnosis and management of sleep problems, 2nd edn. Lippincott Williams & Wilkins, Philadelphia, PA

National Institute of Health, National Institute on Deafness and Other Communication Disorders (2010) Your baby's hearing and communicative development check list. http://www.nidcd.nih.gov/health/hearing/pages/silence.aspx. Accessed 17 June 2014

Ontario Society of Nutrition Professionals in Public Health (2014) Pediatric nutrition guidelines (birth to six years) for health professionals, Ontario, Canada. http://www.healthunit.org/professionals/nutrition/Pediatric%20Nutrition%20Guidelines%20for%20Primary%20Health%20Care%20Providers.pdf. Accessed 28 Aug 2015

Porcher FK (2011) Two-year visit. In: Richardson B (ed) Pediatric primary care: practice guidelines for nurses. Burlington, MA, Jones & Bartlett Learning, pp 109–114. Chapter 14

Potts NL, Mandleco BL (eds) (2012) Pediatric nursing: caring for children and their families, 3rd edn. Delmar Cengage Learning, Clifton Park, NY

Samour PQ, King K (2005) Handbook of pediatric nutrition, 3rd edn. Jones and Bartlett Publishers, Sudbury, MA

Thirty-Month Visit

16

Jerabelle is an active 30-month-old girl who lives with her parents, Mr. and Mrs. Mercado. The grandmother, Mrs. Castro, has come to live with them from the Philippines to help watch Jerabelle and her older sibling Camille, age 6, while the parents work. Jerabelle's current weight is 11.8 kg (25.6 lb). Her height is 87 cm (34.8 in.)—the 25th percentile for height and weight. Her head circumference is 46.4 cm (18.56 in.), the 30th percentile. The Mercados have rent an apartment in a two-family house owned by Mr. Mercado's uncle in a city neighborhood that is home to many Filipinos and near transportation to their jobs. Mrs. Mercado and the grandmother bring Jerabelle to the checkup. Mrs. Mercado is concerned that her daughters fight a lot, with Jerabelle hitting and biting her sister when frustrated. Jerabelle attends regular day care during weekday mornings, taken by her grandmother. The mother says Jerabelle has no interest in toilet training. Mrs. Mercado is concerned about discipline at home and Jerabelle's increasing negative interactions with her sibling. Jerabelle likes to feed herself, but her grandmother is concerned because she makes a mess. Jerabelle takes her socks off by herself but her grandmother would prefer to dress her because it is faster and she has to get Camille to first grade and Jerabelle to day care on time. Jerabelle likes to wear her favorite sleeveless dress even when it is 15 degrees outside. The grandmother asks you what she should do because Jerabelle ends up crying when the grandmother insists that Jerabelle wear the clothes she wants, not what grandma picked.

- **Are Jerabelle's height and weight appropriate for her?**

Yes, she is consistently on the 25th percentile. The health care provider should address the grandmother's feeding concerns during the visit. At 30 months of age, Jerabelle should be given low-fat milk, iron-fortified cereals, and iron-rich foods, such as green leafy vegetables, dried fruits and beans, lean red meats and poultry, and fish (American Academy of Pediatrics 2008; American Academy of Pediatrics 2009). Children this age need at least 700 mg of calcium, which they can get from milk, cheese, beans, broccoli, collard greens and kale, as well as blueberries. Jerabelle needs 600 units of vitamin D,

D. Kramer, *Primary Well-Being: Case Studies for the Growing Child*,
DOI 10.1007/978-3-319-56708-2_16

as well as some sun exposure each day (National Institute of Health 2012). Sources of vitamin D include salmon, canned tuna (1 oz), and ½ large egg yolk. Vitamin C will enhance the absorption of iron and can be found in foods such as citrus fruits and cabbage (American Academy of Pediatrics Undated; American Academy of Pediatrics 2012; American of Pediatrics 2014; Hagan et al. 2008; Hockenberry and Wilson 2011; Ontario Society of Nutrition Professionals in Public Health 2014; Samour and King 2005).

- **Assess Jerabelle's current stage of psychosocial development and how her parents and grandmother can help her master this stage.**

According to Erickson Jerabelle is in the autonomy versus shame and doubt stage of development. Toddlers at this stage want to feel that they have a choice to do what they can on their own, or at least try. During the health visit, the health care provider should observe the communication between parents and Jerabelle: Is there active communication going on? Is Jerabelle asking questions and using phrases appropriate for her age? When given a book, do the parents and Jerabelle look at it together, talk about its contents, and interact? If there is an upset during the visit, how well do the parents calm Jerabelle down? Do Jerabelle and her parents appear to have their feelings under control?

- **Assess the cognitive development of a 30-month-old child.**

According to Piaget, Jerabelle is in the preoperational stage of development. Vocally, Jerabelle can give her first and last names. Her language can be understood about 50% of the time. She uses two–four-word phrases and will have a large language burst soon. She refers to herself by the appropriate pronoun and uses plurals. She can name one color. She can point to six body parts. She shows increased use of imaginary play, such as with dolls and toys. She enjoys rhyming games and social interactions. Her play starts to include other children, such as doing pretend tea parties together. She likes having the same story read over and over to her. She enjoys acting out what others in the household do, such as serving food and sweeping the floor.

This is a good time for parents to discuss what type of play setting or child care/early education would be best for Jerabelle. Since she is already in day care, it would be a good time to go over the program components and assess its quality using a standard checklist (Child Care Aware 2011; Alkon et al. 2008). One such checklist is online from the National Association of Child Care Resource & Referral Agencies (NACCRRA) and it can be downloaded and copied for each child care facility under consideration (see http://ccapub.childcareaware.org/docs/pubs/121e.pdf for a reusable template).

- **What milestones of gross and fine motor development could Jerabelle be expected to display?**

Gross Motor: Jerabelle can jump with both feet. She jumps up and down in place and can jump from chair or step. She can stand on one foot for a short time and take a few steps on tiptoe. Jerabelle can brush her teeth with help and also puts on clothes with help.

Fine Motor: Jerabelle can build a tower up to eight cubes. She can add a chimney to a train of cubes. She has good hand-finger coordination and can hold a crayon with fingers rather than in her fist. She moves her fingers independently. When drawing, Jerabelle imitates vertical and horizontal strokes and makes two or more strokes for a cross. See box "Helping Your Child's Development Two-to-Three Year Olds" on page 152 for suggestions to provide to parents (Hurley 2000).

- **Assess the social behaviors that Jerabelle may exhibit at this age.**

Jerabelle has fears of unexplained changes in her physical environment and unexpected events. But she separates more easily from her mother now. In play, she helps put things away. She may soon start to demonstrate interest in toilet training. Jerabelle is at a point where she wants choices and to assert her own autonomy. Suggest to the grandmother and parents that Jerabelle be given a choice between acceptable clothing each day and choices of food and activities, so she will feel autonomous and help her develop a positive self-esteem.

- **Describe immunization needs for this age.**

For immunizations at this age, consult the CDC, ACIP, or AAP web sites for the current immunization schedule recommendations (Centers for Disease Control 2011):

- CEC National Immunization Program (NIP): http://www.cdc.gov/vaccines
- American Academy of Pediatrics *Red Book:* http://www.aapredbook.org

- **Assess visual and hearing development to the parents.**

At this age, a limited amount of words may indicate a hearing problem or fluid in the ears, which can sound like hearing under water. The child should also be combining words at 30 months. Limited vocabulary and using one-word answers would be cause for an auditory test referral. Hearing evaluations can include conditioned play audiometry and pure tone audiometry, administered by an audiologist, and tympanometry, which can be done by the primary care provider (National Institute of Health 2010).

- **What information can be given concerning discipline and negative sibling interactions, including biting, pushing, and hitting?**

The primary care provider can share with Jerabelle's parents that this is an age of testing limits, including striking other children. They need to use words like "not hitting," give time out, and distract the child when this occurs. Advise the family to help Jerabelle find words for her feelings and also try to anticipate the situation—Does it happen more when Jerabelle is bored, when her sister takes over the play area or has grabbed a favorite object, or when she is angry or in transition? Zero to Three says toddlers are still limited with their words and rely on actions to express their feelings (Parlakian and Lerner 2014). Those with bigger reactions may have a harder time expressing their feelings. It will take time and patience over the next months and years to change aggressive behavior on Jerabelle's part. Advise the parents and grandma on how to help minimize aggressive behavior. See box Discipline Pearls for the 30-Month-Old below and the box: Discipline of the Young Child (page 137). Also the section on bibliotherapy in Chap. 6 can be helpful.

Discipline Pearls for the 30-Month-Old

1. First stay calm to help your child calm down more quickly.
2. Think about whether it is only happening in one setting.
3. Is it toward a particular person?
4. Try to plan ahead, such as when introducing to new person in the family—go over photos in advance of the person or tell a story about them.
5. Use words and gestures to introduce alternative behavior.
6. Distraction and also taking a break may help.
7. Point out to the child the consequences of her behavior, such as "your sister was sad; she didn't want to play with you anymore."
8. Ask "what can we do besides hitting"?
9. Offer a different object or negotiate time using the object.
10. Remove the child from the situation if necessary.
11. Remember to give lots of positive feedback (Parlakian and Lerner 2014).
12. Read books to child and any siblings about appropriate behavior. These books can be found in the library or purchased online. Suggested titles appropriate for toddlers and 3-year-olds include Agassi's (2006) Hands are not for hitting and Spelman and Cote's (2000) When i feel angry.

Sources

Agassi, M. (2006). Hands are not for hitting (Best Behavior). Minneapolis, MN: Free Spirit Publishing.

Burns, C.E., et al. (2009). Pediatric primary care: A handbook for nurse practitioners, 4th ed. Philadelphia, PA: W.B. Saunders.

Joyce, B.A. (2011). Three-year visit. In: Richardson, B. (Ed.), Pediatric primary care: Practice guidelines for nurses. Burlington, MA: Jones & Bartlett Learning. Chapter 15, pp. 115–118.

Parlakian, R. and Lerner, C. (2014). Aggressive behavior in toddlers. Zero to Three. Accessed online June 23, 2014 at http://www.zerotothree.org/child-development/challenging-behavior/aggressive-behavior.html

Spelman, C.M. and Cote, N. (2000). When I feel angry. Morton Grove, IL: Albert Whitman & Company.

- **What would you advise concerning the dressing and eating issues?**

This is an age of seeking autonomy, especially in dressing and eating. Getting Jerabelle dressed in the morning could start at an earlier time to give her time to assert her independence and skills. She could be given a choice of either wearing a sweater over the sleeveless dress or a long sleeve shirt under it to maintain her independence while still addressing her grandmother's concerns. In terms of her messy self-feeding, Jerabelle should be praised for eating herself and should be allowed to self-feed (Casamassimo and Hold 2014; Centers for Disease Control and Prevention 2001). She will get neater as time goes by as she learns to use the spoon and fork more successfully. In the meantime, perhaps the grandmother could put a plastic cloth under the high chair to make the mess easier to clean up (Dixon and Stein 2006).

- **Assess the anticipatory guidance that would be helpful for a 30-month-old child.**

All previous safety concerns are still important: water, car, and household safety (American Academy of Pediatrics 2011). Matches, medication bottles, and other hazards should be kept out of sight and even locked up. Review the box General Safety & Hygiene with the family (page 115).

Look for quality preschool or childcare for Jerabelle. The local childcare resource and referral organization can help with this as well as the checklist guide mentioned above.

Routines in general are important, including enjoyable family activities such as reading and playing, eating and bedtime activities, and potty routines. Getting along with others and consistent discipline are also important at this age (Hagan et al. 2008; Hockenberry and Wilson 2011; Marcdante et al. 2011; McInerny et al. 2009; Potts and Mandleco 2012).

Limit TV, video, and other screen viewing (tablet, smartphone) to no more than 1–2 h a day. Be careful to monitor what Jerabelle watches. When she speaks to her family members, they should listen attentively. Jerabelle's family should provide play opportunities with other children her age and continue to offer choices to encourage autonomy.

References

Agassi M (2006) Hands are not for hitting (Best Behavior). Free Spirit Publishing, Minneapolis, MN

Alkon A, To K, Wolff M, Mackie JF, Bernzweig J (2008) Assessing health and safety in early care and education programs: development of the CCHP health and safety checklist. J Pediatr Health Care 22(6):368–377. http://childcareawaremn.org/sites/default/files/attachments/jphc_hs_checklist.pdf. Accessed 23 Dec 2014

American Academy of Pediatrics (2008) Starting solid foods. Updated 28 May 2013. www.healthychildren.org/. Accessed 25 Mar 2014

American Academy of Pediatrics (2012) Kids and vitamin D deficiency. http://www.aap.org/en-us/about-the-aap/aap-press-room/Pages/Kids-and-Vitamin-D-Deficiency.aspx. Accessed 22 Dec 2014

American Academy of Pediatrics (2014) Healthy active living for families. healthychildren.org/growinghealthy. Accessed 16 Dec 2014

American Academy of Pediatrics (n.d.) Infant-food and feeding. http://www.aap.org/en-us/advocacy-and-policy/aap-health-initiatives/HALF-Implementation-Guide/Age-Specific-Content/Pages/Infant-Food-and-Feeding.aspx. Accessed 18 June 2014

American Academy of Pediatrics, Committee on Injury and Poison Prevention (2001) Injuries associated with infant walkers. Pediatrics 108(3):790–792. http://pediatrics.aappublications.org/content/108/3/790.full. (Reaffirmed in 2005). Accessed 11 Dec 2014

American Academy of Pediatrics, Committee on Nutrition (2009) Pediatric nutrition handbook, 6th edn. American Academy of Pediatrics, Elk Grove Village, IL

American Academy of Pediatrics. Task Force on Sudden Infant Death Syndrome. (2011). SIDS and other sleep-related infant deaths: Expansion of recommendations for a safe infant sleeping environment. *Pediatrics, 128*, 1030–1039

Burns CE et al (2009) Pediatric primary care: a handbook for nurse practitioners, 4th edn. W.B. Saunders, Philadelphia, PA

Casamassimo P, Hold K (2014) Bright futures in practice: oral health, pocket guide, 2nd edn. National Maternal and Child Oral Health Resource Center, Georgetown University, Washington, DC. http://www.mchoralhealth.org/pocket.html. Accessed 18 Dec 2014

Centers for Disease Control and Prevention (2001) Recommendations for using fluoride to prevent and control dental caries in the United States. Morb Mortal Weekly Rep 50:RR-14

Centers for Disease Control and Prevention (2011) Recommendations and guidelines: childhood and adolescent immunization schedules. http://www.cdc.gov/vaccines/schedules/index.html. Accessed 11 Dec 2014

Child Care Aware (2011) Is this the right place for my child? 38 research-based indicators of quality child care. National Association of Child Care Resource & Referral Agencies (NACCRRA). http://ccapub.childcareaware.org/docs/pubs/121e.pdf. Accessed 23 Dec 2014

Dixon SD, Stein MT (2006) Encounters with children: pediatric behavior and development, 4th edn. Mosby, St. Louis, MO

Hagan JF, Shaw JS, Duncan P (eds) (2008) Bright futures: guidelines for health supervision of infants, children, and adolescents, 3rd edn. American Academy of Pediatrics, Elk Grove Village, IL

Hockenberry MJ, Wilson DW (2011) Wong's nursing care of infants and children, 9th edn. Elsevier/Mosby, New York, NY

Hurley DS (2000) Developing fine and gross motor skills: birth to three. PRO-ED, Inc, Austin, TX. www.proedinc.com. Accessed 11 Dec 2014

Joyce BA (2011) Three-year visit (Chapter 15). In: Richardson B (ed) Pediatric primary care: practice guidelines for nurses. Jones & Bartlett Learning, Burlington, MA, pp 115–118

Marcdante KJ, Kliegman RM, Jenson HB et al (eds) (2011) Nelson essentials of pediatrics, 6th edn. Saunders, Philadelphia, PA

McInerny TK, Adam HM, Campbell DE, Kamat DM, Kelleher KJ (eds) (2009) Textbook of pediatric care. American Academy of Pediatrics, Elk Grove Village, IL

National Institute of Health, National Institute on Deafness and Other Communication Disorders (2010) Your baby's hearing and communicative development check list. http://www.nidcd.nih.gov/health/hearing/pages/silence.aspx. Accessed 17 June 2014

National Institute of Health, Osteoporosis and Related Bone Diseases National Resource Center (2012) Calcium and vitamin D: important at every age. http://www.niams.nih.gov/Health_Info/Bone/Bone_Health/Nutrition/. Accessed 23 Dec 2014

Ontario Society of Nutrition Professionals in Public Health (2014) Pediatric nutrition guidelines (birth to six years) for health professionals, ON, Canada. http://www.healthunit.org/professionals/nutrition/Pediatric%20Nutrition%20Guidelines%20for%20Primary%20Health%20Care%20Providers.pdf. Accessed 28 Aug 2015

Parlakian R, Lerner C (2014) Aggressive behavior in toddlers. Zero to three. http://www.zerotothree.org/child-development/challenging-behavior/aggressive-behavior.html. Accessed 23 June 2014

Potts NL, Mandleco BL (eds) (2012) Pediatric nursing: caring for children and their families, 3rd edn. Delmar Cengage Learning, Clifton Park, NY

Samour PQ, King K (2005) Handbook of pediatric nutrition, 3rd edn. Jones and Bartlett Publishers, Sudbury, MA

Spelman CM, Cote N (2000) When I feel angry. Albert Whitman & Company, Morton Grove, IL

Three-Year Visit

17

Tao Fernandez lives with his mother in an inner-city neighborhood in subsidized housing. Their elevator often breaks down and another family shares the apartment. His mother Melinda Costa never finished high school in El Salvador because her parents needed her to help take care of her younger siblings. When she became pregnant, Ms. Costa had no one to help her. The father occasionally drops by to take Tao to the park or bring a present when he has money. Tao weighs 12.5 kg (27.5 lb), stands 91 cm (36.4 in.), and head circumference is 47 cm (21.3 in.). He is in the 10th percentile for physical growth. He is scared when the doctor takes his blood pressure and screams when blood is drawn and at vaccination. He talks deliberately and has understandable speech. His vocabulary has about 500 words. He knows his name and he can speak two to three sentences together. A neighbor watches Tao when the mother goes to work part time in a bakery sweeping the floors or attends GED classes, but this time is mostly spent watching TV. Tao likes to help at home but doesn't always listen. The mother says she has a hard time disciplining Tao and admits sometimes losing her temper and yelling at her son. Tao feeds himself and mostly sits still at the table for his meals. Tao has been toilet trained for a couple of months but has many accidents. He doesn't get to play with many other children.

- **Are Tao's height and weight appropriate for him?**

Yes, he is small, but on the 10th percentile consistently. He needs 1000–1100 calories per day or 100 kcal/kg/day. This should be obtained in three small meals, two snacks, and 16–24 oz of 2% low-fat milk. Tao should be eating seven grains, three vegetables, two fruits, and two proteins (meat, dairy, eggs, or fish) over the course of the day.

- **Assess Tao's current stage of psychosocial development and how his parent can help him master this stage.**

According to Erikson, Tao is still in the Autonomy versus Shame and Doubt stage. Tao has the lower end of normal range of language—it should be 900 words—but he has 500 words. Tao knows his name, but his vocabulary is limited, although

D. Kramer, *Primary Well-Being: Case Studies for the Growing Child*,
DOI 10.1007/978-3-319-56708-2_17

he talks in sentences. This is typical of children in very low-income families who are not attending preschool and have limited social experiences. Also Tao spends much of his time when he is watched by a neighbor while his mother works in viewing television. He likes to help at home and mimic the routines he sees his mother doing, such as setting the table or sweeping the floor. His mother says she has a hard time disciplining Tao, and admits that she loses her temper and yells at him.

The health care provider can identify programs that Tao and his mother may be eligible for that would provide social and learning opportunities in preparation for school for Tao and his mother. The primary care provider can also include a social worker and/or psychologist as part of the team to advocate appropriate service for Ms. Costa and Tao. Ms. Costa should be encouraged to read to Tao, limit television time, and send him to a formal child care/early learning facility so he can interact with children his age and develop his language in a good quality setting. He would be a good candidate for the local Head Start program that includes classes for parents, health care, and quality activities for the children, and is especially for low-income families. See the U.S. Department of Health and Human Services, Administration for Children and Families, Early Childhood Learning and Knowledge Center, *Head Start Locator*—http://eclkc.ohs.acf.hhs.gov/hslc/HeadStartOffices—to help Ms. Costa find a Head Start program near this family. Tao needs opportunities to play outside to explore his physical development and gross motor skills. He needs to be encouraged to play, use imaginative play, and sing with his mother—especially rhyming songs. Local libraries may also have programs for this age group where books are read and group games are offered. Also, the health clinic can investigate signing up for free book distribution programs like "Reach Out and Read," http://www.reachoutandread.org/, that provide personnel and books in health centers and doctor's offices to give out to children after each doctor's visit. The Hippy program (Home Instruction for Parents of Preschool Youngsters, http://www.hippyusa.org/, offers free home reading visits to preschoolers and their families in many states and Ms. Costa could learn many ways to stimulate Tao's cognitive development from the visits.

- **Assess the cognitive development of a 3-year-old child.**

Tao is still in Piaget's Preoperational phase and is egocentric in thought and behavior. He is beginning to understand the concept of time: he uses many time-oriented expressions and talks about past and future as much as present. Tao pretends to tell time. He has an improved concept of space and demonstrates understanding of prepositions. He can follow directional commands and is beginning to be able to view concepts from more than one perspective. He shows increased use of language as mental symbols. Tao is slowly increasing his vocabulary. He can carry a conversation with 2–3 sentences spoken together, but leaves out verbs in sentences (telegraphic speech); but his speech is understandable to others 75% of the time. He can identify his name and age, and use a cup and folk and spoon. Tao should be talking more, regardless of whether anyone is paying attention. He should be repeating sentences of six syllables and asking many questions. He is beginning to sing songs. His vocabulary of 500 words could be higher. His current flat cognitive ability would improve with a quality preschool program for Tao.

- **What milestones of gross and fine motor development could Taos be expected to display?**

Tao should be achieving many milestones, but his experience sitting in front of a television for great parts of the day is limiting his development and he has been told not to make too much noise because of the small living space Tao and his mother share with another family.

Gross Motor: Tao should be able to ride a tricycle at this age. He uses alternate feet to go up a flight of stairs, but comes down using both feet on each the step. He should be jumping off the bottom step and standing on 1 foot for 1 or 2 s and also leap like a broad jump. He does sometimes try to dance when his mother puts on music but cannot always stay on balance. He rides a tricycle competently.

Fine motor: Tao can build a tower of six to eight cubes and a bridge with three cubes. Tao spends time drawing and he can copy a circle, imitate a cross, and draw a person with two body parts. He can name what he has drawn (Hurley 2000).

- **Assess the social behaviors that Tao may exhibit at this age.**

Tao is in Erikson's stage of Initiative versus Guilt. He makes things and plays. He is in Freud's Oedipal stage (ages 3–5), which means he wants the parent of the opposite sex—but he is missing a father figure in his daily life to identify with and move him to the next stage. Tao and his mother can be referred to a local community center that has big brother type programs to provide Tao with a frequent male role model in his life.

Tao can dress himself with a little help on back buttons and shoes. His attention span is increasing and he feeds himself. He can help himself to cereal and milk in the morning and helps his mother to set the table and dry the dishes. He expresses a little fear of the dark and fights going to bed. Tao is clear on his own gender and the gender of others. He likes to please his mother and is always happy to see his father when he occasionally comes to visit. He needs other children to play with too. Advice Ms. Costa that it is important to praise Tao's drawings, building efforts, and positive behaviors such as helping in the apartment and being polite to others.

- **Assess the characteristics of play at this age and suggest appropriate play-things and activities to encourage Tao's development and safety.**

Tao plays mostly alongside other children but is also beginning to play with others (associative play). He is beginning to learn simple games that he shares with his mother, but he often makes up his own rules. He is beginning to share with others.

- **Describe immunization needs for this age.**

For immunizations at this age, consult the CDC, ACIP, or AAP web sites for the current immunization schedule recommendations:

- CEC National Immunization Program (NIP): http://www.cdc.gov/vaccines
- American Academy of Pediatrics *Red Book:* http://www.aapredbook.org (Centers for Disease Control 2011)

- **Assess dental needs, injuries, and sleep needs at this age.**

Tao should be sleeping in a regular bed at this age. He should have been receiving regular dental care but now is a good time to check for evidence of tooth cavities and encourage a visit to the dentist. Tao should be brushing 2 times a day and seeing the dentist two times a year. For guidelines on oral health, see *Bright Futures in Practice: Oral Health, pocket guide* by Paul Casamassimo and Katrina Hold, Ed., Washington, DC: National Maternal and Child Oral Health Resource Center, Georgetown University (Casamassimo and Hold 2014; Centers for Disease Control and Prevention 2001).

The health care provider should look for any bruises or other injuries that might indicate abuse, neglect, or inadequate supervision of Tao. Ask if Ms. Costa has talked to Tao about good touch and bad touch and recommend some books Ms. Costa can read to her son about this topic and about going to the dentist. Titles to suggest include: Rogers, Fred (1985) *Going to day care* (First Experiences); Rogers, Fred (1989) *Going to the dentist*; Lory Britian (1982) *It's MY Body: A Book to Teach Young Children How to Resist Uncomfortable Touch* (Children's Safety Series & Abuse Prevention) Seattle, WA: Parenting Press.

- **Ms. Costa is concerned about her own short fuse and disciplining Tao. What advice would you offer?**

Preschoolers can behave one moment and want to please the parents or other adult, but can also be unreasonable and resist being examined. When Tao misbehaves, Ms. Costa needs to take time out for herself to calm down before she yells at Tao; she should take several deep breaths and count from 1 to 100 to calm herself. Learning to cool off so she can speak to Tao without yelling is important for both of them. Then she can tell Tao what she doesn't like about his behavior very specifically so it is not about Tao as a person. Share with Ms. Costa the box: Discipline of the Young Child (page 137) and Discipline Pearls for a 30-Month-Old on page 158. Ms. Costa might also be referred to a family counselor for some therapy and parenting education, as well as emotional support for her. There may also be community single-parent support groups that Ms. Costa can attend to overcome her isolation and help her control her negative behavior with Tao. Groups can be found at community centers, local clinics and hospitals, and faith-based institutions such as churches, temples, and broader umbrella organizations (Parlakian and Lerner 2014; Porcher 2011; Joyce 2011; Dixon and Stein 2006).

- **What information can be given concerning toileting accidents?**

Having toileting accidents is normal at this age. It is important for Ms. Costa to be nonpunitive, to matter-of-factly change Tao's clothes, and to not get upset. Having accidents is a normal part of toilet training (Burns et al. 2009; Dixon and Stein 2006; Hagan et al. 2008; Hockenberry and Wilson 2011; Marcdante et al. 2011; McInerny et al. 2009; Porcher 2011).

- **What information can be given concerning sleep terrors and nightmares?**

Sleep Terrors: While common in preschoolers, sleep terrors are very frightening to parents. They are defined as a partial arousal from a very deep sleep. The child will scream and thrash about while still asleep but will be calm once awake. Sleep Terrors usually occur 1–4 h into sleep. When this happens to Tao, he sits up and sometimes even runs about, moans or screams, seems confused, and is not aware of his mother. She finds it difficult to comfort him and is worried he will run out of the apartment. Suggest to Ms. Costa that she remain calm and observe Tao for a few minutes, without interfering, until he becomes quiet or wakes fully. She should intervene only to protect Tao from injury, than guide him back to bed. Reassure Ms. Costa that this is a normal, common phenomenon in preschoolers that requires little intervention (Mindell and Owens 2009).

Nightmares: Tao may also have occasional nightmares. These usually occur in the second half of the night and are followed by complete awakening, crying, and expressions of fear. It may be difficult to fall back to sleep and Tao may remember the nightmare and want to talk about it in the morning. Ms. Costa should reassure Tao, stay with him, and offer comfort and a sense of protection. She should not force Tao back to his bed. If the nightmares recur frequently, professional counseling may be advised.

- **Assess the anticipatory guidance that would be helpful for a 3-year-old child.**

Socialization: Advise the mother to spend more time with her child: Ms. Costa should be encouraged to spend more time with Tao, taking him out to the playground, and reading and playing imaginatively with him. Also the father should try to spend more time with his son. Just looking at pictures and talking about them is good for both parents—they don't need to always "read" the story. It is the time together that is important and the building of their parent-child relationship.

Food: Ms. Costa should be sharing meal times together and chatting with Tao; or at least feeding Tao first and then letting him play. Avoid fights over food. If Tao does not want to eat at meal time, let him get down and do not offer food or drink until the next meal. The health provider should check with Ms. Costa on the nutritional quality of Tao's meals and snacks and advise limiting fast food to less than once a week (American Academy of Pediatrics Undated; American Academy of Pediatrics 2012; American Academy of Pediatrics 2014; Hagan et al. 2008; Hockenberry and Wilson 2011; Ontario Society of Nutrition Professionals in Public Health 2014; Samour and King 2005).

Play and Screens: TV viewing should be limited to 1–2 h a day. Tao should have opportunities to play with other children, perhaps by attending a preschool program, and be taken to the playground regularly to promote socialization and gross motor development. He should be using active toys, play with balls, and do other physical activities. The primary care provider will share information about play facilities in the community that Ms. Costa can take Tao to.

Used consistently, discipline is a way to learn rules, not just for punishment. Ms. Costa should set realistic limits for Tao and make sure he knows them so he can relax (see box: Disciplining the Young Child.) Even as she disciplines him, Ms. Costa should find ways to praise Tao. Encouraging him to make choices and linking them with consequences, being patient as he tries things for himself, will also help Tao develop self-confidence and independence.

Safety and Babyproofing: Tao is still a small child and needs constant supervision, even if the apartment has been baby proofed already, for example, cover outlets, remove wires from floor, store matches, and poisons under lock and key. Have working smoke detectors. Good safety practices include: never leave Tao alone in the bathtub, dress him on a low surface, keep ladders locked up, and small items stored in high drawers. Advise Ms. Costa how to teach about "good touch/bad touch." If there are any guns in the house, keep them out of reach, locked, and unloaded. Tell Ms. Costa to store ammunition and guns separately. When Tao has a play date at another child's house, ask if there are any guns in the house and if yes, ask for them to be locked up. (Review the chart: *General Safety & Hygiene* (page 115) with the parent) (American Academy of Pediatrics 2011)

Travel: Ms. Costa should use a car seat when taking Tao in a moving vehicle and put him in the back seat of the car. Tao should wear a helmet when riding tricycles, scooters, or other toys with wheels.

Sun exposure: When out in the sun, Ms. Costa should apply sunscreen of SPF 15 or higher to Tao and herself.

References

Alkon A, To K, Wolff M, Mackie JF, Bernzweig J (2008) Assessing health and safety in early care and education programs: development of the CCHP health and safety checklist. J Pediatr Health Care 22(6):368–377. http://childcareawaremn.org/sites/default/files/attachments/jphc_hs_checklist.pdf. Accessed 23 Dec 2014

American Academy of Pediatrics (n.d.) Infant food and feeding. http://www.aap.org/en-us/advocacy-and-policy/aap-health-initiatives/HALF-Implementation-Guide/Age-Specific-Content/Pages/Infant-Food-and-Feeding.aspx. Accessed 18 June 2014

American Academy of Pediatrics (2011) Task Force on Sudden Infant Death Syndrome. SIDS and other sleep-related infant deaths: Expansion of recommendations for a safe infant sleeping environment. Pediatrics, 128, 1030–1039

American Academy of Pediatrics (2012) Kids and vitamin D deficiency. http://www.aap.org/en-us/about-the-aap/aap-press-room/Pages/Kids-and-Vitamin-D-Deficiency.aspx. Accessed 22 Dec 2014

American Academy of Pediatrics (2014) Healthy active living for families. healthychildren.org/growinghealthy. Accessed 16 Dec 2014

American Academy of Pediatrics, Committee on Injury and Poison Prevention (2001) Injuries associated with infant walkers. Pediatrics 108(3):790–792. http://pediatrics.aappublications.org/content/108/3/790.full. (Reaffirmed in 2005). Accessed 11 Dec 2014

American Academy of Pediatrics (2008) Starting solid foods. www.healthychildren.org/. Updated 28 May 2013, Accessed 25 Mar 2014

American Academy of Pediatrics, Committee on Nutrition (2009) Pediatric nutrition handbook, 6th edn. American Academy of Pediatrics, Elk Grove Village, IL

Burns CE et al (2009) Pediatric primary care: a handbook for nurse practitioners, 4th edn. W.B. Saunders, Philadelphia, PA

Casamassimo P, Hold K (2014) Bright futures in practice: oral health, pocket guide, 2nd edn. National Maternal and Child Oral Health Resource Center, Georgetown University, Washington, DC. http://www.mchoralhealth.org/pocket.html. Accessed 18 Dec 2014

Centers for Disease Control and Prevention (2011) Recommendations and guidelines: childhood and adolescent immunization schedules. http://www.cdc.gov/vaccines/schedules/index.html. Accessed 11 Dec 2014

Centers for Disease Control and Prevention (2001) Recommendations for using fluoride to prevent and control dental caries in the United States. Morb Mortal Weekly Rep 50:RR-14

Child Care Aware (2011) Is this the right place for my child? 38 research-based indicators of quality child care. National Association of Child Care Resource & Referral Agencies (NACCRRA). http://ccapub.childcareaware.org/docs/pubs/121e.pdf. Accessed 23 Dec 2014

Dixon SD, Stein MT (2006) Encounters with children: pediatric behavior and development, 4th edn. Mosby, St. Louis, MO

Hagan JF, Shaw JS, Duncan P (eds) (2008) Bright futures: guidelines for health supervision of infants, children, and adolescents, 3rd edn. American Academy of Pediatrics, Elk Grove Village, IL

Hockenberry MJ, Wilson DW (2011) Wong's Nursing care of infants and children, 9th edn. Elsevier/Mosby, New York, NY

Hurley DS (2000) Developing fine and gross motor skills: birth to three. PRO-ED, Inc, Austin, TX. www.proedinc.com. Accessed 11 Dec 2014

Joyce BA (2011) Three-year visit (preschool). In: Richardson B (ed) Pediatric primary care: practice guidelines for nurses. Burlington, MA, Jones & Bartlett Learning

Marcdante KJ, Kliegman RM, Jenson HB et al (eds) (2011) Nelson essentials of pediatrics, 6th edn. Saunders, Philadelphia, PA

McInerny TK, Adam HM, Campbell DE, Kamat DM, Kelleher KJ (eds) (2009) Textbook of pediatric care. American Academy of Pediatrics, Elk Grove Village, IL

Mindell JA, Owens JA (2009) A clinical guide to pediatric sleep: diagnosis and management of sleep problems, 2nd edn. Lippincott Williams & Wilkins, Philadelphia, PA

National Institute of Health, National Institute on Deafness and Other Communication Disorders (2010) Your baby's hearing and communicative development check list. http://www.nidcd.nih.gov/health/hearing/pages/silence.aspx. Accessed 17 June 2014

National Institute of Health, Osteoporosis and Related Bone Diseases National Resource Center (2012) http://www.niams.nih.gov/Health_Info/Bone/Bone_Health/Nutrition/. Accessed 23 Dec 2014

Ontario Society of Nutrition Professionals in Public Health (2014) Pediatric nutrition guidelines (birth to six years) for health professionals. ON, Canada. http://www.healthunit.org/professionals/nutrition/Pediatric%20Nutrition%20Guidelines%20for%20Primary%20Health%20Care%20Providers.pdf. Accessed 28 Aug 2015

Parlakian R, Lerner C (2014) Aggressive behavior in toddlers. Zero to three. http://www.zerotothree.org/child-development/challenging-behavior/aggressive-behavior.html. Accessed 23 June 2014

Porcher FK (2011) Thirty-month visit. In: Richardson B (ed) Pediatric primary care: practice guidelines for nurses. Burlington, MA, Jones & Bartlett Learning

Potts NL, Mandleco BL (eds) (2012) Pediatric nursing: caring for children and their families, 3rd edn. Delmar Cengage Learning, Clifton Park, NY

Samour PQ, King K (2005) Handbook of pediatric nutrition, 3rd edn. Jones and Bartlett Publishers, Sudbury, MA

Four-Year Visit 18

Alberto comes to the pediatric clinic with his mother, Mrs. Guayas-Cardozo, for his 4-year checkup in their suburban community outside a major urban area. Mrs. Guayas-Cardozo brings along Alberto's 6-month old brother Jose for the checkup. Alberto weighs 14.5 kg (31.9 lb), which is above the 40th percentile in weight but stands 94 cm (37.6 in.) which is in the 10th percentile for height. His father is a contractor and his mother, who appears obese, is a domestic worker. She brings Alberto after day care for the checkup. His mother is concerned that Alberto is not eating enough. Alberto has a body mass of 16.4 which is in the 75th percentile for BMI. He is not very active at home or in the playground at school. He doesn't always take time to go to the bathroom when he needs to so he has many accidents during the day. Alberto knows his first and last name and that he is a boy. He can describe events and tell a story. Developmentally, he can skip and hop on one foot and go upstairs with alternating feet. He can catch a bounced ball and can identify several colors and numbers. Alberto enjoys playing with other children in school and has friends in the day care center. He likes singing rhyming songs and counting. He is able to dress himself, wash his hands, and brush his teeth. His parents remind him to spit out the toothpaste. There are no safe parks nearby in their neighborhood. When he comes home from day care, Alberto tells his mother that his friend Raphael takes out all the toys and makes a mess. Mrs. Guayas-Cardozo was told by the teacher that no such child is in the class and she is concerned. Alberto usually watches television for about 2.5 h; then he plays with his toys. He especially likes his fire engine and blocks that his father made for him. Mrs. Guayas-Cardozo is still concerned that Alberto has temper tantrums when he does not get what he wants. Mrs. Guayas-Cardozo is also concerned that Alberto complains to her that she spends too much time with his new brother and Alberto wants more of her attention.

18.1 Are Alberto's Height and Weight Appropriate for Him?

Alberto's weight is in the 40th percentile while his height is much lower, which places him in the 75th percentile for his BMI. This is of concern as he is at increased risk for becoming overweight as a Mexican American and also by

D. Kramer, *Primary Well-Being: Case Studies for the Growing Child*,
DOI 10.1007/978-3-319-56708-2_18

having one or both parents obese. Families in poverty often have food insecurities that lead them to eat high-fat, nutrient-light foods, such as those sold at McDonalds. It is important for the health care provider to assess the perceptions of height, weight, and body image from the perspective of the child and parent in order to encourage motivation to change dietary patterns (Society of Nutrition Professionals in Public Health 2014; Samour and King 2005; American Academy of Pediatrics Undated; American Academy of Pediatrics 2012, 2014; Hagan et al. 2008; Hockenberry and Wilson 2012; Ontario Society of Nutrition Professionals in Public Health 2014; American Academy of Pediatrics, Committee on Nutrition 2009; Potts and Mandleco 2012).

Alberto's mother is concerned about him not eating enough, which is common in parents who don't assess their children's weight appropriately; also the child may not accurately report what he is eating. The treatment course is to change the eating patterns to nutrient-dense foods, and increase physical activity. It is important to emphasize the role of the parent and encourage them to be the role models for Alberto. Families can engage in physical activity together—aim for at least an hour a day, going for walks after dinner, playing in the playground, and reducing sedentary and screen-time activities to less than 2 h a day. It is important that Alberto not skip breakfast. When possible the family should eat meals together, drinking water or zero calorie beverages, and use low-fat milk. The family may also be eating a lot of high-fat, inexpensive take-out meals. Eating home cooked fresh food and holding family mealtime is another weight maintenance strategy. Alberto should have three meals a day with healthy snacks, including five servings of fruits and vegetables per day and two cups of low-fat milk (National Institute of Health, Osteoporosis and Related Bone Diseases National Resource Center 2012).

Special times with the family should involve activities that are not sedentary or revolve around food. The diet should be high in calcium and fiber, with balanced fat, carbohydrates, and proteins. Alberto should not be rewarded with food for good behavior. Refer to the newly revised USDA http://www.choosemyplate.gov/ for guidelines. For more information on children's nutrition and educational resources, see: http://www.choosemyplate.gov/kids/. The goal for the child is to maintain the same weight so as Alberto grows his BMI will decrease.

- **Assess Alberto's current stage of psychosocial development and how his parents can help him master this stage.**

  According to Erikson, Alberto is in the Initiative versus Guilt stage of development. The parents should encourage and praise all of Alberto's work and play activities. They should use time-out with verbal limit setting for discipline.

- **Assess the cognitive development of a 4-year-old child.**

  According to Piaget, Alberto is still in the preoperational phase of development, but has also begun the Intuitive Thought phase. For him causality is still related to the proximity of events. Alberto understands time better, especially in terms of the sequence of daily events. He still judges everything according to one dimension, such as width, heights, or order. The immediate perceptual clues dominate his judgment. He is beginning to develop less egocentrism and more social awareness. Alberto can name four colors. He is aware of his gender and others. He can play simple board or card games. He can draw a person with three parts. He can tell us what will happen next in a book. He may count correctly but has poor mathematical concepts of numbers. Alberto obeys because his parents have set limits—not because of his understanding of right and wrong (Burns et al. 2009; Dixon and Stein 2006; Hagan et al. 2008; Hockenberry and Wilson 2011; Marcdante et al. 2011; McInerny et al. 2009; Porcher 2011).

- **What milestones of gross and fine motor development could Alberto be expected to display?**

Gross motor: Alberto skips and hops on one food. He catches a ball reliably and can throw the ball overhand. He balances on his foot for 2 s and can walk downstairs alternating footing.

Fine Motor: Alberto uses scissors successfully to cut out picture following an outline. He can close his shoes with Velcro, but has difficulty with making a bow. Alberto likes to dress himself, including buttons. He puts on his shoes and socks. When drawing, he can copy a cross and square, and trace a cross and diamond. He draws a person with three body parts (Hurley 2000).

- **Assess the social behaviors that Alberto may exhibit at this age.**

Children at 4 years of age want to be independent. They also tend to be egocentric and impatient. They can be aggressive physically as well as verbally, including biting and hitting. Alberto takes pride in his accomplishments, but he also has mood swings. He can show off dramatically, but also enjoys entertaining others. He tells family tales to others with no restraint. Alberto still has many fears, such as going to sleep. His play is associative and imaginary playmates are common. He uses dramatic, imaginative, and imitative devices. His sexual exploration and curiosity is demonstrated through play, such as being a doctor or nurse and giving an examination (Richardson 2011; Taylor 2001; Parlakian and Lerner 2014; Hockenberry and Wilson 2011; Dixon and Stein 2006).

- **Assess the characteristics of play at this age and suggest appropriate playthings and activities to encourage Alberto's development and safety. How would you address his imaginary friend?**

Alberto attends preschool but doesn't have many friends there. But he has an imaginary friend. Alberto's imaginary friend is in his class at preschool and he also talks about his "friend" at home. The health care provider should tell Alberto's parents that 4-year-olds typically have an imaginary friend—65% of children under the age of seven have one at some point (Taylor 2001). When a child doesn't have a lot of friends they often create imaginary ones. It is normal and part of the child's make-believe play. Reassure the parents that this is normal and that the imaginary friend will help Alberto in times of loneliness and also to work out what he is feeling. Parents can call the imaginary friend by name; however, the child cannot blame the imaginary friend for doing a behavior that the child would be responsible for, such as making a mess.

Alberto needs to be encouraged to have friends over in order to learn to socialize. The parents will want to promote active play for Alberto: including an imagination station, cars and trucks, pretend stove, dishes, and pots and foods. Items should indicate they are appropriate for his age group. He should be playing outdoors with balls and jump ropes, and be climbing walls and structures in the park (American Academy of Pediatrics 2011; Alkon et al. 2008).

- **The mother is concerned about Alberto's attitude toward his younger brother. What would you advise?**

  It's very common for children to be jealous of younger or older siblings. This can be expressed in different ways. Some children become aggressive toward there sibling; some become withdrawn and quiet. Others can say how they feel, such as "You gave more to her," or "you give more attention to him." An effective way to deal with sibling rivalry issues is to express: "oh, would you like more" or "shall we plan a special time for you and me," or "would you like special kisses." This validates the child's experience and offers them what they were looking for instead of the parents being defensive (Dixon and Stein 2006; Goodard 2011; Parlakian and Lerner 2014; Richardson 2011). Identifying appropriate storybooks that describe situations of sibling rivalry with helpful solutions will help Alberto and his parents deal with this situation in a sensitive way. Hearing the story will help Alberto share his feelings about being in a similar situation. Spending time in reading to children is a safe way to explore feelings and attitudes, increases children's self-esteem, and provides comfort (Goddard 2011). Books that addresses sibling rivalry include Mister Fred Rogers' book: *The New Baby,* (reissued by Puffin in 1998), and also Martha Alexander's *Nobody Asked Me If I Wanted a Baby Sister* (published by Dial in 1971).

- **Describe immunization needs at this age.**

  For immunizations at this age, consult the CDC, ACIP, or AAP web sites for the current immunization schedule recommendations (Centers for Disease Control and Prevention 2001, 2011):

– CEC National Immunization Program (NIP): http://www.cdc.gov/vaccines
– American Academy of Pediatrics *Red Book*: http://www.aapredbook.org

- **Mrs. Guayais-Cardozo is concerned about Alberto's temper tantrums and disciplining him. What advice would you offer?**

  Remind the mother about setting clear guidelines and not using time-out for more than 4 min (1 min/year). She should praise Alberto for accomplishments and his cooperation, whether helping around the house or in the community. She should spend positive time with him at home and in the community—reading, rhyming, singing, and playing simple games like "Chutes and Ladders." Suggest that Alberto be taken to the library and to parks where he can run around and be with other children; also take him to other places that might be interesting that they could talk about together, such as a visit to the zoo or local museum during free hours—almost every institution like this has a free time for entry. Praise Alberto when he runs and jumps and climbs. The family can become involved in a place of worship or cultural group if they are interested to give Alberto a sense of a more extensive community, or join their local community center or ethnic organization.

- **What information can be given concerning toileting accidents and nightmares?**

  Both of these are normal in the preschool-age child. For the toileting accidents, suggest that Mrs. Guayais-Cardozo treat it matter-of-factly, clean Alberto up, and watch for signs of when he has to go to the toilet next time. For nightmares, offer comfort and he will soon go back to sleep (Burns et al. 2009; Dixon and Stein 2006; Hagan et al. 2008; Hockenberry and Wilson 2011; Marcdante et al. 2011; McInerny et al. 2009; Porcher 2011; Mindell and Owens 2009).

- **Assess the anticipatory guidance that would be helpful for a 4-year-old child.**

  Four-year-olds are more aggressive in their motor activity, including biting and hitting and pushing. They may resist authority and require limit setting on their behaviors using time-out.

  At this age, Alberto will have an active imagination that includes some fantastic tales and imaginary friends. Children at this age might also have nightmares and night terrors. If Alberto has a nightmare, wake the child to calm him. Alberto may be experimenting with language, such as calling his parent by her first name and using offensive language that he has heard; appropriate limit setting is important in these situations. Alberto needs to know what the guidelines are in advance on expected behavior, and they should be enforced consistently using patient instruction and time-out, talking to him respectfully in a calm voice (Taylor 2001).

References

Alkon A, To K, Wolff M, Mackie JF, Bernzweig J (2008) Assessing health and safety in early care and education programs: development of the CCHP health and safety checklist. J Pediatr Health Care 22(6):368–377. http://childcareawaremn.org/sites/default/files/attachments/jphc_hs_checklist.pdf. Accessed 23 Dec 2014

American Academy of Pediatrics. Task Force on Sudden Infant Death Syndrome. (2011). SIDS and other sleep-related infant deaths: Expansion of recommendations for a safe infant sleeping environment. Pediatrics, 128, 1030–1039

American Academy of Pediatrics (2012) Kids and vitamin D deficiency. http://www.aap.org/en-us/about-the-aap/aap-press-room/Pages/Kids-and-Vitamin-D-Deficiency.aspx. Accessed 22 Dec 2014

American Academy of Pediatrics (2014) Healthy active living for families. healthychildren.org/growinghealthy. Accessed 16 Dec 2014

American Academy of Pediatrics (n.d.) Infant food and feeding. http://www.aap.org/en-us/advocacy-and-policy/aap-health-initiatives/HALF-Implementation-Guide/Age-Specific-Content/Pages/Infant-Food-and-Feeding.aspx. Accessed 18 June 2014

American Academy of Pediatrics, Committee on Injury and Poison Prevention (2001) Injuries associated with infant walkers. Pediatrics 108(3):790–792. http://pediatrics.aappublications.org/content/108/3/790.full. Accessed 11 Dec 2014 (Reaffirmed in 2005)

American Academy of Pediatrics, Committee on Nutrition (2009) Pediatric nutrition handbook, 6th edn. American Academy of Pediatrics, Elk Grove Village, IL

Burns CE et al (2009) Pediatric primary care: a handbook for nurse practitioners, 4th edn. W.B. Saunders, Philadelphia, PA

Centers for Disease Control and Prevention (2001) Recommendations for using fluoride to prevent and control dental caries in the United States. In: Morbidity and Mortality Weekly Report, vol 50(RR-14)

Centers for Disease Control and Prevention (2011) Recommendations and guidelines: childhood and adolescent immunization schedules. http://www.cdc.gov/vaccines/schedules/index.html. Accessed 11 Dec 2014

Dixon SD, Stein MT (2006) Encounters with children: pediatric behavior and development, 4th edn. Mosby, St. Louis, MO

Goodard AT (2011) Children's books for use in bibliotherapy. J Pediatr Health Care 25:57–61

Hagan JF, Shaw JS, Duncan P (eds) (2008) Bright futures: guidelines for health supervision of infants, children, and adolescents, 3rd edn. American Academy of Pediatrics, Elk Grove Village, IL

Hockenberry MJ, Wilson DW (2011) Wong's nursing care of infants and children, 9th edn. Elsevier/Mosby, New York, NY

Hurley DS (2000) Developing fine and gross motor skills: birth to three. PRO-ED, Inc, Austin, TX. www.proedinc.com. Accessed 11 Dec 2014

Marcdante KJ, Kliegman RM, Jenson HB et al (eds) (2011) Nelson essentials of pediatrics, 6th edn. Saunders, Philadelphia, PA

McInerny TK, Adam HM, Campbell DE et al (eds) (2009) Textbook of pediatric care. American Academy of Pediatrics, Elk Grove Village, IL

Mindell JA, Owens JA (2009) A clinical guide to pediatric sleep: diagnosis and management of sleep problems, 2nd edn. Lippincott Williams & Wilkins, Philadelphia, PA

National Institute of Health, Osteoporosis and Related Bone Diseases National Resource Center (2012) Calcium and vitamin D: important at every age. http://www.niams.nih.gov/Health_Info/Bone/Bone_Health/Nutrition/. Accessed 23 Dec 2014

Ontario Society of Nutrition Professionals in Public Health (2014) Pediatric nutrition guidelines (birth to six years) for health professionals. ON, Canada. http://www.healthunit.org/professionals/nutrition/Pediatric%20Nutrition%20Guidelines%20for%20Primary%20Health%20Care%20Providers.pdf. Accessed 28 Aug 2015

Parlakian R, Lerner C (2014) Aggressive behavior in toddlers. Zero to three. http://www.zerotothree.org/child-development/challenging-behavior/aggressive-behavior.html. Accessed 23 June 2014

Porcher FK (2011) Two-year visit. In: Richardson B. (Ed.), Pediatric primary care: Practice guidelines for nurses. Burlington, MA: Jones & Bartlett Learning. Chapter 14, pp. 109–114

Potts NL, Mandleco BL (eds) (2012) Pediatric nursing: caring for children and their families, 3rd edn. Delmar Cengage Learning, Clifton Park, NY

Richardson B (ed) (2011) Pediatric primary care: practice guidelines for nurses. Jones & Bartlett Learning, Burlington, MA

Samour PQ, King K (2005) Handbook of pediatric nutrition, 3rd edn. Jones and Bartlett Publishers, Sudbury, MA

Taylor M (2001) Imaginary companions and the children who create them. Oxford University Press, New York, NY

Five-Year Visit 19

Mina Asad is coming to the pediatric clinic with her mother Mrs. Asad and her paternal grandmother. They live in a small urban city around the corner from the local mosque. They immigrated to America when Mina was 3 years old. Mina has been attending a preschool at the mosque and her mother is concerned about Mina starting kindergarten at the public school a few blocks away in the fall. Mina weighs 16 kg (35.2 lb) (25th percentile) and stands 108 cm (43.2 in.) in the 50th percentile. Her blood pressure is 91/53. Her BMI is 13.7 (in the 3rd percentile). Mina is a quiet girl at home with her older brothers. Her grandmother is concerned that in the public school Mina will be encouraged to speak up to boys, not only girls. This would not be considered respectful for a woman's behavior in their culture. Mina wears a head veil, like her mother and grandmother. Mina can tell a story in full sentences, count to ten, and name six colors. She can draw a person with six body parts and can copy squares and triangles. She also can hop, skip, and likes to climb in the playground. Recently a fire erupted in Mina's building and she has become fearful of noises. The grandmother is also concerned that Mina does not eat enough foods. She eats fruits and vegetables and dairy products but she is a very picky eater. She doesn't like meat, fish, or eggs. She eats only white pita bread with humus for many meals, but won't eat the falafel balls her grandma fries especially for her.

- **Are Mina's height and weight appropriate for her?**

Mina is in the 50th percentile for height and 25 percentile for weight. She has alterations in nutrition as revealed by her BMI in the 3rd percentile. Mina needs three meals a day and three healthy snacks per day. It is important to get a three-day diet history on Mina to assess her caloric and nutritional intake. A behavioral assessment to determine Mina's energy level should be included in her thorough physical exam. Blood work should include electrolytes and a protein panel, thyroid screen, and a CBC with differential. Also check Mina's iron and lead levels (Society of Nutrition Professionals in Public Health 2014; Samour and King 2005; American Academy of Pediatrics Undated; American Academy of Pediatrics 2012; American

D. Kramer, *Primary Well-Being: Case Studies for the Growing Child*,
DOI 10.1007/978-3-319-56708-2_19

of Pediatrics 2014; Hagan et al. 2008; Hockenberry and Wilson 2012; Ontario Society of Nutrition Professionals in Public Health 2014).

Children need 34 servings of calcium-rich foods per day. An 8-oz glass of milk provides 300 mg of calcium. Her parents should encourage Mina to drink low-fat milk, 1–2%, and no more than 4–6 oz of 100% fruit juice. She should be eating appropriate amounts of protein, carbohydrates, fruits, and vegetables. Mina needs 90 kcal/kg/day divided into three meal and three snacks. Fluid requirements are 100 mL/kg/day, with increased needs based on activity levels and climate. Mina needs 13–19 g of protein a day (American Academy of Pediatrics, Committee on Nutrition, 2009). Advise Mina's parents to go to My Pyramid for Preschoolers, which is for children ages 3–5 (United States Department of Agriculture 2014). (See: http://www.choosemyplate.gov/preschoolers.html.)

Regarding the families' concern about Mina's sporadic eating, the health care provider can advise Mrs. Asad and her grandmother to provide Mina with small quantities of food six times a day, making sure she has breakfast. She should get two cups of low-fat milk each day and can combine humus with whole wheat pita bread, brown rice, quinoa, or beans as alternate sources of protein.

- **Assess Mina's current stage of psychosocial development and how her family can help her master this stage.**

According to Erickson, Mina is still in the Initiative versus Guilt phase of development. She needs praise for what she is doing, whether physical activities, art projects, quiet play, or helping with chores. At this age, Mina is less rebellious and argumentative and more calm and eager to focus on what she is doing. She will have better manners and be able to take care of herself in terms of dress and hygiene. Mina brushes her teeth twice a day and sees the dentist every 6 months. She occasionally needs supervision and prodding in these areas and this is normal.

Mina has developed a fear of loud noises because of a fire in her building and she should be evaluated for post-traumatic stress disorder (PTSD) to see if she needs counseling. Usually 5-year-olds have fewer fears. The family should provide reassurance for Mina that she is safe. They can institute a safety plan and have drills so everyone will know what to do in case of a fire, such as the exit to use, the place to meet, and how to leave by staying low to the floor (stop, drop, and roll). The parents should remain calm and praise Mina for even normal behavior but not over-respond when it is negative.

Mina is more settled and eager to do things, but not as open and accessible in thoughts and behavior as earlier ages. She can be independent but trustworthy; take more responsibility, and is less foolhardy. In general, she relies on outer authority to control her world. She is eager to do things right and to please and tries to "live by the rules." Her play is associative; she tries to follow rules but may cheat to avoid losing. It is important for her to be active and to get together with other children, at home and in the park. She should have at least an hour of physical activity daily, which can be split into several periods in the course of the day (Terry 2011; Nickell 2011).

- **Assess the cognitive development of a 5-year-old child.**

According to Piaget a 5-year-old is in the preoperational stage of development. Mina has good, clear diction. She can tell a simple story using complete sentences. She uses appropriate pronouns and her sentences contain 6–8 words and include all parts of speech—verbs, adjectives, nouns, pronouns. She can count up to 20 and name 4 or more colors and match 10 or more colors. She can match letters but not necessarily read them. She is good at sorting shapes and she can name coins. Her family speaks Arabic at home, and Mina speaks both English and Arabic. She has an English vocabulary of about 2100 words. She can talk about her drawings or make comments and enumerate. She knows the days of the week, months, and other time-associated words and what things are made of. She can follow three commands in succession and has a greater understanding of others' perspectives. Mina can be inquisitive and want factual information about the world.

Mina is not ready for concentrated close work or small print because of slight farsightedness and still unrefined eye-hand coordination (Burns et al. 2009; Dixon and Stein 2006; Hagan et al. 2008; Hockenberry and Wilson 2011; Marcdante et al. 2011; McInerny et al. 2009; Porcher 2011).

- **What milestones of gross and fine motor development could Mina be expected to display?**

Gross motor: Mina can balance on 1 foot for a few seconds. She skips and hops on alternate feet. She can throw and catch a ball well. She likes to jump rope and can skate with good balance. She can walk front and backward heel to toe and balance on alternate feet with her eyes closed.

Fine motor: Mina has a mature grasp of a pencil. She can tie shoelaces and use scissors, simple tools, or a pencil competently. She can print some letters and numbers, and write her first name. She can copy squares and triangles and draw a person with at least six body parts. At the table she can cut her food with a knife (Hurley 2000).

- **Describe immunization needs for this age.**

For immunizations at this age, consult the CDC, ACIP, or AAP web sites for the current immunization schedule recommendations (Centers for Disease Control 2011):

- CEC National Immunization Program (NIP): http://www.cdc.gov/vaccines
- American Academy of Pediatrics *Red Book*: http://www.aapredbook.org

- **What culturally is the role of Mina in her family and how would a health professional discuss this with her family**?

Mina's family has only been in the United States for a few years and is adjusting to a society with different values, which includes gender relationships, patterns of communication, and observance of holidays—both religious and secular, as well as different dress patterns and expectations for behavior. The health care provider can help the family clearly define their beliefs and values for and what they want to communicate to her. They should be encouraged to discuss openly what is happening in school. They will want to nurture a relationship with Mina so that she feels comfortable discussing anything with her parents and grandmother. At this age her church group of friends will also be in school with her when she makes the transition to public school and will be her primary circle for friendship in the new school. There should also be someone in the new school whom they can approach with their concerns such as a guidance counselor, teacher, or principal (Child Care Aware 2011).

- **What anticipatory guidance would you offer Mina's family?**

Mina's mother and grandmother are concerned about her going to public school in the fall. The health care provider should assess whether Mina's family understands the local educational system and whether they understand English sufficiently to interact with the school—filling out forms and attending meetings and school functions, such as open school night and parent-teacher meetings. Stress that it is important for Mina's parents to attend these meetings and become knowledgeable about their child's learning experiences and her teacher. If they can, the parents should request a tour of the school with Mina to allay any fears and answer any questions. Getting familiar with her new surroundings before the first day of school is also helpful to transition from her private preschool to the public one in the community. Encourage Mina to talk to her family every day about her experiences at school, what she did, what she liked, and anything that may worry her. Also if anyone is not nice to her, she should tell her teacher and her parents so they can help her deal with this.

Explain that children of this age, while they have friends and should be open to them, the family is still the main authority in their lives. There are differences and it would be helpful to talk with Mina concerning how the rules about how young girls or young woman behave in home and church need to remain respectful. While in public school, girls talk to boys and vice versa. Indicate that you understand the grandmother's concerns about her granddaughter's reputation as a young woman and keep the doors open to discuss the situation again with the health provider at future visits (Alkon et al. 2008; Potts and Mandleco 2012; Terry 2001; Dixon and Stein 2006).

References

Alkon A, To K, Wolff M, Mackie JF, Bernzweig J (2008) Assessing health and safety in early care and education programs: development of the CCHP health and safety checklist. J Pediatr Health Care 22(6):368–377. http://childcareawaremn.org/sites/default/files/attachments/jphc_hs_checklist.pdf. Accessed 23 Dec 2014

American Academy of Pediatrics (2012) Kids and vitamin D deficiency. http://www.aap.org/en-us/about-the-aap/aap-press-room/Pages/Kids-and-Vitamin-D-Deficiency.aspx. Accessed 22 Dec 2014

American Academy of Pediatrics (2014) Healthy active living for families. healthychildren.org/growinghealthy. Accessed 16 Dec 2014

American Academy of Pediatrics (n.d.) Infant food and feeding. http://www.aap.org/en-us/advocacy-and-policy/aap-health-initiatives/HALF-Implementation-Guide/Age-Specific-Content/Pages/Infant-Food-and-Feeding.aspx. Accessed 18 June 2014

American Academy of Pediatrics, Committee on Nutrition (2009) Pediatric nutrition handbook, 6th edn. American Academy of Pediatrics, Elk Grove Village, IL

Burns CE et al (2009) Pediatric primary care: a handbook for nurse practitioners, 4th edn. W.B. Saunders, Philadelphia, PA

Centers for Disease Control and Prevention (2011) Recommendations and guidelines: childhood and adolescent immunization schedules. http://www.cdc.gov/vaccines/schedules/index.html. Accessed 11 Dec 2014

Child Care Aware (2011) Is this the right place for my child? 38 research-based indicators of quality child care. National Association of Child Care Resource & Referral Agencies (NACCRRA). http://ccapub.childcareaware.org/docs/pubs/121e.pdf. Accessed 23 Dec 2014

Dixon SD, Stein MT (2006) Encounters with children: pediatric behavior and development, 4th edn. Mosby, St. Louis, MO

Hagan JF, Shaw JS, Duncan P (eds) (2008) Bright futures: guidelines for health supervision of infants, children, and adolescents, 3rd edn. American Academy of Pediatrics, Elk Grove Village, IL

Hockenberry MJ, Wilson DW (2011) Wong's nursing care of infants and children, 9th edn. Elsevier/Mosby, New York, NY

Hurley DS (2000) Developing fine and gross motor skills: birth to three. PRO-ED, Inc, Austin, TX. www.proedinc.com. Accessed 11 Dec 2014

Marcdante KJ, Kliegman RM, Jenson HB et al (eds) (2011) Nelson essentials of pediatrics, 6th edn. Saunders, Philadelphia, PA

McInerny TK, Adam HM, Campbell DE et al (eds) (2009) Textbook of pediatric care. American Academy of Pediatrics, Elk Grove Village, IL

Nickell PM (2011) Six-year visit (school readiness). In: Richardson B (ed) Pediatric primary care: practice guidelines for nurses. Burlington, MA, Jones & Bartlett Learning

Ontario Society of Nutrition Professionals in Public Health (2014) Pediatric nutrition guidelines (birth to six years) for health professionals. ON, Canada. http://www.healthunit.org/professionals/nutrition/Pediatric%20Nutrition%20Guidelines%20for%20Primary%20Health%20Care%20Providers.pdf. Accessed 28 Aug 2015

Porcher FK (2011) Two-year visit. In: Richardson B. (Ed.), Pediatric primary care: Practice guidelines for nurses. Burlington, MA: Jones & Bartlett Learning. Chapter 14, pp. 109–114

Potts NL, Mandleco BL (eds) (2012) Pediatric nursing: caring for children and their families, 3rd edn. Delmar Cengage Learning, Clifton Park, NY

Samour PQ, King K (2005) Handbook of pediatric nutrition, 3rd edn. Jones and Bartlett Publishers, Sudbury, MA

Terry EG (2011) Seven- to ten-year visit (school age). In: Richardson B (ed) Pediatric primary care: practice guidelines for nurses. Burlington, MA, Jones & Bartlett Learning

United States Department of Agriculture (2014) Choose My Plate.gov. Daily food plan for preschoolers. http://www.choosemyplate.gov/preschoolers/Plan/. Accessed 31 Dec 2014

20 Six-Year Visit

Jamar comes to the pediatric clinic with his mother, Mrs. Campbell, who was born in Jamaica and is in her mid-30s. Mrs. Campbell completed her bachelor's degree in accounting and works for a small local accounting firm. Jamar's paternal grandmother helps out with picking Jamar up after school and lives nearby. Jamar's father was killed by a stray bullet during a shooting in their neighborhood. The mother says Jamar is worried about who his teacher will be in school, and if she will be nice. The grandmother is concerned about Jamar playing in sports activities because he might get hurt. Jamar is friendly and enjoys playing with other kids and playing sports. Jamar weighs 26.34 kg (58 in.) and stands 123.5 cm (48.5 in.), putting him in the 95th percentile for weight and height. His blood pressure is 96/55. His BMI is 17.3, which is in the 90th percentile. Mrs. Campbell signed Jamar up for T-ball in the local community afterschool program but the grandmother disapproved. The mother is more concerned that her son should have social experiences after school. Jamar asks if he could go to school by himself, like some of his friends, and his mother is worried that she might be overprotective but told him he may not go to school by himself until he is 9 years old. Jamar has had regular visits to the dentist and likes brushing his teeth.

- **Are Jamar's height and weight appropriate for him?**

  Yes. Jamar is in the 95 percentile for both height and weight and his BMI is in the 90th percentile. His average weight gain/year is now: 1.8–2.7 kg (4–6 lbs). His average linear growth/year: 5 cm (2 in.). Jamar continues to need 90 kcal/kg/day divided into three meals with two nutritious snacks (Ontario Society of Nutrition Professionals in Public Health 2014). Mrs. Campbell should limit Jamar's non-nutritious (junk food) intake. The health provider should refer Mrs. Campbell to Choose My Plate.gov for serving size and food group recommendations (Society of Nutrition Professionals in Public Health 2014; Samour and King 2005; American Academy of Pediatrics 2014; Hagan et al. 2008; Hockenberry and Wilson 2012; Ontario Society of Nutrition Professionals in Public Health 2014; United States Department of Agriculture 2014). Whenever possible, advise Mrs. Campbell to

D. Kramer, *Primary Well-Being: Case Studies for the Growing Child*,
DOI 10.1007/978-3-319-56708-2_20

have her family eat together to prevent childhood obesity, and encourage healthy eating habits (Hammons and Fiese 2011). Eating together also has positive psychosocial benefits for the family and has been related to reduced incidence of juvenile delinquency, greater academic achievement, and improved psychological well-being (Cook and Dunifon 2012).

- **Assess Jamar's current stage of psychosocial development and how his family can help him master this stage.**

According to Erikson, Jamar is in the industry versus inferiority stage. He likes to do projects and get praised. Mrs. Campbell should encourage and praise his work at school and at home, for example his art projects, construction projects, team accomplishments, and club achievements.

It is also the latency period of Freud when children try to do everything right and are usually positive about themselves and their relationships with others. They follow adult examples, but want more independence. Mrs. Campbell should be teaching Jamar how to cross the street by stopping at the curb and looking, but not let him go alone yet. Advise Mrs. Campbell that this practice should go on for a long time, until age 10 or older (Hagan et al. 2008; Hockenberry and Wilson 2011), as the street can be very dangerous. If the light is red or yellow he should be instructed to wait until it is green or the white figure appears. Then he should look to the left, then the right, and back to the left. Emphasize to Jamar to never cross the street without a grown-up. If he is going on the school bus, he needs to know where to wait and an adult should supervise getting on and off the bus.

- **Assess the cognitive development of a 6-year-old child.**

According to Piaget a 6-year-old child has moved from magical thinking into the concrete operational phase of cognitive development. Jamar is able to understand conservation of mass, rules of reversibility and decentration—being able to focus on more than one attribute of an object at a time, such as the height and width of a glass he is filling with water, and is linked to the development of short-term memory (Simatwa 2010). He can classify objects and is starting to understand another person's perspective. He should be playing board games, checkers, and simple card games. Jamar reads from memory and enjoys oral spelling games. He knows his right and left hands. He has a well-established vocabulary and can recite his address and phone number. He recognizes most letters of the alphabet and can define at least seven words and identify opposites.

Jamal understands time not only in relation to his own activities such as bed time and bath time. Starting at age six, Jamar begins to understand time as a concept—when something happens, for example, whether it is morning or afternoon. He now also starts to understand the permanence of death. Jamar can articulate his needs but his grammar may be incorrect.

Jamal is in the preconventional stage of moral development. He wants to be a good boy and not ruin any of his relationships with others. Jamar should be encouraged to be independent, including doing age-appropriate chores around the house.

- **What milestones of gross and fine motor development could Jamar be expected to display?**

Jamar uses a knife to spread butter or jam on bread at the table. He can cut, fold, and paste paper. He enjoys trying out his abilities and will gradually increase in dexterity. This will be an active age, with constant activity. Jamar may return often to finger feeding because he is so active. Jamar likes to draw, print, and color; he can draw and copy shapes. He can draw a man with six body parts and can print some letters and numbers. His vision has reached 20/20, which is maturity. Jamar can balance on each foot briefly and walk forward and backward walking heel-to-toe, and hop; he does somersaults and likes playing chasing games such as tag. He can ride a bicycle. He can throw and catch a small ball.

- **Assess the social behaviors that Jamar may exhibit at this age.**

Six-year-olds are typically in the first grade of school and peer relationships have greater importance than they did previously. Jamar will continue to learn about his world through play and developing his skills and knowledge at school. Jamar should be encouraged to be involved with cooperative play and be in team and group activities in and outside of school, especially those involving physical activity. Advise Mrs. Campbell to pick up on the interests of Jamar and seek out activities and classes that will further these interests, such as art classes, gymnastics, swim lessons, sport teams, chess, and other game clubs. Financial assistance can often be arranged and many public facilities have a “free” day each week.

Jamar’s mother should be encouraging social interaction and regular exercise and making play dates for him to promote friendships. Get-togethers don’t necessarily need to be at home—friends can play in the park together with parental supervision, or meet at a mall recreation area or other public facility. Often first graders develop a best friend. Jamar has a great need for children of his own age (Dixon and Stein 2006).

- **Assess the characteristics of play at this age and suggest appropriate playthings and activities to encourage Jamar’s development and safety.**

Jamar can share and cooperate better. He will like to play board games and do projects involving cutting paper, drawing and building with Lego, erector sets, blocks, and other construction sets. He will cheat to win sometimes. He will engage in rough play and may still have occasional temper tantrums. Jamar will copy what the adults are seen doing and frequently boast about his accomplishments. Help Mrs. Campbell and grandma to understand that Jamar wants to be more independent and have his own way of doing things.

- **Describe immunization needs at this age.**

For immunizations at this age, consult the CDC, ACIP, or AAP web sites for the current immunization schedule recommendations (Centers for Disease Control 2011):

- CEC National Immunization Program (NIP): http://www.cdc.gov/vaccines
- American Academy of Pediatrics *Red Book*: http://www.aapredbook.org

- **Assess dental needs for this age.**

This is the age when baby teeth start falling out and permanent teeth erupt. Semiannual dental visits are especially important and Jamar should be brushing his teeth two times a day and flossing at least once daily. If the water is not fluoridated in his city, he should have a fluoride supplement. Remind Jamar that his new teeth need to last him forever and he should take good care of them. Suggest to Jamar's mother that she talk to the dentist about possible use of sealants to protect Jamar's teeth from cavities. For guidelines on Oral health, See: *Bright Futures in Practice: Oral Health, pocket guide* by Paul Casamassimo and Katrina Hold, Ed., Washington, DC: National Maternal and Child Oral Health Resource Center, Georgetown University (Casamassimo and Hold 2014; Centers for Disease Control and Prevention 2001).

- **Assess sleep needs for this age.**

Jamar should be getting 8–12 h of sleep a night and should have a consistent bedtime routine at this age. He may occasionally have nightmares or night terrors/sleepwalking (Mindell and Owens 2009).

- **Assess the anticipatory guidance that would be helpful for a 6-year-old child.**

Elimination: Remind Mrs. Campbell that most 6-year-olds are toilet trained but may have occasional accidents. His timing of bowel movements may vary. Ask Mrs. Campbell what is normal for Jamar: an acceptable range is 1 time every 2–3 days to 1–3 times daily. Jamar will urinate similar to an adult, 5–6 times daily. It is important that when he starts school, Jamar feels comfortable going to the bathroom in school. Jamar may occasionally experience enuresis—the normal rate is 5–7% at this age due to deep sleep or missed cues. Mrs. Campbell should remain matter-of-fact when Jamar has urinary or bowel incontinence and avoid punishment.

General Safety: Remind Mrs. Campbell about using appropriate safety restraints in motor vehicles. She should be reminding Jamar of pedestrian safety rules when they are out in the community. The family should be aware of appropriate protective equipment for all sporting activities such as helmets when biking. This is a good age for him to learn to swim. All sports and play activities should be properly supervised and facilities in safe condition. Jamar is still too young to be left by himself without appropriate supervision. When Mrs. Campbell is at work, she should arrange appropriate, safe supervision for Jamar before and after school. He should know how to operate household appliances safely and not do it alone. Mrs. Campbell should continue to keep all hazards and medicines out of reach/locked up and monitor use. The family should have a safety plan in case of fire. By age 6 Jamar should know his phone number and address and he should be taught to dial 911 for emergencies (American Academy of Pediatrics 2011).

Guns: Mrs. Campbell should teach Jamar about gun safety and to not play with guns or handle them in his own home or when visiting others. Any gun in the house should be stored separately from ammunition and both should be in locked cabinets.

Strangers: Mrs. Campbell should talk to Jamar about strangers. He should never go with a stranger or take things from a stranger. If a stranger says his mother sent them, Jamar should run and tell a teacher or familiar adult that a stranger wanted him to do something. He should also be aware of inappropriate touch or any touch that makes him feel uncomfortable.

Screen Time: At this age, Jamar's time viewing TV and using a computer should be limited to less than 2 h/day. Neither television nor computer should be in Jamar's bedroom (Terry 2011).

School Readiness: The health care provider should assess that all physical, developmental, and psychological milestones needed for school are evident. These include screening for any special needs and appropriate referrals and placements if necessary. Talk with Mrs. Campbell about her comfort level in separating from Jamar and whether Jamar has any difficulty separating. Encourage Mrs. Campbell to have a tour of the school, meet the teachers and administrators, and find out what the rules are in the class, so that she can discuss them with Jamar and prepare him. Explain to Mrs. Campbell that her positive attitude and advocacy for school will have a great influence on Jamar's acceptance regarding school and its rules and routines. Encourage Mrs. Campbell to arrange for Jamar to meet his teacher before the first day of school and obtain a copy of the rules and routines of his class. It is normal for children to have fear or anxiety about the first day of school. Reading books, such as *The First Day of School*, and others that can be found in the library on this topic, is a helpful way to prepare Jamar for school (Nickell 2011).

Bullying: The Health care provider should encourage Mrs. Campbell to talk with Jamar about bullying, what it is, how to defend himself, and when to let other adults know. Find out from Mrs. Campbell if Jamar has ever been bullied or hit by other children or if he has demonstrated bullying or aggression toward others. Bullying is when another person comes to hurt you either physically or emotionally or to force you to do something. In this situation, Jamar should firmly say: "Stop bothering me," leave the situation and go tell a responsible adult, such as his teacher. Mrs. Campbell should practice with Jamar so he can say this with confidence and leave the immediate area. Mrs. Campbell should try to have supervision in situations where there could be bullying and she should talk to the school about whether they have an anti-bullying campaign. If there is no anti-bullying program, she could help to start one. If Jamar is being bullied, he should walk with a responsible adult to school. Mrs. Campbell should actively look for ways to increase Jamar's self-image and self-esteem by developing his talents or interests. The health care provider should give Mrs. Campbell the guide "How to Address Bullying" from Bright Futures found at: http://www.brightfutures.org/mentalhealth/pdf/families/mc/bullying.pdf.

References

American Academy of Pediatrics (2011) Task Force on Sudden Infant Death Syndrome. SIDS and other sleep-related infant deaths: Expansion of recommendations for a safe infant sleeping environment. Pediatrics, 128, 1030–1039

Bright Futures (n.d.) How to address bullying. Bright futures tool for families. http://www.brightfutures.org/mentalhealth/pdf/families/mc/bullying.pdf. Accessed 2 Jan 2015

Burns CE et al (2009) Pediatric primary care: a handbook for nurse practitioners, 4th edn. W.B. Saunders, Philadelphia, PA

Casamassimo P, Hold K (2014) Bright futures in practice: oral health, pocket guide, 2nd edn. National Maternal and Child Oral Health Resource Center, Georgetown University, Washington, DC. http://www.mchoralhealth.org/pocket.html. Accessed 18 Dec 2014

Centers for Disease Control and Prevention (2001) Recommendations for using fluoride to prevent and control dental caries in the United States. Morb Mortal Weekly Rep 50:RR-14

Centers for Disease Control and Prevention (2011) Recommendations and guidelines: childhood and adolescent immunization schedules. http://www.cdc.gov/vaccines/schedules/index.html. Accessed 11 Dec 2014

Cook E, Dunifon R (2012) Parenting in context: do family meals really make a difference? (Parenting in Context). Cornell University, College of Human Ecology, Ithaca, NY. http://www.human.cornell.edu/pam/outreach/upload/Family-Mealtimes-2.pdf. Accessed 2 Jan 2015

Dixon SD, Stein MT (2006) Encounters with children: pediatric behavior and development, 4th edn. Mosby, St. Louis, MO

Hagan JF, Shaw JS, Duncan P (eds) (2008) Bright futures: guidelines for health supervision of infants, children, and adolescents, 3rd edn. American Academy of Pediatrics, Elk Grove Village, IL

Hammons AJ, Fiese BH (2011) Is frequency of shared family meals related to the nutritional health of children and adolescents. Pediatrics 127(6):e1565–e1574

Hockenberry MJ, Wilson DW (2011) Wong's nursing care of infants and children, 9th edn. Elsevier/Mosby, New York, NY

Marcdante KJ, Kliegman RM, Jenson HB et al (eds) (2011) Nelson essentials of pediatrics, 6th edn. Saunders, Philadelphia, PA

McInerny TK, Adam HM, Campbell DE et al (eds) (2009) Textbook of pediatric care. American Academy of Pediatrics, Elk Grove Village, IL

Mindell JA, Owens JA (2009) A clinical guide to pediatric sleep: Diagnosis and management of sleep problems. 2nd ed. Philadelphia, PA: Lippincott Williams & Wilkins

Nickell PM (2011) Six-year visit (school readiness). In: Richardson B (ed) Pediatric primary care: practice guidelines for nurses. Burlington, MA, Jones & Bartlett Learning

Ontario Society of Nutrition Professionals in Public Health (2014) Pediatric nutrition guidelines (birth to six years) for health professionals. ON, Canada. http://www.healthunit.org/professionals/nutrition/Pediatric%20Nutrition%20Guidelines%20for%20Primary%20Health%20Care%20Providers.pdf. Accessed 28 Aug 2015

Potts NL, Mandleco BL (eds) (2012) Pediatric nursing: caring for children and their families, 3rd edn. Delmar Cengage Learning, Clifton Park, NY

Samour PQ, King K (2005) Handbook of pediatric nutrition, 3rd edn. Jones and Bartlett Publishers, Sudbury, MA

Simatwa EMW (2010) Piaget's theory of intellectual development and its implication for instructional management at pre-secondary school level. Educ Res Rev 5(7):366–371. http://www.academicjournals.org/article/article1379610138_Simatwa.pdf. Accessed 2 Jan 2014

Terry EG (2011) Seven- to ten-year visit (school age). In: Richardson B (ed) Pediatric primary care: practice guidelines for nurses. Burlington, MA, Jones & Bartlett Learning

United States Department of Agriculture (2014) Choose My Plate.gov. Daily food plan for preschoolers. http://www.choosemyplate.gov/preschoolers/Plan/. Accessed 31 Dec 2014

Seven-Year Visit

21

Mr. Giotti brings his daughter Rosetta to the pediatric clinic for her annual school checkup before second grade. She weighs 21.85 kg (48.25 lb), and is 120.6 cm (47.5 in. tall), placing her in the 50th percentile for weight and height. Her blood pressure is 96/57and her BMI is 15.0, which is the 40th percentile. Mr. Giotti brags about how Rosetta learned to read in first grade. Rosetta likes school and has a best friend in her class. She is very careful to do the right thing. She waits for her turn in school and at home, and is very helpful to her family, doing many chores each day to help her working parents. She works very hard at trying to be perfect as the only child in her family. Her mother is at work as a medical assistant and can't make the visit. Mr. Giotti runs a small bakery in the community. Rosetta comes to the bakery after school when her mother is at work. Her grandmother, Mrs. Giotti, who lives with them in one apartment of their two-family house, comes and picks Rosetta up after her job in a garment factory to take Rosetta home and start dinner. Mr. Giotti is worried that Rosetta is too hard on herself and she complains when things aren't perfect. The teacher tells Mr. Giotti that Rosetta is doing well at school, gets along well with others, and is eager to learn. Rosetta wants to join the Little League and Mr. Giotti expresses concerns.

- **Is Rosetta's height and weight appropriate for her?**

She is in the 50th percentile for both weight and height and in the 40th for BMI. At this age her height increases a little over 2 in. a year. She is entering middle childhood and the closer she gets to puberty the more she will have spurts of growth. Typically, children at this age gain 2–3 kg per year in weight (4.5–6 lb/year) (Samour and King 2005; American Academy of Pediatrics 2014; Hagan et al. 2008; Cook and Dunifon 2012; Hammons and Fiese 2011).

D. Kramer, *Primary Well-Being: Case Studies for the Growing Child*,
DOI 10.1007/978-3-319-56708-2_21

- **Assess Rosetta's current stage of psychosocial development and how her parents can help her master this stage.**

According to Erikson, Rosetta is in the industry versus inferiority stage of development. She should be encouraged and praised for her work at school, on teams, and in clubs. Her wish to join the Little League for softball is very appropriate for her age, especially if other girls in her class are participating. The health care provider should reassure Mr. Giotti that Rosetta can safely participate in softball. He should make sure that the league has adult supervision and uses appropriate safety equipment. The focus of the game should be on having fun and not on winning. The goal is to learn team cooperation and good sportsmanship as well as have physical exercise and fun (Burns et al. 2009; Dixon and Stein 2006; Hagan et al. 2008; Hockenberry and Wilson 2011; Marcdante et al. 2011; McInerny et al. 2009).

Rosetta is working on competence, independence, and responsibility. She takes learning new things seriously and is in Freud's stage of latency and Erikson's initiative stage. Mr. Giotti should praise everything Rosetta does and continue to be clear about household rules and routines.

- **Assess the cognitive development of a 7-year-old child.**

Rosetta is in second grade. According to Piaget, a 7-year-old is in the stage of concrete operations. Rosetta will notice that certain parts are missing from pictures. She can copy a diamond and repeat three numbers backward. She has a good concept of time and can use a clock for minding the time. She can read a nondigital clock or watch correctly to the quarter hour (Simatwa 2010).

She is reading well but may skip words such as "it," "the," and "he" or not pause at the end of a sentence or comma.

- **What milestones of gross and fine motor development could Rosetta be expected to display?**

Rosetta will get her maxillary central incisors and lateral mandibular incisors. Her jaw will begin to expand to accommodate permanent teeth. She will be more cautious when beginning new activities. As part of her drive for perfection, she practices activities to master them. At meals she uses a table knife for cutting meat; but she may need help with tough or difficult pieces. She brushes and combs her hair acceptably without help.

- **Assess the social behaviors that Rosetta may exhibit at this age.**

Rosetta likes to help and have choices but is less argumentative and stubborn. Some children at this age will steal, but not Rosetta. She is becoming a real member of her family group. She likes to takes part in group play and prefers being with girls. But she also spends time alone and does not require a lot of companionship. She should be encouraged to invite friends over from school and have a best friend (Terry 2011).

- **Describe community resources that could help Rosetta and her family with safe activities and age-appropriate guidelines for independence.**

  Rosetta should be encouraged to attend classes at the local community center or settlement house or other sources of afterschool activities. However, her parents should be careful not to overload her with too many outside activities. Time spent with her grandmother is also nurturing time that can give Rosetta a lifetime of good memories and warm feelings in a positive relationship.

- **Describe immunization needs at this age.**

  For immunizations at this age, consult the CDC, ACIP, or AAP web sites for the current immunization schedule recommendations (Centers for Disease Control 2011):

– CEC National Immunization Program (NIP): http://www.cdc.gov/vaccines
– American Academy of Pediatrics *Red Book:* http://www.aapredbook.org

- **Assess dental needs at this age.**

  At this age, Rosetta should be able to brush her teeth by herself with fluoride toothpaste after each meal but at least twice a day and floss at least once a day. The water supply should contain fluoride, or she should be getting a fluoride supplement (Casamassimo and Hold 2014; Centers for Disease Control and Prevention 2001).

  Permanent teeth will start erupting in the order in which the baby teeth were lost. Dental visits should continue twice a year for exams and cleaning. If Rosetta has many cavities, a sealant may be recommended. It is good that Rosetta is a careful brusher and flosser. For guidelines on oral health, see *Bright Futures in Practice: Oral Health, pocket guide* by Paul Casamassimo and Katrina Hold, Ed., Washington, DC: National Maternal and Child Oral Health Resource Center, Georgetown University.

- **Mr. Giotti is concerned about Rosetta's urge for perfection. What advice would you offer?**

  The health care provider should ask father if there are signs of inflexibility where Rosetta becomes rigid or has meltdowns if she cannot do things the way she wants. Is she self-critical or self-accepting? Her parents and grandmother should encourage Rosetta to be accepting; not everything needs to be perfect. They should remind Rosetta that it is not all or nothing and doing things well takes time and practice. The health care provider should assess Rosetta for anxiety and ask about possible stressors in her daily routine.

- **Assess the anticipatory guidance that would be helpful for a 7-year-old child.**

Good touch, bad touch: It is important for the health care provider to review with Mr. Giotti the rules about touching and being touched by another person. He should explain to Rosetta that any part of her body that is under her bathing suit should not be touched by another person. She is the only one in charge of these parts of her body. No adult or another child should touch them or ask to see them or demand that she not tell her parents what they want or did. Rosetta should go tell her parent or another adult right away if she experiences this situation.

Physical changes: Part of anticipatory guidance is for the health care provider to talk to Rosetta about upcoming changes she will notice in her body. An excellent book to share with her is the 2013 title by Christine Northrup and Tracey Kristinia: *Beautiful Girl*: *Celebrating the Wonders of Your Body (published by Hay House).*

Breast buds may begin to develop by age 8.

Six- and seven-year-olds have similar issues around safety, independence, bullying, and sports participation. See Chap. 20 on the 6-year visit for further anticipatory guidance.

References

American Academy of Pediatrics, Committee on Nutrition (2009) Pediatric nutrition handbook, 6th edn. American Academy of Pediatrics, Elk Grove Village, IL

American Academy of Pediatrics (2014) Healthy active living for families. healthychildren.org/growinghealthy. Accessed 16 Dec 2014

Bright Futures (n.d.) How to address bullying. Bright futures tool for families. http://www.brightfutures.org/mentalhealth/pdf/families/mc/bullying.pdf. Accessed 2 Jan 2015

Burns CE et al (2009) Pediatric primary care: a handbook for nurse practitioners, 4th edn. W.B. Saunders, Philadelphia, PA

Casamassimo P, Hold K (2014) Bright futures in practice: oral health, pocket guide, 2nd edn. National Maternal and Child Oral Health Resource Center, Georgetown University, Washington, DC. http://www.mchoralhealth.org/pocket.html. Accessed 18 Dec 2014

Centers for Disease Control and Prevention (2001) Recommendations for using fluoride to prevent and control dental caries in the United States. Morb Mortal Weekly Rep 50:RR-14

Centers for Disease Control and Prevention (2011) Recommendations and guidelines: childhood and adolescent immunization schedules. http://www.cdc.gov/vaccines/schedules/index.html. Accessed 11 Dec 2014

Cook E, Dunifon R (2012) Parenting in context: do family meals really make a difference? (Parenting in context). Cornell University, College of Human Ecology, Ithaca, NY. http://www.human.cornell.edu/pam/outreach/upload/Family-Mealtimes-2.pdf. Accessed 2 Jan 2015

Dixon SD, Stein MT (2006) Encounters with children: pediatric behavior and development, 4th edn. Mosby, St. Louis, MO

Hagan JF, Shaw JS, Duncan P (eds) (2008) Bright futures: guidelines for health supervision of infants, children, and adolescents, 3rd edn. American Academy of Pediatrics, Elk Grove Village, IL

Hammons AJ, Fiese BH (2011) Is frequency of shared family meals related to the nutritional health of children and adolescents. Pediatrics 127(6):e1565–e1574

Hockenberry MJ, Wilson DW (2011) Wong's nursing care of infants and children, 9th edn. Elsevier/Mosby, New York, NY

Marcdante KJ, Kliegman RM, Jenson HB et al (eds) (2011) Nelson essentials of pediatrics, 6th edn. Saunders, Philadelphia, PA

McInerny TK, Adam HM, Campbell DE, Kamat DM, Kelleher KJ (eds) (2009) Textbook of pediatric care. American Academy of Pediatrics, Elk Grove Village, IL

Northrup C, Kristina T (2013) Celebrating the wonders of your body. Hay House, Carlsbad, CA

Potts NL, Mandleco BL (eds) (2012) Pediatric nursing: caring for children and their families, 3rd edn. Delmar Cengage Learning, Clifton Park, NY

Samour PQ, King K (2005) Handbook of pediatric nutrition, 3rd edn. Jones and Bartlett Publishers, Sudbury, MA

Simatwa EMW (2010) Piaget's theory of intellectual development and its implication for instructional management at pre-secondary school level. Educ Res Rev 5(7):366–371. http://www.academicjournals.org/article/article1379610138_Simatwa.pdf. Accessed 2 Jan 2014

Terry EG (2011) Seven- to ten-year visit (school age). In: Richardson B (ed) Pediatric primary care: practice guidelines for nurses. Jones & Bartlett Learning, Burlington, MA

United States Department of Agriculture (2014) Choose My Plate.gov. Daily food plan for preschoolers. http://www.choosemyplate.gov/preschoolers/Plan/. Accessed 31 Dec 2014

Eight-Year Visit

22

Tito comes to the pediatric clinic with Mrs. Munoz while Mr. Munoz is at work. He weighs 20.40 kg (45 lb), which is in the third percentile, and is 118.1 cm (46.5 in.) tall, putting him in the fifth percentile for height. His tanner stage is 2. His blood pressure is 94/56 and his BMI is 14.6, or third percentile. He is a good boy, doing his work and listening to the teachers in the parochial school in their community but he is lately making excuses to stay home from school, such as having a stomach-ache. Mrs. Munoz is concerned that there is something wrong with Tito. His mother usually walks him to school. Tito does very well in school, but recently he has started not completing his homework and doing poorly on tests, according to the teacher at open school night. He has one good friend but does not have a group that he is connected with.

- **Is Tito's height and weight appropriate for him? Is his nutrition adequate?**

Tito is in the fifth percentile for height and weight and the third percentile for body mass. He is on the slender side but his growth is consistent. As his body size increased, Tito's body fat became relatively stable, giving a slimmer appearance than in his preschool years. He will grow an average of a little over 5 cm/year (2 in.) in the grade school years. Especially for boys, the closer to puberty, the greater the chances for increased growth. Between ages 9 and 14 Tito could start having enlarged testes and getting a small amount of pubic hair and hair under his arms. These are the beginning signs of puberty. If he starts to have these signs earlier, Tito may be in precocious puberty, and he should be evaluated for growth problems. Tito's appetite tends to vary due to growth fluctuations, but he should not be losing weight (Samour and King 2005; American Academy of Pediatrics 2014; Hagan et al. 2008; Cook and Dunifon 2012; Hammons and Fiese 2011).

The health care provider should encourage Mr. and Mrs. Munoz to have honest, age-appropriate discussions about sex with Tito using accurate terminology. They should listen carefully to Tito's questions and try to only give as much information as Tito requires to answer them.

D. Kramer, *Primary Well-Being: Case Studies for the Growing Child*,
DOI 10.1007/978-3-319-56708-2_22

Tito should be eating between 1600 and 2400 calories/day. His diet should consist of nutrient-dense foods with a wide variety of fruits, vegetables, whole grains, and nonfat or low-fat dairy foods. The health care provider should stress to Mrs. Munoz the importance of parents being good role models and that families that eat together tend to share more nutritious meals. Another good rule to model is no snacking in front of the television.

When Tito sees his parents enjoying a wide variety of nutritious food he is more likely to want them too. Tito should have a nutritious breakfast each day. Having Tito help in meal preparation is another strategy to encourage healthy eating; usually children want to eat what they have prepared.

When shopping for food, the health provider should encourage Mrs. Munoz to read food labels carefully, noting in particular the calories from fat, type of fat, sodium, cholesterol, vitamins, minerals, and serving size. Tito should be reading the labels too. He should also be encouraged to make healthy choices when eating out. Refer the family to choosemyplate.gov for age-appropriate nutrition planning. Videos and materials on the web site are available in Spanish and English.

Tito may need a multivitamin if he is not eating enough to get essential nutrients but Mrs. Munoz says that he is not particularly picky, which can be typical of this age. In that case, Mrs. Munoz would want to slightly adjust Tito's portions or food groups in order to ensure adequate intake and perhaps have him eat more at snack times than at regular meals.

For his one to two snacks a day, Tito can eat fresh, canned, or frozen vegetables or fruits. Suggest that Mrs. Munoz can keep cut-up vegetables such as celery sticks, cucumber slices, carrot sticks, green or red pepper slices, or broccoli in the refrigerator. Bananas are also a good snack—especially frozen and whipped in the blender. Other snack ideas to share with the family include cold skim or 1% milk with whole-grain sugar-free cereal, peanut butter sandwich, or crackers with hummus, or fruit smoothie made with fresh fruit, skim milk, ice, and a dash of vanilla or cinnamon. Nonfat or low-fat yogurt or cheese, air-popped or unbuttered popcorn, baked tortillas or pretzels with salsa, chocolate skim milk made at home to control the amount of sugar, and low-fat frozen yogurt fruit juice bars (without added sugar) are also suitable for snacks. Basically, a snack is anything that is healthy and nutritious to eat in a smaller than normal portion size.

- **Assess Tito's current stage of psychosocial development and how his parents can help him master this stage.**

According to Erikson, Tito is in the industry versus inferiority stage of development. Tito usually likes to do his school homework and is easy to get along with at home. He likes being rewarded for doing well and for his chores. He can be dramatic but is also more sociable and better behaved. He is playing only with other boys by this age. Tito should be encouraged to participate in activities that build his self-confidence and increase his network of friends. Making friends is extremely important at this age (Burns et al. 2009; Dixon and Stein 2006; Hagan et al. 2008; Hockenberry and Wilson 2011; Marcdante et al. 2011; McInerny et al. 2009; Potts and Mandeleco 2012).

- **Assess the cognitive development of an 8-year-old child.**

An 8-year-old is in the concrete operation stage of development. He can go from specific to general reasoning. He knows concrete concepts such as conservation of mass and liquids but doesn't understand abstract or hypothetical concepts yet. He can give similarities and differences between two things from memory, count backwards from 20 to 1, and repeat days of the week and months in order. He knows the date and can describe common objects in detail, not merely their use. Tito is better able to express emotions and ideas, but does not always understand the abstract terms he may be using. He is learning to communicate clearly with friends (Simatwa 2010).

This is also the collection age. Tito will likely have a collection such as cards, or rocks or miniature racecars, or other items that are special to him and that he keeps in a special area or container in his bedroom.

- **What milestones of gross and fine motor development could Tito be expected to display?**

Tito is growing about 5 cm a year. His lateral incisors (maxillary) and mandibular cuspids will erupt. His movement is fluid, often graceful, and poised and he is confident in his body. Children at this age are typically always moving—for example, jumping, chasing, skipping, doing cartwheels, and standing upside-down, but their development is slowing down. Tito's motor skills have improved in strength, balance, and coordination.

Screening for scoliosis is important at this age.

- **Assess the social behaviors that Tito may exhibit at this age.**

This is an age that focuses on peer relationships. Tito is currently having difficulty establishing these relationships and not wanting to go to school is a symptom. Making friends is one of the most important mid-childhood tasks. If Tito has siblings, they may be replacing his need for many outside friends. Usually friends will have similar temperament and interests. Tito's one friend may be more satisfactory for him than a larger group of friends. It is normal to seek friends from his age group but cliques may be present. Tito's teacher should be able to give information about cliques in the class to Mrs. Munoz and parent-teacher communication should be encouraged. Tito also should be encouraged to be part of teams, have more friends over, and participate in a few afterschool activities.

Tito is concerned about his bad grades and being embarrassed. Mrs. Munoz will want to help Tito find an area that he has an interest or aptitude in and nurture it—either by doing it together, providing expert lessons, or doing it with friends or in a group. These interests can include a musical instrument, a sport, study of one subject, singing with a choir, and many more. Involvement in these activities will also help Tito master the balance between success and failure in life and begin to understand that the effort is often the reward. Tito's self-concept—of his body, his sociability, and his intellect—will affect his ability to feel successful in his activities and relationships. He needs to have a positive self-image in his abilities to do most day-to-day activities, skills, and chores.

Tito's parents and teachers are important significant others and will influence his behavior and self-concept. The health care provider should encourage Mr. and Mrs. Munoz to share unscheduled spontaneous time with Tito to talk, listen, or do an activity together. Having time to talk will help Tito deal with fears, disappointments, and stress.

Tito is still not ready to stay at home alone, but he should be learning safety, security, and emergency procedures for when he is old enough to be left alone for short times such as after school (Terry 2011).

- **Assess the characteristics of play at this age and appropriate playthings.**

Tito can use common tools such as a hammer, saw, screwdriver, and household and sewing utensils. He helps with routine household tasks such as dusting and sweeping. He can take food himself, use serving utensils, and pour a beverage for himself and others.

- **Describe immunization for this age.**

For immunizations at this age, consult the CDC, ACIP, or AAP web sites for the current immunization schedule recommendations (Centers for Disease Control 2011):

- CEC National Immunization Program (NIP): http://www.cdc.gov/vaccines
- American Academy of Pediatrics *Red Book:* http://www.aapredbook.org

- **What would you suggest to Tito's parents concerning vision at this age.**

Vision at 8 years should be 20/20, but sometimes at this age, myopia-nearsightedness starts to occur and school difficulty may be the only sign—a symptom that Tito is experiencing. Tito should be evaluated for visual acuity and ocular alignment annually at his health care visits and routine school checks. If he is having trouble completing assignments in school or sits close to the television screen, a vision screen should also be done. Children who fail to pass the screening test should have a complete ophthalmological examination.

Also the health care provider should consider a hearing screening for Tito, especially if he has a history of frequent ear infections or there is a concern about speech development.

- **Mrs. Munoz is concerned about Tito's declining interest in school and lack of friendships. What advice would you offer?**

The health care provider can guide Mrs. Munoz in finding out why Tito is suddenly not performing in school and seems disinterested in attending. If Tito seems distracted in school or home, if he is having trouble completing schoolwork or keeping up with the pace in school, or if he is misbehaving at school or getting into trouble with other children, the health care provider should consider whether he has a learning disability or is being bullied by another student at school. Children with presumed or diagnosed learning disabilities should have a comprehensive pediatric medical eye exam to identify and treat any undiagnosed vision impairment as well as a hearing exam, especially if he has a history of ear infections. Referrals should be made for appropriate medical, psychological, and educational evaluation and treatment of the learning disability.

Perhaps Tito is not getting enough sleep at night—he needs 10–11 h at night. If he is feeling stress and anxiety, it could be contributing to insomnia. Stress may be caused by another student bullying Tito. If he is snoring it could be sleep apnea. Perhaps Tito has been receiving peer pressure to abuse substances, especially alcohol. The physical exam is the first place to start. Suggest to Mrs. Munoz that she discuss with Tito's teacher how he presents in the classroom. Mrs. Munoz can also speak to the school's psychologist to gather more information. Questions should be asked about Tito's Internet and social media contacts; filters need to be on the computer he uses as well as any smartphone for permissible and nonpermissible sites, whether at home, or in public settings such as the library.

- **Assess the anticipatory guidance that would be helpful for an 8-year-old child.**

See box "General Safety and Hygiene" (page 115) for points of discussion to review with Mrs. Munoz. Specific guidance for this age includes topics such as sleep, activity level, fireworks, media, substance abuse, and sexual abuse.

Sleep: Remind Mrs. Munoz of the importance of sleep for Tito and maintaining daily routines. He should use his bed only for sleeping and not have a television or computer in his room. She can allow Tito to read quietly to himself before sleep or read to him, sing a lullaby, or do other soothing activities. Make Mrs. Munoz aware that Tito may have occasional nightmares or sleep disturbances such as night terrors or sleepwalking. Other concerns at this age interfering with sleep may be fear of the dark or being alone; experiencing stress or anxiety about something that happened during the day also impacts sleep.

General activity: Tito needs a variety of daily physical activities, including team/individual sports, family activities, free play, walking, bicycling, chores, and walking up and down stairs. Mr. and Mrs. Munoz should model and promote regular physical activity; he should wear appropriate protective sports gear but also consume adequate calcium to decrease the risk of fractures. Tito will tend to put on weight as he approaches puberty.

Fire safety: The health care provider should warn Tito and his mother about the dangers of fireworks to eyes, limbs, and body injuries. Tito can enjoy firework displays put on by professionals.

Media: Remind the parents about limiting screen time on television, computers, smartphones, tablets, and other electronic media. His TV/computer time should be less than 2 h a day. His parents should also monitor what social media Tito may use and take care to select appropriate material on the Internet or television. Mr. and Mrs. Munoz should become knowledgeable about what Tito watches and uses and consider keeping the computer in a place where its use can be monitored and not in Tito's bedroom. Point out that there are online programs for monitoring usage and controlling computer activity. The parents should talk often with Tito about online and social media safety and responsibility. Encourage Mr. and Mrs. Munoz to set a good example by limiting their own viewing time and doing other healthy activities together.

Sexual abuse. Point out to Mrs. Munoz that most sexual abuse occurs between the ages of 8 and 12, and in a majority of cases the abuser is known to the child. The health care provider and the parents should speak to Tito about "good touch/bad touch" concepts and the possible scenarios that may occur. They should support abuse prevention programs at school and listen carefully to Tito if he may have a concern, particularly of a sexual nature.

Substance abuse: This is the age when experimentation and casual use may begin, often through peer pressure, and now is the time for the parents to talk to Tito about drinking and drug use as well as exposure to second-hand smoke. Point out that children exposed to smoke are at risk of developing asthma, bronchitis, middle-ear disease, pneumonia, wheezing and coughing spells, and behavioral/cognitive problems. If Mr. or Mrs. Munoz smokes, it is more likely that Tito will too. Now would be a good time for them to stop smoking and set a good example for Tito.

References

American Academy of Pediatrics, Committee on Nutrition (2009) Pediatric nutrition handbook, 6th edn. American Academy of Pediatrics, Elk Grove Village, IL

American Academy of Pediatrics (2014) Healthy active living for families. healthychildren.org/growinghealthy. Accessed 16 Dec 2014

Bright Futures (n.d.) How to address bullying. Bright futures tool for families. http://www.brightfutures.org/mentalhealth/pdf/families/mc/bullying.pdf

Burns CE et al (2009) Pediatric primary care: a handbook for nurse practitioners, 4th edn. W.B. Saunders, Philadelphia, PA

Centers for Disease Control and Prevention (2011) Recommendations and guidelines: childhood and adolescent immunization schedules. http://www.cdc.gov/vaccines/schedules/index.html. Accessed 11 Dec 2014

Cook E, Dunifon R (2012) Parenting in context: do family meals really make a difference? (Parenting in context). Cornell University, College of Human Ecology, Ithaca, NY. http://www.human.cornell.edu/pam/outreach/upload/Family-Mealtimes-2.pdf. Accessed 2 Jan 2015

Dixon SD, Stein MT (2006) Encounters with children: pediatric behavior and development, 4th edn. Mosby, St. Louis, MO

Hagan JF, Shaw JS, Duncan P (eds) (2008) Bright futures: guidelines for health supervision of infants, children, and adolescents, 3rd edn. American Academy of Pediatrics, Elk Grove Village, IL

Hammons AJ, Fiese BH (2011) Frequency of shared family meals related to the nutritional health of children and adolescents. Pediatrics 127(6):e1565–e1574

Hockenberry MJ, Wilson DW (2011) Wong's nursing care of infants and children, 9th edn. Elsevier/Mosby, New York, NY

Marcdante KJ, Kliegman RM, Jenson HB et al (eds) (2011) Nelson essentials of pediatrics, 6th edn. Saunders, Philadelphia, PA

McInerny TK, Adam HM, Campbell DE, Kamat DM, Kelleher KJ (eds) (2009) Textbook of pediatric care. American Academy of Pediatrics, Elk Grove Village, IL

Potts NL, Mandleco BL (eds) (2012) Pediatric nursing: caring for children and their families, 3rd edn. Delmar Cengage Learning, Clifton Park, NY

Samour PQ, King K (2005) Handbook of pediatric nutrition, 3rd edn. Jones and Bartlett Publishers, Sudbury, MA

Simatwa EMW (2010) Piaget's theory of intellectual development and its implication for instructional management at pre-secondary school level. Educ Res Rev 5(7):366–371. http://www.academicjournals.org/article/article1379610138_Simatwa.pdf. Accessed 2 Jan 2014

Terry EG (2011) Seven- to ten-year visit (school age). In: Richardson B (ed) Pediatric primary care: practice guidelines for nurses. Burlington, MA, Jones & Bartlett Learning

United States Department of Agriculture (2014) Choose My Plate.gov. Daily food plan for preschoolers. http://www.choosemyplate.gov/preschoolers/Plan/. Accessed 31 Dec 2014

Nine-Year Visit

23

Monique is brought to her school's health clinic for her school checkup by her mother, Mrs. Despre. Mr. and Mrs. Despre have been in America for 2 months and Monique has just been registered for public school. They live with her mother's brother and his family. Her mother speaks Creole and French and the pediatric office has an interpreter for the visit. Monique weighs 40.64 kg (89.5 lb), and stands 142.9 cm tall (56.25 in.), putting her in the 95th percentile for weight and height. Monique's BMI is 19.9, which is in the 90th percentile. Her blood pressure is 103/61. Her tanner stage is 2. She is quiet during the visit. Monique avoids looking the pediatrician in the eye, stays near her mother, and looks to her for approval. Mother states this is her first child and she is not sure how to talk about the changing body with her daughter. Mrs. Despre is thinking it is time to introduce foods that will promote good health and in keeping with her belief in hot and cold and light and heavy foods; she is worried that the foods Monique needs at this age will not be available in her neighborhood or in school lunches. Monique talks Creole to her cousins and says some words in English.

- **Is Monique's height and weight appropriate for her? Address her mother's diet concerns in the context of her culture.**

Monique weighs 27 kg (59.4 lb), and stands 137 cm tall (54.8 in.), putting her in the 50th percentile for weight and height. Monique's BMI is 14.38, which is in the tenth percentile. Monique is balanced in terms of her height and weight.

The health care provider should be aware that in the Haitian culture, lunch is typically the largest meal. Breakfast consists of bread and butter and coffee, and supper is superhot cereal. Heavy foods are cornmeal mush and broiled plantains and potatoes. Light foods include bread and soup because they are easy to digest. Haitians drink a lot of homemade fruit juices. As the family gets used to living in a new country, there may be tension over what foods Monique wants to eat as she learns about the American diet.

D. Kramer, *Primary Well-Being: Case Studies for the Growing Child*,
DOI 10.1007/978-3-319-56708-2_23

The health care provider can help parents to talk with their child about food: Encourage Mrs. Despre to initiate a conversation with Monique about diet and nutrition. This is the age when children are at risk of overweight or obesity; where meals begin to be skipped more often; and where the child will eat snacks and not be hungry at mealtimes, and substitute high-fat quick foods for good nutrition. The health care provider should try to explain the child's weight and height in relation to the balance between the child's food intake and the calories they need to be healthy and grow and address the child directly in the conversation. It is important every day to have breakfast and to eat healthy foods, which include fruits, vegetables, whole grains and cereals, low-fat dairy products, and lean meats. Monique should be encouraged to choose low-fat milk or water instead of soda and sugared drinks. She should limit fruit juices to 4–6 oz/day. Remind Monique that eating healthy helps promote healthy growth and prevents weight problems. Tell Monique that her body is growing at a faster rate during puberty. If Monique ever wants to consider dieting or taking dietary supplements, advise her to discuss it first with her health care provider. Dieting is almost never a good idea and the health care provider wants to make sure that any supplements are safe and therapeutic and will really help Monique to achieve her goals (American Academy of Pediatrics 2009; Samour and King 2005; American of Pediatrics 2014; Hagan et al. 2008; Hockenberry and Wilson 2012; Cook and Dunifon 2012; Hammons and Fiese 2011; United States Department of Agriculture 2014).

- **Assess Monique's current stage of psychosocial development and how her parents can help her master this stage.**

  According to Erikson Monique is in industry versus inferiority stage of development. As she enrolls in a new school and gets used to a new life she will need additional supports to help her thrive in school and in the community. She will want to achieve social skills, technological skills, and interpersonal and personal skills and have a sense of accomplishment as opposed to a sense of inferiority. She may be placed in an English as a Second Language class with a bilingual staff member to help her with the transition from Haiti to the USA. Her community will hopefully have resources to help, such as after-school classes in English and homework help, sport clubs, and other social group activities, so that Monique can feel comfortable and adjust in positive ways. At this age, she will want to be more independent. For Freud, this is the stage of latency. Monique will want to have same-sex friends and be part of a group of friends to do activities with. At the same time, her parents need to strengthen her against peer pressure for negative behaviors, such as experimenting with smoking or drinking alcohol (Dixon and Stein 2006).

- **Assess the cognitive development of a child this age.**

  According to Piaget Monique is in the concrete operation stage of development. She has many accomplishments from her upbringing in Haiti, but will need support in her transition to third or fourth grade in the USA. She knows about using money. She likes to read and can do fractions in math. She is more aware of time and has been reliable in getting to school on time in Haiti. She is very concerned about doing well in school in the USA.

Monique grasps the concepts of parts and whole, and understands cause and effect, and concepts of conservation. She can classify objects by more than one quality. She likes to collect seashells and has brought some of her collection from Haiti. She makes elaborate paintings using watercolors, and likes to do detailed drawings (Simatwa 2010).

- **What milestones of gross and fine motor development could Monique be expected to display?**

At this age, Monique will have increased smoothness and speed in her fine motor control. She has increased fine motor control. Her mother says that she writes very neatly. Monique can dress herself completely. She likes to jump, skip, and run and is an active child (Potts and Mandelico 2012).

- **Assess the social behaviors that Monique may exhibit at this age.**

A 9-year-old is usually much more sociably tuned in with peers and outside activities. Monique will need help to find her place in her new American community. According to Mrs. Despre, in Haiti, Monique exercised choice in making purchases and helped her mother buy groceries at the local store in the morning and ran errands. She liked school in Haiti and enjoyed answering questions. She wanted good grades and was afraid of failing. She was a very good student and had become more self-critical recently. She played a lot of soccer and played well. She likes playing games and being part of a team. She had particular friends and groups. She is beginning to be modest and have increased body awareness.

It is important for the health care provider to understand that in Haitian culture, it is considered disrespectful to look in the eyes of authority figures or to speak out to them. The health care provider should explain to Monique and her mother that in Western cultures, it is respectful to make eye contact with people you are talking to, including authorities. It is also important to speak up if she doesn't understand something, for example a question by a health worker or teacher (Burns et al. 2009; Dixon and Stein 2006; Hagan et al. 2008; Hockenberry and Wilson 2011; Marcdante et al. 2011; McInerny et al. 2009).

- **Describe immunization for this age.**

The health care provider needs to help Monique catch up with her immunizations to be ready for school. The provider should also find out whether Monique has had BCG in Haiti. Consult the CDC guidelines for catching up at the CDC, ACIP, or AAP web sites for the current immunization schedule recommendations (Centers for Disease Control 2011):

- CEC National Immunization Program (NIP): http://www.cdc.gov/vaccines
- American Academy of Pediatrics *Red Book*: http://www.aapredbook.org

- **Mrs. Despre is concerned about Monique' secondary sexual characteristics and how she should talk to her daughter about her changing body. What advice would you offer?**

The health care provider should suggest that Mrs. Despre talk to her daughter about the way people's bodies change as they grow up. Monique can start noticing her body changing: her skin may become oilier, she may need to bath daily and use deodorant, and she will want to wash her face in the morning and at night (Terry 2011).

Mrs. Despre should point out to Monique that her breasts will start to get bigger (they are already budding), and as they grow she will need to wear a bra. Tell Monique about other changes she will be experiencing: you will get hair in your underarms and pubic area but also start to grow taller. Monique's body will start to prepare a place for a baby to be born eventually. Point out that women wear sanitary napkins or pads in their underwear because they can have some shedding of their uterus and have some blood coming from the vagina. Pads can be changed and thrown out and it is important to wash her hands well after changing pads. When Monique first starts this shedding—called menstruation—it may not come regularly every month. Suggest that it is a good idea to have a pad in Monique's bag in case her body starts to change when she is away from home.

Mrs. Despre should remind Monique that it is never ok for another person to show her their private parts or to ask to touch or view hers. Monique should go away from those people and go to an adult for help.

The health care provider should give the family a resource booklet for parent and child, preferable in Creole: American Academy of Pediatrics: *What's Happening to my Body?* See: http://www.healthychildren.org/English/ages-stages/gradeschool/puberty/Pages/Whats-Happening-to-my-Body.aspx.

- **Assess the anticipatory guidance that would be helpful for a child this age.**

Talk about the same general safety and hygiene guidelines that you would of previous ages. See box "General Safety and Hygiene" (page 115).

Monique will need assistance in transitioning from Haitian to American culture. It is important to help her transition but also to help her maintain her own positive identity. Is her family going to a church that is mostly Haitian? Is there a local group or community center that has many Haitians as members and/or on the staff? Monique will need help with English as well as her parents. She will need positive feedback to continue her strong commitment to learning and her values of friendship and competencies in sports. The foods in school will be different from what she is used to (Dunn 2002).

References

American Academy of Pediatrics, Committee on Nutrition (2009) Pediatric nutrition handbook, 6th edn. American Academy of Pediatrics, Elk Grove Village, IL

American Academy of Pediatrics (2014) Healthy active living for families. healthychildren.org/growinghealthy. Accessed 16 Dec 2014

Burns CE et al (2009) Pediatric primary care: a handbook for nurse practitioners, 4th edn. W.B. Saunders, Philadelphia, PA

Centers for Disease Control and Prevention (2011) Recommendations and guidelines: childhood and adolescent immunization schedules. http://www.cdc.gov/vaccines/schedules/index.html. Accessed 11 Dec 2014

Cook E, Dunifon R (2012) Parenting in context: do family meals really make a difference? (Parenting in context). Cornell University, College of Human Ecology, Ithaca, NY. http://www.human.cornell.edu/pam/outreach/upload/Family-Mealtimes-2.pdf. Accessed 2 Jan 2015

Dixon SD, Stein MT (2006) Encounters with children: pediatric behavior and development, 4th edn. Mosby, St. Louis, MO

Dunn AM (2002) Culture, competence, and the primary care provider. J Pediatr Health Care 1(3):105–111

Hagan JF, Shaw JS, Duncan P (eds) (2008) Bright futures: guidelines for health supervision of infants, children, and adolescents, 3rd edn. American Academy of Pediatrics, Elk Grove Village, IL

Hammons AJ, Fiese BH (2011) Frequency of shared family meals related to the nutritional health of children and adolescents. Pediatrics 127(6):e1565–e1574

Hockenberry MJ, Wilson DW (2011) Wong's nursing care of infants and children, 9th edn. Elsevier/Mosby, New York, NY

Marcdante KJ, Kliegman RM, Jenson HB et al (eds) (2011) Nelson essentials of pediatrics, 6th edn. Saunders, Philadelphia, PA

McInerny TK, Adam HM, Campbell DE, Kamat DM, Kelleher KJ (eds) (2009) Textbook of pediatric care. American Academy of Pediatrics, Elk Grove Village, IL

Potts NL, Mandleco BL (eds) (2012) Pediatric nursing: caring for children and their families, 3rd edn. Delmar Cengage Learning, Clifton Park, NY

Samour PQ, King K (2005) Handbook of pediatric nutrition, 3rd edn. Jones and Bartlett Publishers, Sudbury, MA

Simatwa EMW (2010) Piaget's theory of intellectual development and its implication for instructional management at pre-secondary school level. Educ Res Rev 5(7):366–371. http://www.academicjournals.org/article/article1379610138_Simatwa.pdf. Accessed 2 Jan 2014

Terry EG (2011) Seven- to ten-year visit (school age). In: Richardson B (ed) Pediatric primary care: practice guidelines for nurses. Jones & Bartlett Learning, Burlington, MA

United States Department of Agriculture (2014) Choose My Plate.gov. Daily food plan for preschoolers. http://www.choosemyplate.gov/preschoolers/Plan/. Accessed 31 Dec 2014

24 Ten-Year Visit

Ten-year-old Pat Masca is brought by his grandfather to the Indian Reservation's pediatric clinic for his annual physical. His father is working on an oil rig. Pat's mother is a domestic helper in the nearby town. Pat weighs 31.4 kg (69.25 pounds), and stands 137.5 cm (54.25 in.) tall, putting him in the 50th percentile for weight and height. His BMI is 16.6 (45th percentile). His blood pressure is 102/61. His tanner stage is 1. Pat's grandfather is concerned about the way Pat rides his bike in the street. Pat doesn't like wearing a helmet, and recently someone else on the reservation had a serious bike accident. His grandfather also sees other children using alcohol and drugs and he wants to know how to talk to his grandson about it before Pat is tempted to try this. Pat also sees other kids about his age smoking. His grandfather also thinks it is time to talk about becoming a man and the changes that are taking place in Pat's body.

- **Is Pat's height and weight appropriate for him?**

Yes: Pat weighs 31.4 kg (69.25 pounds), and stands 137.5 cm (54.25 in.) tall putting him in the 50th percentile for weight and height. His BMI is 16.6 (45th percentile). Pat's growth has slowed in height as expected but his weight gain may speed up at this age and he may become a little overweight briefly until he begins his postpuberty growth spurt. His remaining teeth will emerge and become fully developed, except for wisdom teeth. The family should be encouraged to eat meals together at least three times a week. These meals are a pleasant time for communication and will model good choices in eating habits, especially as the grandfather is worried about risky behavior tempting his grandson. Research reports that children in families that eat together have decreased risky behaviors (Cook and Dunifon 2012; American Academy of Pediatrics 2009; Samour and King 2005; American Academy of Pediatrics 2014; Hagan et al. 2008; Hockenberry and Wilson 2012; Hammons and Fiese 2011; United States Department of Agriculture 2014).

D. Kramer, *Primary Well-Being: Case Studies for the Growing Child*,
DOI 10.1007/978-3-319-56708-2_24

- **Assess Pat's current stage of psychosocial development and how his family can help him master this stage of social behavior.**

According to Erikson, Pat is in the industry versus inferiority stage of development. He should be encouraged and praised in his schoolwork, participate in teams, and join clubs in his school and community. Pat is still in Freud's latency stage. He has a strong focus on achieving his schoolwork and accomplishing on his teams and clubs that he attends (Dixon and Stein 2006).

Pat is very social at this age. He has two close friends that he does everything with. He is starting to be interested in girls. He interacts respectfully with adults and peers. He likes family members and wants to please them in many ways, and likes to demonstrate affection. He enjoys board games and going to organized groups such as scouting groups or chess club at school.

Pat has also gained mastery over himself and his world. He can make useful articles or do easy repairs. He can groom himself and take responsible care for a pet. The health care provider should advise Pat's grandfather to support Pat in his activities to develop positive self-esteem: asking Pat what he thinks and helping him develop self-confidence. The family should encourage Pat to do regular chores and consider giving him a weekly allowance. This can help foster Pat's need for independence and self-respect.

Pat should be encouraged to join teams and after-school activities at the Native American Community Center serving the community as well as off the reservation (Burns et al. 2009; Dixon and Stein 2006; Hagan et al. 2008; Hockenberry and Wilson 2011; Marcdante et al. 2011; McInerny et al. 2009; Potts and Mandleco 2012).

- **Assess the cognitive development of a child of this age.**

According to Piaget, Pat is in the concrete operation stage. He is in the sixth grade. Pat likes books and writing. He can write brief stories. He uses the phone to call and text family members. He is influenced by the media and peer pressure (Simatwa 2010).

- **Assess community resources that could help Pat and his family with safe activities and age-appropriate guidelines for preventing addictive negative social behaviors such as alcohol and drug use.**

Pat's grandfather is very concerned about preventing addictive negative social behaviors. This is a common concern as children approach puberty. At the same time, Pat still has great respect for his family. This is a good time for the parents and grandfather to talk to Pat about negative social behaviors and their impact on Pat's future. Within Native American culture, there are rituals to draw on to help Pat through this transition to adolescence. One is a retreat to the forest for an individual spiritual experience, usually at age 12 or 13. During this retreat, fasting is used to teach patience and discipline and isolation is used to help the boy have a dream or vision; prayers are offered (Garwick and Auger 2000). Learning his tribe's special ritual dances and other customs is also important. Sharing family meals and spending time together with family as well as being involved in supervised group activities, such as teams and clubs, will help Pat resist tempting negative behaviors.

- **Describe immunization for this age.**

For immunizations at this age, consult the CDC, ACIP, or AAP web sites for the current immunization schedule recommendations (Centers for Disease Control 2011):

- CEC National Immunization Program (NIP): http://www.cdc.gov/vaccines
- American Academy of Pediatrics *Red Book:* http://www.aapredbook.org

- **Mr. Masca is concerned about talking to his grandson about sexual development? What advice would you offer?**

The health care provider should suggest that Mr. Masca talk to Pat about how people's bodies change as they grow up. Pat can start noticing his body changing; his skin may become oilier; he may need to bath daily and use deodorant and wash his face upon awakening and before bedtime. His testicles will begin to grow larger and the penis will become longer and wider. Other changes Pat will notice are that he will get hair under his underarms and pubic area and it will become thicker and curlier over time.

Pat will also have a growth spurt and start to grow taller at a very fast rate. His voice will change as the voice box (larynx) grows longer and his voice will start to crack and deepen.

Pat may experience a wet sticky discharge on his pajama bottoms or bed linen, called wet dreams. This discharge will contain sperm and special fluid caused by hormone surges that occur in Pat's sleep.

Remind Pat that it is never OK for another person to show him their private parts or to ask to touch or view theirs. Pat should go away from those people and tell his parents or grandfather.

A good resource is the booklet for parent and child: American Academy of Pediatrics: *What Happening to my Body?* See http://www.healthychildren.org/English/ages-stages/gradeschool/puberty/Pages/Whats-Happening-to-my-Body.aspx.

The health care provider should talk to the family about any rites of passage that the family is anticipating for their child in the next couple of years.

- **Assess the anticipatory guidance that would be helpful for a child this age.**

General issues for this age are bike safety, wearing helmets, gun safety, bullying, and exercise (Terry 2011).

Substance abuse: Grandfather should talk to Pat about not smoking tobacco or marijuana, using drugs, or drinking alcohol. These substances can diminish the capacity of Pat's lungs and cause cancer. They also alter the neurotransmitters in the brain that enable clear thinking and concentrated functioning and destroy brain cells. If Pat is smoking or using drugs, the health care provider should talk with Pat about getting help for quitting. The grandfather and parents should know who Pat's friends are and how he spends his time with them, and be very clear about his families' expectations regarding not smoking, drinking, or using drugs. Pat's grandfather should praise him for not using these substances and encourage Pat to support friends who also choose not to smoke, or use drugs or alcohol. Pat's grandfather should consider locking the liquor cabinet and putting prescription drugs in a place where Pat cannot get them.

It is important for parents and health care providers to understand that children are constantly being exposed through the media to people smoking and drinking. The clear message by the family should be that any "substance use is substance abuse" (Hagan et al. 2008). They should model good behavior, and if they smoke, they should try to quit. If alcohol is drunk at home, it should be done responsibly and discussed with Pat. Directly ask Pat if any of his friends smoke, drink, or use alcohol or beer, and whether the child will ever do that.

Bicycle safety: This a very real issue at this age as Pat is seeking more independence and is feeling more grown up. The health care provider should review the following rules with Pat and his grandfather: Wear helmets at all times that meet the safety standards of the Consumer Product Safety Commission (www.cpsc.gov) and fit properly. It is important for parents to wear helmets as well to serve as good role models. Pat should know the basic traffic rules and follow them, such as signs/lights. He should be reminded to stop and look both ways at all intersections, ride in single file or on bike paths, and ride in the same direction as traffic. Pat should be sure to tie his shoelaces and not wear any clothing with strings that could get caught in the bike chain. He should not use earphones while riding.

Gun safety: Guns and ammunition need to be stored and locked separately. Pat should be told to never touch a gun, to assume that all guns are loaded and to stay away from them, and to tell his parents if anyone shows him a gun whether a stranger or someone they know.

Bullying: Children of this age can sometimes be the target of bullies. Pat needs to know strategies for dealing with bullying such as strong friendships. Advise Pat that if someone bullies him, he can say to them "you can't talk that way to me" and then leave the situation and go find an adult to tell (Bright Futures undated).

Exercise: Pat should be getting at least 60 min of exercise a day, including sports, running, walking, gymnastics, swimming, and bike riding. Gardening and hunting are also beneficial.

References

American Academy of Pediatrics, Committee on Nutrition (2009) Pediatric nutrition handbook, 6th edn. American Academy of Pediatrics, Elk Grove Village, IL

American Academy of Pediatrics (2014) Healthy active living for families. healthychildren.org/growinghealthy. Accessed 16 Dec 2014

Bright Futures (undated) How to address bullying. Bright Futures Tool for Families. http://www.brightfutures.org/mentalhealth/pdf/families/mc/bullying.pdf

Burns CE et al (2008) Pediatric primary care: a handbook for nurse practitioners, 4th edn. W.B. Saunders, Philadelphia, PA

Centers for Disease Control and Prevention (2011) Recommendations and guidelines: Childhood and adolescent immunization schedules. http://www.cdc.gov/vaccines/schedules/index.html. Accessed 11 Dec 2014

Cook E, Dunifon R (2012) Parenting in context: Do family meals really make a difference? (parenting in context). Cornell University, College of Human Ecology, Ithaca, NY. Accessed 2 Jan 2015. http://www.human.cornell.edu/pam/outreach/upload/Family-Mealtimes-2.pdf

Dixon SD, Stein MT (2006) Encounters with children: pediatric behavior and development, 4th edn. Mosby, St. Louis, MO

Garwick A, Auger S (2000) What do providers need to know about American Indian culture? Recommendations from urban Indian caregivers. Family Syst Health 18:177–189

Hagan JF, Shaw JS, Duncan P (eds) (2008) Bright futures: guidelines for health supervision of infants, children, and adolescents, 3rd edn. American Academy of Pediatrics, Elk Grove Village, IL

Hammons AJ, Fiese BH (2011) Frequency of shared family meals related to the nutritional health of children and adolescents. Pediatrics 127(6):e1565–e1574

Hockenberry MJ, Wilson DW (2011) Wong's nursing care of infants and children, 9th edn. Elsevier/Mosby, New York, NY

Marcdante KJ, Kliegman RM, Jenson HB et al (eds) (2011) Nelson essentials of pediatrics, 6th edn. Saunders, Philadelphia, PA

McInerny TK, Adam HM, Campbell DE, Kamat DM, Kelleher KJ (eds) (2009) Textbook of pediatric care. American Academy of Pediatrics, Elk Grove Village, IL

Potts NL, Mandleco BL (eds) (2012) Pediatric nursing: caring for children and their families, 3rd edn. Delmar Cengage Learning, Clifton Park, NY

Samour PQ, King K (2005) Handbook of pediatric nutrition, 3rd edn. Jones and Bartlett Publishers, Sudbury, MA

Simatwa EMW (2010) Piaget's theory of intellectual development and its implication for instructional management at pre-secondary school level. Educ Res Rev 5(7):366–371. http://www.academicjournals.org/article/article1379610138_Simatwa.pdf. Accessed 2 Jan 2014

Terry EG (2011) Seven- to ten-year visit (school age). In: Richardson B (ed) Pediatric primary care: practice guidelines for nurses. Burlington, MA, Jones & Bartlett Learning

United States Department of Agriculture (2014) Choose My Plate.gov. Daily food plan for preschoolers. http://www.choosemyplate.gov/preschoolers/Plan/. Accessed 31 Dec 2014

25 Eleven-Year Visit

Nancy is a third-generation American and is brought for her annual camp checkup by her mother, Mrs. Jones. Nancy weighs 54 kg (119 pounds); her height is 156.2 cm (61.5 in.), putting her in the 95th percentile for both. Her blood pressure is 107/63. Her BMI is 22.1 putting her in the 93rd percentile. Her tanner stage is 3. Nancy lives in a suburb of a large city with a noted school system and expensive homes. Her parents belong to the local county club and Mrs. Jones is a member of the Junior League. Mrs. Jones is concerned that Nancy is exposed to the wrong children in the community and wants to know more about her friends and what they do together. Mrs. Jones is concerned that Nancy is not spending as much time on her school work as she used to and wants to be out with her friends more often. Nancy also is not doing all her chores lately. Mrs. Jones is proud of how Nancy has become classroom president and headed up a project to collect clothes for the homeless. But she is worried that Nancy sometimes seems disappointed in how difficult it is to organize some activities with her classmates.

- **Is Nancy's height and weight appropriate for her and what physical development can be expected?**

  Nancy weighs 54 kg (119 pounds); her height is 156.2 cm (61.5 in.), putting her in the 95th percentile for both. Her BMI is in the 93rd percentile, which is appropriate for her age. She is in a period of rapidly accelerating growth and her secondary sex characteristics have become evident. At this age she should be eating more dairy, 1200–1500 mg of calcium a day, equivalent to 3–4 servings along with 600 IU daily of vitamin D and some sun exposure. She should also have more iron in her diet from dark green leafy vegetables, meats, and egg yolks. Nancy should be eating three nutritious meals a day and be snacking on healthy foods such as fruits, vegetables, nuts, and low-fat dairy. She should choose foods rich in calcium and iron (American Academy of Pediatrics 2009; Samour and King 2005; American of Pediatrics 2014; Hagan et al. 2008; Hockenberry and Wilson 2011; Cook and Dunifon 2012; Hammons and Fiese 2011; United States Department of Agriculture 2014).

D. Kramer, *Primary Well-Being: Case Studies for the Growing Child*,
DOI 10.1007/978-3-319-56708-2_25

The health care provider should encourage Nancy to maintain a healthy weight through exercise and appropriate eating habits. This will also help reduce stress and may help relieve Nancy's moodiness. Moderate to vigorous exercise for 30–60 min at least three times a week will benefit Nancy during this stressful time.

At this age, girls are often taller than boys because girls have their growth spurt about 6–12 months before menarche and boys have their growth spurt later, after their puberty changes start. At age 11, Nancy is experiencing sweating, and her skin is oily. As part of her secondary sexual development, her breasts have continued to develop and she has pubic hair and axillary hair. Menarche may begin soon for Nancy as she is already at Tanner stage 3 (Terry 2011).

It is important for the health care provider to review the menstrual cycle with Nancy. This should include education regarding self-care and the anticipation of developing womanhood. The provider may decide to do this separately with Nancy first, and then review it when the parent and child are together. This is a sensitive time in the development of the adolescent and a good time to meet alone with the child.

As Nancy goes through the physical changes of early adolescence, she should know that her peers are changing in the same way too, each at their own pace. This may lead to increased self-consciousness and a focus on external characteristics, but reassure Nancy that all girls go through these changes, and that her physical exam findings are normal (Burns et al. 2009; Dixon and Stein 2006; Hagan et al. 2008; Hockenberry and Wilson 2011; Marcdante et al. 2011; McInerny et al. 2009; Potts and Mandleco 2012).

- **Assess Nancy's current stage of psychosocial development and how her parents can help her master this stage.**

As Nancy heads toward her teen years, she will be testing her boundaries with her parents, trying to define her independence and detach yet still wishing to be dependent on them. Mr. and Mrs. Jones will begin to have conflicts with Nancy over her behavior and limit setting. At the same time, Nancy will seek closer ties to her peers to counter the instability she feels caused by rapid changes in her body and her feelings. She will idealize close friendships with her girlfriends and struggle to find her place among her peers.

According to Erikson, Nancy is in the industry versus inferiority stage of development. Socially, Nancy needs to be part of a peer group and she is, as evidenced by being elected class president. Adolescents at this age seek independence; they want to be with friends of their own choosing. Often they will wear t-shirts, hairstyles, and accessories to fit in with peers. Early adolescence is a time of being included in social networks. Nancy will want to hang out with friends in shopping malls, movie theatres, music concerts, and parks. Since young people do not have a driver's license usually until age 16, they depend on public transportation, such as walking, biking, and car rides from family and friends. Mr. and Mrs. Jones need to continue to monitor what Nancy is doing and with whom she is doing it so she remains safe while becoming more independent.

The health care provider should assess how Nancy is developing in her thinking. Is Nancy able to think logically and abstractly? Does she have idealistic thoughts about what she thinks ought to be? She now has many different teachers and many different classes in which there are different children. Sixth grade brings increased expectations in school and course work, and greater social demands of all the different groups of friends in each class. This could be very exciting because Nancy may find she especially likes learning a particular area or topic. But sometimes she will find the increased academic and social expectations difficult. If this is the case, the situation should be discussed with Nancy's teachers, Mr. and Mrs. Jones, and supportive professionals.

As Nancy matures, she is spending more time without adult supervision and may be attracted to risky behaviors with this new freedom. Recent brain research tells us that adolescent brains are still maturing and teens do not always make the best decisions to not engage in alcohol and drugs (Hagan et al. 2008). Being involved in organized and supervised activities will help reduce this risk as well as positive parental dialogue and presence (Resnick et al. 1997; Belcher and Shinitzky 1998).

The health care provider should ask Nancy about friends, family, and school. Does she have a best friend? A supportive adult? Nancy's relationship with her parents is changing. Nancy is seeking independence and having mood swings. She may challenge rules and be argumentative. She will be more dependent at times as well as seeking independence at others. The parenting style that is most successful with adolescents is the "authoritative parent"–one who sets clear boundaries, expresses unconditional love, and offers consistent discipline. Advise Mrs. Jones to identify a consistent caring adult outside the family that Nancy can talk to as her own personal confidant but whom the family can trust as well (Dixon and Stein 2006).

The health care provider can advise the parents that it is normal for Nancy to be preoccupied with rapid bodily changes at this age. Nancy will try out various roles, testing her values and behaviors. She will feel more or less attractive by the acceptance or rejection of her peers; her parents and other adults in her life will need to help her develop her own positive self-image. Nancy may strive to conform to group norms, to obtain a feeling of belonging and self-worth to build her social competence. But Nancy may also experience mood swings and daydreaming. She may show anger outwardly expressed with moodiness, temper outbursts, and verbal insults.

The health care provider should ask Mrs. Jones and Nancy how well they connect as a family and whether they discuss the rules and expectations of their household together. Some families set aside special time each week for family meetings to air these topics. Other issues to discuss as a family include getting to know Nancy's friends, curfew issues, being in charge of an organization at school, and community issues. The family can help Nancy understand that difficult times and disappointments are usually temporary. They should give Nancy ways to cope when she is feeling sad, depressed, nervous, or overwhelmed by her responsibilities and prepare her for what to expect in the future. If any of these challenges continue to be overwhelming to Nancy, the family should seek professional help and guidance.

The health care provider should help her parents anticipate Nancy's need for greater privacy. Nancy's involvement in school activities allows her wider exposure to peers and interests. If Nancy starts being socially isolated, it is a warning sign for depression and should be taken seriously. Mrs. Jones should be advised to monitor Nancy's self-esteem and watch for excessive stress or depression, including signs of social isolation.

According to Freud, Nancy is in the latency period of psychosexual development. She is increasingly exploring her thoughts and feelings. She may begin to date, usually in a group, and experience limited intimacy, such as holding hands and kissing. Her family can help support her through this period with positive praise and open communication. During the health care provider's time alone with Nancy, the provider should ask about any physical, emotional, or sexual abuse.

- **Assess the cognitive development of a child this age.**

As the brain continues to develop into early adulthood, Nancy will begin to transition from concrete to abstract thinking, making variable and inconsistent progress. She may be able to think abstractly about math concepts and other academic subject. Nancy's ability to think abstractly can give her better reasoning but not always better decision making related to her choices when under peer pressure. Nancy will display a better ability to see other points of view.

The health care provider could suggest to Mrs. Jones that she help Nancy organize her time and activities as she has taken on a large leadership role. As schoolwork gets more complex, this is especially important. Ask Mrs. Jones and Nancy about Nancy's school performance—her academic, athletic, and personal goals. Nancy should be encouraged to have responsibilities at home even while participating more in school and the community. She should take on new responsibilities with adult supervision.

Nancy is involved in some extracurricular activities. This is a healthy development. Advise Mrs. Jones to encourage Nancy's involvement in groups that interest her and help Nancy talk through her problems. Mrs. Jones should give Nancy words for her feelings and thoughts. She should offer Nancy different options so she feels independent. Group discussions with her peers will help Nancy learn to express herself. Warn the family about too much screen time that will interfere with communication opportunities with Nancy's peers, family, and other adults. Also point out unhealthy behaviors such as smoking and drinking and abusing drugs (Alvardo and Richardson 2011).

- **How would you address Mrs. Jones' concerns about Nancy's friendships and activism?**

The health care provider should encourage Mr. and Mrs. Jones to get to know Nancy's friends and help her to make good decisions about choosing friends and activities. Nancy should still be supervised by her parents or another responsible adult. The family should spend time every day to talk about different things, including successes and difficulties and making a positive effort, and the importance of school, friendships, and other people in Nancy's life. The parents should reassure Nancy of their love and monitor and guide Nancy as she takes more charge of her school work. Dinner time is a good time of day to have these family discussions.

Nancy may need more help with organizing and setting priorities as she moves through middle school into high school. Her parents should continue to encourage reading books and also help her obtain magazines on subjects that interest her. The health care provider should suggest that Nancy bring a book when she may have to wait somewhere or is in a situation needing patience. With modern technology, a book can be always ready on her cell phone.

- **Describe immunization needs:**

For immunizations at this age, consult the CDC, ACIP, or AAP web sites for the current immunization schedule recommendations (Centers for Disease Control 2011):

- CEC National Immunization Program (NIP): http://www.cdc.gov/vaccines
- American Academy of Pediatrics Red Book: http://www.aapredbook.org

Note that the human papillomavirus (HPV) is for males and females.

- **Assess the anticipatory guidance that would be helpful for a child this age.**

Safety Issues: The health care provider should go over safety issues with Mrs. Jones and Nancy. The teenage years are an era of high rates of unintentional injury leading to disability and often death. Remind Mrs. Jones and Nancy about accident prevention through the use of seat belts, helmets, proper sports equipment, water-safety instruction, and learning CPR. Tell them that firearms should be locked up and ammunition kept in a separate place (Resnick et al. 1997).

Substance Abuse: Talk to Nancy about the dangers of drug use, both ingested and inhaled, and give her strategies to resist negative peer pressure. These include building her own self-esteem and interests, staying away from peers who use drugs, and staying connected to her parents even if they don't agree with her—the parents can help in difficult situations and talk through problems with Nancy (Belcher and Shinitzy 1998).

Dating: Talk to Nancy about being pressured on dates to behave in ways that are not comfortable to her to prevent date rape, such as intimate physical contact. Suggest ways to prevent this, such as going out in groups, not being alone in isolated places, not being together behind a locked door, and doing activities in public that both enjoy. Dating is about respecting each other and being concerned about each other, not about crossing a physical intimacy line. Nancy should be encouraged to speak up to her date that she doesn't want this kind of contact right now; she should call for help if things get dangerous. Mr. and Mrs. Jones should praise her and reinforce this decision with positive and open conversations about this issue and about difficult situations in life. They can also do role-playing to help Nancy feel comfortable with speaking up to her boyfriends about her feelings. Getting to know Nancy's friends and dates will also help.

Depression: It is important to screen Nancy for depression, especially as her school work and activity level have changed recently. She could use some help organizing with her increased volunteerism. She should also be screened in case she is using alcohol or drugs. Nancy could be at risk for suicide due to her extreme stress as class president and being an overachiever. The health care provider should encourage Nancy to call when she needs advice or is seeking information about the changes going on in her life or whenever she feels stressed. The health care provider should always be looking for signs of physical, emotional, and sexual abuse as well.

School: Education is the main focus of Nancy's life now. Mr. and Mrs. Jones should be encouraged to praise Nancy's positive efforts, but also prepare her for the often difficult transition to high school. Nancy may need help with the transition after achieving so much in leadership in middle school and she may need to alter her priorities. Nancy's parents should support her leadership role in after-school activities that interest her.

Sexuality: The health care provider should counsel Nancy to practice sexual abstinence. She should offer accurate information and invite Nancy to call the office for advice/information as needed. The health care provider should reassure Nancy of her privacy when talking to her. Nancy should also be encouraged to have another trusted adult to talk to about sexuality issues. This can include a parent.

Electronic devices/Internet: The health care provider should talk about safe use of the Internet and online social networks. Remind Nancy not to send pictures, especially revealing ones, over the Internet or phone, and to use caution when sharing personal information, photos, videos, and live audio and video chats by Internet and phone.

References

Alvardo MJ, Richardson B (2011) Eleven to thirteen year visit (preadolescent). In: Richardson B (ed) Pediatric primary care: practice guidelines for nurses. Jones & Bartlett Learning, Burlington, MA

American Academy of Pediatrics, Committee on Nutrition (2009) Pediatric nutrition handbook, 6th edn. American Academy of Pediatrics, Elk Grove Village, IL

American Academy of Pediatrics (2014) Healthy active living for families. healthychildren.org/growinghealthy. Accessed 16 Dec 2014

Belcher HM, Shinitzky HE (1998) Substance abuse in children: prediction, protection, and prevention. Arch Pediatr Adolesc Med 152(10):952–960

Burns CE et al (2009) Pediatric primary care: a handbook for nurse practitioners, 4th edn. W.B. Saunders, Philadelphia, PA

Centers for Disease Control and Prevention (2011) Recommendations and guidelines: childhood and adolescent immunization schedules. http://www.cdc.gov/vaccines/schedules/index.html. Accessed 11 Dec 2014

Cook E, Dunifon R (2012) Parenting in context: do family meals really make a difference? (parenting in context). Cornell University, College of Human Ecology, Ithaca, NY. http://www.human.cornell.edu/pam/outreach/upload/Family-Mealtimes-2.pdf. Accessed 2 Jan 2015

Dixon SD, Stein MT (2006) Encounters with children: pediatric behavior and development, 4th edn. Mosby, St. Louis, MO

Hagan JF, Shaw JS, Duncan P (eds) (2008) Bright futures: guidelines for health supervision of infants, children, and adolescents, 3rd edn. American Academy of Pediatrics, Elk Grove Village, IL

Hammons AJ, Fiese BH (2011) Frequency of shared family meals related to the nutritional health of children and adolescents. Pediatrics 127(6):e1565–e1574

Hockenberry MJ, Wilson DW (2011) Wong's nursing care of infants and children, 9th edn. Elsevier/Mosby, New York, NY

Marcdante KJ, Kliegman RM, Jenson HB et al (eds) (2011) Nelson essentials of pediatrics, 6th edn. Saunders, Philadelphia, PA

McInerny TK, Adam HM, Campbell DE, Kamat DM, Kelleher KJ (eds) (2009) Textbook of pediatric care. American Academy of Pediatrics, Elk Grove Village, IL

Potts NL, Mandleco BL (eds) (2012) Pediatric nursing: caring for children and their families, 3rd edn. Delmar Cengage Learning, Clifton Park, NY

Resnick MD, Bearman PS, Blum RW et al (1997) Protecting adolescents from harm. Findings from the National Longitudinal Study on Adolescent Health. JAMA 278(1):823–832

Samour PQ, King K (2005) Handbook of pediatric nutrition, 3rd edn. Jones and Bartlett Publishers, Sudbury, MA

Simatwa EMW (2010) Piaget's theory of intellectual development and its implication for instructional management at pre-secondary school level. Educ Res Rev 5(7):366–371. http://www.academicjournals.org/article/article1379610138_Simatwa.pdf. Accessed 2 Jan 2014

Terry EG (2011) Seven- to ten-year visit (school age). In: Richardson B (ed) Pediatric primary care: practice guidelines for nurses. Burlington, MA, Jones & Bartlett Learning

United States Department of Agriculture (2014) Choose My Plate.gov. Daily food plan for preschoolers. http://www.choosemyplate.gov/preschoolers/Plan/. Accessed 31 Dec 2014

Twelve-Year Visit

26

Charles is a young man of communion age whose family belongs to the Church of the Angels. He comes to the pediatric clinic for his school checkup with his parents, Mr. and Mrs. Iglesias. His parents came from the Dominican Republic before he was born and his father runs a small electronics store. They are proud of how well Charles does in school. Charles weighs 39.78 kg (87.85 pounds) and stands 149.7 cm tall (59 in.), representing the 50th percentile for weight and height; his BMI is 17.8 (52nd percentile). His blood pressure is 106/62. His tanner stage is 2. Mrs. Iglesias is worried that Charles is filling up on junk food. His parochial school has dances for his grade and Charles is concerned that the girl he wants to ask to the dance will not go with him and also that his parents want to chaperone him. Charles will have his communion at the church in a few months and his parents are worried that he is not spending enough time preparing for it, preferring to watch television and play games on the Internet.

- **Is Charles's height and weight appropriate for him?**

Yes, they are both on the 50th percentile. But Charles is filling up on junk food. He needs to be reminded about good nutrition and his family should be referred to http://www.choosemyplate.gov/kids/index.html for specific guidelines to encourage good nutrition. The health care provider can remind the Iglesias that the way to manage weight is through healthy eating and physical activity and that parents are still the best role models for their children despite peer pressures. During the adolescent years, much of the child's diet includes irregular eating patterns and one-fourth of the daily caloric intact is often eaten through snacks. However, the health care provider should still screen Charles for a potential eating disorder, especially if Charles' weight has changed recently or if another family member has had an eating disorder. Symptoms may include new restrictive food patterns, eating fewer meals, taking smaller portion sizes, preoccupation with body appearance, and preoccupation with exercise. The health care provider can ask the parents questions pertaining to these symptoms (Rosen 2010; Cotton et al. 2003; DeSocio et al. 2007).

D. Kramer, *Primary Well-Being: Case Studies for the Growing Child*,
DOI 10.1007/978-3-319-56708-2_26

The health care provider should talk to the Iglesias and Charles about supporting a healthy weight—the balance between a healthy diet and physical activity—and a healthy self-image, by commenting positively on things Charles does rather than his physical appearance. Research has supported that eating together as a family helps children choose healthier foods (Cook and Dunifon 2012).

Charles needs 1300 milligrams of calcium. He is about to go through another growth spurt. Good sources of calcium are low-fat milk, yogurt, cheese, dark green leafy vegetables, cooked dried beans, and canned salmon. Some foods are fortified with calcium (American Academy of Pediatrics 2009; Samour and King 2005; American of Pediatrics 2014; Hagan et al. 2008; Hockenberry and Wilson 2012; Cook and Dunifon 2012; Hammons and Fiese 2011; United States Department of Agriculture 2014).

The health care provider should remind the family that a healthy diet includes lots of fruits and vegetables of varying colors, three or more servings of dairy products, whole grain cereals or breads, and foods with protein and iron like fish, chicken, and lean meats. Charlie should limit high-fat or low-nutrient foods such as candy, chips, and sodas. Easy-to-take nutritious snacks should always be in the refrigerator such as carrot and celery sticks, cucumbers, peanut or other nut butter spreads, cheese sticks, and bean spreads. These can also be taken to school. Also Charles should drink plenty of water and limit fruit juice and sugared beverage intake (Burns et al. 2009; Dixon and Stein 2006; Hagan et al. 2008; Hockenberry and Wilson 2011; Marcdante et al. 2011; McInerny et al. 2009; Potts and Mandleco 2012). For further food and nutrition ideas, refer the family to http://www.choosemyplate.gov/kids/index.html.

- **Assess Charles's current stage of psychosocial development and how his parents can help him master this stage.**

According to Erikson, Charles is in the identity versus role confusion stage of development. In this stage, Charles is developing a sense of self and will be planning for his future work and education. While participating in sports, teams, and clubs is important, cementing Charles' identity is key to successfully completing this stage (Dixon and Stein 2006).

Mr. and Mrs. Iglesias should show Charlie their concerns about Charlie's social life. They need to work together to give Charlie the ability to solve problems, make good decisions, and cope with stress as he moves through adolescence. Perhaps they can role play together about asking the girl to the dance and practice different responses to potential answers. Ask Mr. Iglesias whether he thinks Charles worries too much or seems overly anxious and to think about how he helps Charlie cope with stress, make decisions, and solve problems.

The health care provider should ask Charlie, "Do you worry a lot or feel overly stressed out? How do you cope with stress?" The family should involve Charlie in family decision making as appropriate so he has experience in problem solving. They should ask Charlie to help think through solutions and brainstorm together rather than giving the answers to Charlie. This will help boost Charles' self-esteem.

The health care provider and Mr. and Mrs. Iglesias can reassure Charles that all people have stress at some point in their lives, from daily school deadlines to occasional friendship blowups. It is important for Charles to figure out himself how to deal with daily stress in ways that work for him. The health care provider can say to Charles: "If you would like some help with this, I would be happy to give you some ideas." The health care provider should be asking Charles how he feels about his upcoming communion, what extra stress it may be placing on him, and talk together with his family about reducing the stress.

The health care provider would want to ask Charles if he is feeling bored or sad and whether he had any difficulty sleeping. Does he find conflicts between his parents and their culture and what his friends are doing? Everyone has a hard time some times, but usually they are able to continue to do well in school and keep up with friends and family. Sometimes, people feel too sad, nervous, hopeless, or angry. If Charles feels that way, it is important that he speak to the health expert, his parent, or another adult. Ask Charles if he ever feels so upset that he wishes he weren't alive or if he keeps remembering something that is unpleasant. These are suicide warnings and should be taken very seriously.

Advise Mr. and Mrs. Iglesias to keep Charles' television viewing, computer time, and video games to less than 2 h per day. These activities interfere with opportunities to engage in social activities and communication with peers and family.

Charlie is at home much of the time. He may be watching television so much out of boredom or depression. Worsening academic performance may be one sign of depression. Stress and conflicts with his parents, especially over cultural issues, may also be a factor. The health care provider will want to make sure that Charles is not depressed and explore with him the options for spending his time, including outside with friends, on a sports team, at after-school recreation, and pursuing an interest such as taking music lessons.

- **Assess Charles' moral development and its consequences for adolescence.**

Adolescents in the early teen years are in the conventional level of moral reasoning according to Kohlberg (Kohlberg and Gilligan 1972). Charles will have moral standards that are governed by concrete rules of what is right and wrong. These behaviors are used to gain the approval of parents and teachers by demonstrating that he upholds and respects the social order.

- **Assess the cognitive development of a child this age.**

According to Piaget, Charles is in the formal operations stage. Charles is beginning to think abstractly. He can think about possibilities and formulate a hypothesis. This is important in helping to support Charles in being able to plan for the future and understanding the consequences of behaviors such as healthy eating, substance abuse, doing well in school, and finding areas of interest. The health care provider should suggest to Charles' parents that they engage him in discussing ideas for his communion and any other aspects of daily life that Charles is involved in with them to acknowledge his cognitive growth and maturing decision-making abilities (Simatwa 2010).

- **Assess the social behaviors that Charles may exhibit at this age and any cultural issues.**

Charles should be increasingly spending time with his friends and peers instead of his parents. As he works toward an independent identity, Charles may experience cultural tensions with his parents, especially his striving for independence and his greater connection to the general American culture. He may speak English better than his parents and be embarrassed by their accents. The family's church and parochial school community are clearly important to them and will be resources for helping guide Charles to other safe and appropriate community agencies to spur his independence in a protected environment (Alvardo and Richardson 2011).

- **Describe immunization needs.**

For immunizations at this age, consult the CDC, ACIP, or AAP web sites for the current immunization schedule recommendations (Centers for Disease Control 2011):

- CEC National Immunization Program (NIP): http://www.cdc.gov/vaccines
- American Academy of Pediatrics *Red Book:* http://www.aapredbook.org

- **Assess the anticipatory guidance that would be helpful for a child this age.**

See **General Safety & Hygiene** box (page 115) and guidance for the 11-Year-Old Visit for topics to cover in anticipatory guidance. Also review Adolescent Section of Physical Exam chapter above. Below are a few highlights to cover.

Safety: Remind Mr. and Mrs. Iglesias and Charles about using appropriate safety equipment and measures and getting plenty of physical activity for at least 1 h a day total.

Screen time: Suggest that Charles cut back on screen time to less than 2 h a day aside from school work.

References

Alvardo MJ, Richardson B (2011) Eleven to thirteen year visit (preadolescent). In: Richardson B (ed) Pediatric primary care: practice guidelines for nurses. Burlington, MA, Jones & Bartlett Learning

American Academy of Pediatrics, Committee on Nutrition (2009) Pediatric nutrition handbook, 6th edn. American Academy of Pediatrics, Elk Grove Village, IL

American Academy of Pediatrics (2014) Healthy active living for families. healthychildren.org/growinghealthy. Accessed 16 Dec 2014

Burns CE et al (2009) Pediatric primary care: a handbook for nurse practitioners, 4th edn. W.B. Saunders, Philadelphia, PA

Centers for Disease Control and Prevention (2011) Recommendations and guidelines: Childhood and adolescent immunization schedules. http://www.cdc.gov/vaccines/schedules/index.html. Accessed 11 Dec 2014

Cook E, Dunifon R (2012) Parenting in context: do family meals really make a difference? (Parenting in context). Cornell University, College of Human Ecology, Ithaca, NY. http://www.human.cornell.edu/pam/outreach/upload/Family-Mealtimes-2.pdf. Accessed 2 Jan 2015

Cotton MA, Ball C, Robinson P (2003) Four simple questions can help screen for eating disorders. J Gen Intern Med 18(1):53–56

DeSocio JE, O'Toole JK, Memirow SJ et al (2007) Screening for childhood eating disorders in primary care. Prim Care Companion J Clin Psychiatry 9(1):16–20

Dixon SD, Stein MT (2006) Encounters with children: pediatric behavior and development, 4th edn. Mosby, St. Louis, MO

Hagan JF, Shaw JS, Duncan P (eds) (2008) Bright futures: guidelines for health supervision of infants, children, and adolescents, 3rd edn. American Academy of Pediatrics, Elk Grove Village, IL

Hammons AJ, Fiese BH (2011) Frequency of shard family meals related to the nutritional health of children and adolescents. Pediatrics 127(6):1565–1154

Hockenberry MJ, Wilson DW (2011) Wong's nursing care of infants and children, 9th edn. Elsevier/Mosby, New York, NY

Kohlberg L, Gilligan C (1972) The adolescent as a philosopher: the discovery of the self in a post-conventional world. In: Kagan J, Coles R (eds) 12 to 16: early adolescence. Norton, New York, NY, pp 148–155

Marcdante KJ, Kliegman RM, Jenson HB et al (eds) (2011) Nelson essentials of pediatrics, 6th edn. Saunders, Philadelphia, PA

McInerny TK, Adam HM, Campbell DE, Kamat DM, Kelleher KJ (eds) (2009) Textbook of pediatric care. American Academy of Pediatrics, Elk Grove Village, IL

Potts NL, Mandleco BL (eds) (2012) Pediatric nursing: caring for children and their families, 3rd edn. Delmar Cengage Learning, Clifton Park, NY

Rosen DS (2010) Clinical report: identification and management of eating disorders in children and adolescents. Pediatrics 111(1):204

Samour PQ, King K (2005) Handbook of pediatric nutrition, 3rd edn. Jones and Bartlett Publishers, Sudbury, MA

Simatwa EMW (2010) Piaget's theory of intellectual development and its implication for instructional management at pre-secondary school level. Educ Res Rev 5(7):366–371. http://www.academicjournals.org/article/article1379610138_Simatwa.pdf. Accessed 2 Jan 2014

United States Department of Agriculture (2014) Choose My Plate.gov. Daily food plan for preschoolers. http://www.choosemyplate.gov/preschoolers/Plan/. Accessed 31 Dec 2014

Thirteen-Year Visit

27

David is brought into the clinic for his school checkup by his mother, Mrs. Horowitz. They live in a bustling section of a big city in a community with many resources that meet their religious and cultural needs. David weighs 29.85 kilo (65.75 pounds) and stands 137.6 cm tall (54.25 in.) and is in the 5th percentile. His BMI is 15.8, which is in the 7th percentile. His blood pressure is 101/59. His tanner stage is 2. David has told his mother that he is embarrassed about being shorter than the girls as his bar mitzvah is approaching. He is also nervous about performing the readings in the temple in their community in front of friends and relatives and the big party afterward to celebrate. David is a quiet young man and is looking forward to his party. He has carefully selected the activities that he and his friends will be playing with the DJ and is concerned that some of his school friends might be disappointed in the kosher food that will be served.

- **Is David's height and weight appropriate for him?**

  David is in the 5th percentile for height and weight and the 7th for body mass. At this age most girls have already had their growth spurt. Boys do not have their growth spurt until after puberty, which for boys is usually between ages 15 and 19. The health care provider should explain to David that boys' and girls' bodies change at different times, with girls changing earlier than boys. He should continue eating a healthy diet and avoid foods high in fat and low in nutrition (American Academy of Pediatrics, Committee on Nutrition 2009; Samour and King 2005; American Academy of Pediatrics 2014; Hagan et al. 2008; Hockenberry and Wilson 2011; Cook and Dunifon 2012; Hammons and Fiese 2011; United States Department of Agriculture 2014).

- **Assess David's current stage of psychosocial development and how his parents can help him master this stage.**

  According to Erikson this stage is identity versus role confusion. Adolescents are usually trying to figure out their identity in the world, who they are and what kind of person they will be. David's parents have helped to encourage independence by

D. Kramer, *Primary Well-Being: Case Studies for the Growing Child*,
DOI 10.1007/978-3-319-56708-2_27

letting him plan activities for his special day. They should talk to him about what he is thinking and feeling and praise him for the decision-making process he is going through and trying to balance his cultural family with his social environment. The health practitioner should tell David that this is a good time to think about what interests him and makes him happy. It is a time of making friends and keeping them. At the same time it is important to stay connected to family members. David's relationship with his family, his Rabbi, his teachers, and his peers are all impacting his sense of self. Especially at this time of his Bar Mitzvah, he is exploring the cultural expectations of his home and his peers in society. Having positive cultural connections and strong family support and understanding will help foster a healthy sense of identity in David and help him bridge his Jewish cultural and social worlds. The interactions David has with the different people in his life and the success and achievement he has socially is what will help foster his development into a self-confident adult (Dixon and Stein 2006).

- **Assess the cognitive development of a child this age.**

  David is in Piaget's formal operations stage. David can solve hypothetical problems and use scientific reasoning. This is a good age for David to talk things out and use his reason, and to discover his own opinions and thoughts about the world. David will also be exploring his relationships to other people and how to think about and respond to different situations that arise. He will be looking at the different role models in his life and the competing pressures between his family values and those of his peers. He will begin to think about what he wants to believe and how he will behave (Simatwa 2010).

- **Assess the social behaviors that David may exhibit at this age.**

  David will want to be with groups of friends at this age. His focus will be on friends, social networks, school performance, and team performance. He may spend more time with boys in groups than girls. According to Kohlberg, David is at the postconventional level. Morally, he wants to follow the rules of society and be good to all people. He will see taking care of himself as a part of adult standard behavior and want to be responsible for himself. The health care provider should encourage David to take on new responsibilities at home, school, and in the community. In David's spiritual community, these obligations are traditional with the celebration of his Bar Mitzvah and part of the passage to manhood. David will want to choose volunteer opportunities that appeal to him as part of this process.

- **Assess community resources that could help David and his family with safe activities and age-appropriate guidelines for independence.**

  David and his parents will want to seek out their local religious institution and communal leaders, including their spiritual leader, for guidance, as well as other communal facilities and appropriate activities. The general community will also have organized activities, such as boys clubs, scouting, and sport networks that can benefit David.

- **Assess dental needs for this age.**
  This is the age when David should be assessed by his dentist for orthodontia needs. Hopefully David has been going to the dentist twice a year as recommended by the American Dental Association and the American Academy of Pediatrics. He should be brushing and flossing his teeth twice a day after meals and before bedtime (Casamassimo and Hold 2014; Centers for Disease Control and Prevention 2001). For guidelines on oral health, see *Bright Futures in Practice: Oral Health, pocket guide* by Paul Casamassimo and Katrina Hold, Ed., Washington, DC: National Maternal and Child Oral Health Resource Center, Georgetown University.

- **Describe immunization and dental needs for this age.**
  For immunizations at this age, consult the CDC, ACIP, or AAP web sites for the current immunization schedule recommendations (Centers for Disease Control 2011):

– CEC National Immunization Program (NIP): http://www.cdc.gov/vaccines
– American Academy of Pediatrics Red Book: http://www.aapredbook.org

- **Mr. and Mrs. Horowitz are concerned about David' social life and self-image. What is David's psychosexual stage? What advice would you offer? How would you talk to David and his parents about their concerns about his Bar Mitzvah?**
  David is in Freud's genital stage of development and will be exploring relationships. David is at the age where he enjoys being in groups; however he is working on finding his own identity. A Bar Mitzvah is a rite of passage ceremony for a Jewish male in which a young man takes on religious responsibilities as an adult and is publically acknowledged by his family and community. David will have increased value among his peers after this ceremony. David will feel more confident if he can select the foods and participate in planning the event with his parents. He knows what his friends will like. The health care provider should encourage David and his parents to work together on planning his Bar Mitzvah and preference should be given as much as possible to David's desires for this special day. Specific restrictions due to finances, family issues, and other limits should be discussed with David so he can understand why everything he wants may not be possible. By the parents making David a full partner in the planning process, they are showing David he is becoming an adult in their eyes. This will enhance his self-image of being responsible and competent.

- **Assess the anticipatory guidance that would be helpful for a child this age.**
  David is at the cusp of adolescent development. This is a time of changing emotions and unpredictable behavior. David may at times be extra sensitive to others behavior or perceive a different message than what was meant by his parents and friends. The health care provider should point out to the parents that David is going

to develop greater independence from them and his family and may go back and forth on being dependent or independent. His friends will become very important and he will show a strong need to belong to the group.

The health care provider should advise Mr. and Mrs. Horowitz to accept David as a unique individual and respect his ideas, inclinations, dislikes and desires. They should be involved with David's school and attend activities and events that he participates in. They should listen respectfully to David's ideas even when they differ from theirs and avoid criticizing David, especially on no-win issues. This is a time when David will be learning by being allowed to choose options and accept the natural consequences of his own choices, even when the choices are not ones his parents would make. David may test authority at home and school. Having a consistent, caring adult who he feels comfortable communicating with will help David get through this period of development.

The health care provider should emphasize to David and his parents the value of clear house rules and what happens when they are broken. Outside the home, the rules of society and natural consequences will also teach David about responsibility. The parents should always keep the channels of communication open and while allowing increasing independence, keep within the limits of safety and stability for David. His privacy should be respected, but the parents should try to sense, share and respond to his feelings and statements, and be generally available for questions, information and companionship. The parents should avoid comparing David to others in the family, and welcome his friends. When parents realize they made a mistake, they should apologize (Burns et al. 2009; Dixon and Stein 2006; Hagan et al. 2008; Hockenberry and Wilson 2011; Marcdante et al. 2011; McInerny et al. 2009; Potts and Mandleco 2012; Alvardo and Richardson 2011).

Also review guidance given to 12-year-old above and give David a copy of the fact sheet: *Bright Futures Patient Handout Early Adolescent Visit*. (2010). https://brightfutures.aap.org/pdfs/Visit%20Forms%20by%20Age%20110/11-14%20Year/D.Adol.PATH.EA.pdf

David's parents can be given the fact sheet: *Bright Futures Parent Early Adolescent Visits*. (2010). https://brightfutures.aap.org/pdfs/Visit%20Forms%20by%20Age%20110/11-14%20Year/D.Adol.PH.EA.pdf

References

Alvardo MJ, Richardson B (2011) Eleven to thirteen year visit (preadolescent). In: Richardson B (ed) Pediatric primary care: practice guidelines for nurses. Burlington, MA, Jones & Bartlett Learning

American Academy of Pediatrics, Committee on Nutrition (2009) Pediatric nutrition handbook, 6th edn. American Academy of Pediatrics, Elk Grove Village, IL

American Academy of Pediatrics (2010a) Bright Futures patient handout early adolescent visits. https://brightfutures.aap.org/pdfs/Visit%20Forms%20by%20Age%20110/11-14%20Year/D.Adol.PATH.EA.pdf. Accessed 15 Jan 2015

American Academy of Pediatrics (2010b) Bright Futures parent handout early adolescent visits. https://brightfutures.aap.org/pdfs/Visit%20Forms%20by%20Age%20110/11-14%20Year/D.Adol.PH.EA.pdf. Accessed 15 Jan 2015

American Academy of Pediatrics (2014) Healthy active living for families. healthychildren.org/growinghealthy. Accessed 16 Dec 2014

Burns CE et al (2009) Pediatric primary care: a handbook for nurse practitioners, 4th edn. W.B. Saunders, Philadelphia, PA

Casamassimo P, Hold K (2014) Bright futures in practice: oral health, pocket guide, 2nd edn. National Maternal and Child Oral Health Resource Center, Georgetown University, Washington, DC. http://www.mchoralhealth.org/pocket.html. Accessed 18 Dec 2014

Centers for Disease Control and Prevention (2001) Recommendations for using fluoride to prevent and control dental caries in the United States. Morb Mortal Wkly Rep 50(RR-14):1–42

Centers for Disease Control and Prevention (2011) Recommendations and guidelines: Childhood and adolescent immunization schedules. http://www.cdc.gov/vaccines/schedules/index.html. Accessed 11 Dec 2014

Cook E, Dunifon R (2012) Parenting in context: do family meals really make a difference? (parenting in context). Cornell University, College of Human Ecology, Ithaca, NY. http://www.human.cornell.edu/pam/outreach/upload/Family-Mealtimes-2.pdf. Accessed 2 Jan 2015

Dixon SD, Stein MT (2006) Encounters with children: pediatric behavior and development, 4th edn. Mosby, St. Louis, MO

Hagan JF, Shaw JS, Duncan P (eds) (2008) Bright futures: guidelines for health supervision of infants, children, and adolescents, 3rd edn. American Academy of Pediatrics, Elk Grove Village, IL

Hammons AJ, Fiese BH (2011) Frequency of shared family meals related to the nutritional health of children and adolescents. Pediatrics 127(6):e1565–e1574

Hockenberry MJ, Wilson DW (2011) Wong's nursing care of infants and children, 9th edn. Elsevier/Mosby, New York, NY

Marcdante KJ, Kliegman RM, Jenson HB et al (eds) (2011) Nelson essentials of pediatrics, 6th edn. Saunders, Philadelphia, PA

McInerny TK, Adam HM, Campbell DE, Kamat DM, Kelleher KJ (eds) (2009) Textbook of pediatric care. American Academy of Pediatrics, Elk Grove Village, IL

Potts NL, Mandleco BL (eds) (2012) Pediatric nursing: caring for children and their families, 3rd edn. Delmar Cengage Learning, Clifton Park, NY

Samour PQ, King K (2005) Handbook of pediatric nutrition, 3rd edn. Jones and Bartlett Publishers, Sudbury, MA

Simatwa EMW (2010) Piaget's theory of intellectual development and its implication for instructional management at pre-secondary school level. Educ Res Rev 5(7):366–371. http://www.academicjournals.org/article/article1379610138_Simatwa.pdf. Accessed 2 Jan 2014

United States Department of Agriculture (2014) Choose My Plate.gov. Daily food plan for preschoolers. http://www.choosemyplate.gov/preschoolers/Plan/. Accessed 31 Dec 2014

28 Fourteen-Year Visit

Reimi Maki is brought to the pediatric clinic by her mother for her school checkup. Reimi weighs 37.76 kilo (83.25 pounds), and stands 148.7 cm tall (58.5 in.), putting her in the 5th percentile. Her BMI is 17.1, or the 12th percentile for BMI. Her blood pressure is 106/63. Her tanner stage is 3. Her mother was born in Japan but the family moved to the USA when Mrs. Maki was 4. They live in a major city where Japanese food and supplies are available. Mrs. Maki has become aware of some disturbing issues in Reimi's school such as use of pornography and teen suicides. She sees that Reimi is not sharing as much information about her activities with her mother as she used to. Mrs. Maki believes in strict control of her daughter at this age and is disturbed by the pressures from school friends. Reimi has many responsibilities besides her school work. She is expected to practice her violin for an hour every evening and to study her parent's language in addition to another language in school.

- **Is Reimi's height and weight appropriate for her?**

  Reimi is in the 5th percentile for weight and height, which is within normal limits for this age. She eats a balanced diet with small portions and enjoys sitting with her family during meals. The family eats a mostly traditional Japanese diet with lots of soy, rice, fish, and vegetables. They eat healthy snacks such as nuts and fruits (Samour and King 2005; American Academy of Pediatrics 2014; Hagan et al. 2008; Hockenberry and Wilson 2011; United States Department of Agriculture 2014; Cook and Dunifon 2012; Hammons and Fiese 2011).

- **Assess Reimi's current stage of psychosocial development and how her parents can help her master this stage.**

  According to Erikson Reimi is in the identity versus role confusion stage. Adolescents are trying to figure out their identity in the world. This is an age that is vulnerable to suicidal ideation. The health care provider should talk to Mrs. Maki about how to create an environment to help protect Reimi from suicide. Positive

D. Kramer, *Primary Well-Being: Case Studies for the Growing Child*,
DOI 10.1007/978-3-319-56708-2_28

steps include creating a warm and caring family environment, building Reimi's self-esteem and confidence, fostering her social and problem-solving skills, and allowing her to participate in decision making by offering choices and seeking out her ideas. It's wonderful that Reimi's family has high expectations but they need to be realistic. The parents need to demonstrate to Reimi that they care about her and her feelings. Reimi seems to have a supportive cultural group with her language lessons and is dedicated to her violin practice. She also needs time for nurturing friendships and to feel that her family respects her as an individual.

The parents should try to help Reimi to work through disappointments and give her skills to cope with frustration and negative feelings. They should make time to listen to her and to celebrate the good things with Reimi and try to have a supportive relationship with her (Burns et al. 2009; Dixon and Stein 2006; Hagan et al. 2008; Hockenberry and Wilson 2011; Marcdante et al. 2011; McInerny et al. 2009; Potts and Mandleco 2012; Alvardo and Richardson 2011).

- **Assess the social behaviors that Reimi may exhibit at this age. Mrs. Maki is concerned about Reimi's friends and shifting attention away from her parents' guidance. How should she talk to her daughter about her changing attitudes. What advice would you offer?**

Reimi wants to get together with her peers and be in a group. She is very responsible. She takes responsibility for getting her homework done and to school on time. She also practices her violin and studies her parent's native language in addition to school studies. It is important parents to discuss with her that everyone has stresses, deadlines, and difficulties. It is important for Reimi and her family to recognize when she is feeling stressed and to help her figure out how to deal with it in the best way that works for her. If the stress becomes overwhelming for Reimi or is impacting her in other areas, she should seek professional guidance or be taken to a professional counselor by her parents.

The health care provider can remind Mrs. Maki to provide opportunities for Reimi to socialize with her peers. Discuss with the family when would be the best time to do that. Point out to Mrs. Maki the importance of helping Reimi to incorporate peer time with her violin and language studies schedule.

- **Describe immunization needs for this age**

For immunizations at this age, consult the CDC, ACIP, or AAP web sites for the current immunization schedule recommendations (Centers for Disease Control and Prevention 2011):

- CEC National Immunization Program (NIP): http://www.cdc.gov/vaccines
- American Academy of Pediatrics *Red Book:* http://www.aapredbook.org

- **How would you talk to Reimi and Mrs. Maki about concerns of pornography and suicide in her peers?**

Both Mr. and Mrs. Maki need to talk with Reimi about what Reimi should do when asked to do unusual things with friends or strangers. For example if she is on the Internet and is asked to turn on her web cam by someone she doesn't usually Skype with or have face-to-face computer time, Reimi should refuse and tell her parents or a trusted adult. Similarly, if she is asked to allow someone else's computer to enter hers, she should reject the offer (American Academy of Pediatrics 2013; American Academy of Pediatrics 2006; Joffe and Blythe 2009; Neinstein 2007).

Mrs. Maki should talk to Reimi about her use of technology and get familiar with it herself. For example, open a Facebook profile if Reimi has one. Telling Reimi about her own daily use of the social media is a good way for Mrs. Maki to start a daily conversation about Reimi's online habits. Mrs. Maki should tell Reimi that she writes on Facebook is public to everyone. Reimi needs to use discretion in what she posts to her Facebook page. Mrs. Maki can ask Reimi if anyone has sent any disturbing chats or statements to her.

Mrs. Maki can emphasize that everything sent over the Internet or a cell phone can be shared with the entire world. Good judgment is important in sending messages and pictures. The parent can discuss what good judgment is with Reimi and the possible consequences of poor judgment (minor punishment to legal action for sexting and bullying). Mrs. Maki can help Reimi set privacy settings on social media sites appropriately.

The health care provider and Mr. and Mrs. Maki can talk to Reimi about the dangers of Chat rooms, bullying and sexting. It is helpful to keep the computer in a public part of the Maki household, such as the family room or kitchen, so Mrs. Maki can check on what Reimi is doing on line and how much time she spends. The Maki's can also talk to other parents in Reimi's class about their children's use of social media.

For more guidelines on using social media and adolescence, see American Academy of Pediatrics. *Talking to kids and teens about social media and sexting*. http://www.aap.org/en-us/about-the-aap/aap-press-room/news-features-and-safety-tips/pages/Talking-to-Kids-and-Teens-About-Social-Media-and-Sexting.aspx#sthash.Vi05nMhk.dpuf. Updated May 31, 2013.

Also check for legal guidelines in your state regarding Internet access and use for teenagers. The health care provider can offer Reimi an opportunity to meet alone without her parents present and go over some of these sensitive issues from Reimi's point of view.

References

Alvardo MJ, Richardson B (2011) Fourteen to seventeen year visit (adolescent). In: Richardson B (ed) Pediatric primary care: practice guidelines for nurses. Jones & Bartlett Learning, Burlington, MA

American Academy of Pediatrics (2014) Healthy active living for families. healthychildren.org/growinghealthy. Accessed 16 Dec 2014

American Academy of Pediatrics (2013) Talking to kids and teens about social media and sexting, updated ed. http://www.aap.org/en-us/about-the-aap/aap-press-room/news-features-and-safety-tips/pages/Talking-to-Kids-and-Teens-About-Social-Media-and-Sexting.aspx#sthash.Vi05nMhk.dpuf. Accessed 15 Jan 2015

American Academy of Pediatrics (2006) The teen driver. Pediatrics 126(2):404

Burns CE et al (2009) Pediatric primary care: a handbook for nurse practitioners, 4th edn. W.B. Saunders, Philadelphia, PA

Centers for Disease Control and Prevention (2011) Recommendations and guidelines: Childhood and adolescent immunization schedules. http://www.cdc.gov/vaccines/schedules/index.html. Accessed 11 Dec 2014

Cook E, Dunifon R (2012) Parenting in context: do family meals really make a difference? (Parenting in context). Cornell University, College of Human Ecology, Ithaca, NY. http://www.human.cornell.edu/pam/outreach/upload/Family-Mealtimes-2.pdf. Accessed 2 Jan 2015

Dixon SD, Stein MT (2006) Encounters with children: pediatric behavior and development, 4th edn. Mosby, St. Louis, MO

Hagan JF, Shaw JS, Duncan P (eds) (2008) Bright futures: guidelines for health supervision of infants, children, and adolescents, 3rd edn. Elk Grove Village, IL, American Academy of Pediatrics

Hammons AJ, Fiese BH (2011) Frequency of shared family meals related to the nutritional health of children and adolescents. Pediatrics 127(6):e1565–e1574

Hockenberry MJ, Wilson DW (2011) Wong's nursing care of infants and children, 9th edn. Elsevier/Mosby, New York, NY

Joffe A, Blythe MJ (eds) (2009) Handbook of adolescent medicine. Hanley and Belfus, Philadelphia, PA

Marcdante KJ, Kliegman RM, Jenson HB et al (eds) (2011) Nelson essentials of pediatrics, 6th edn. Saunders, Philadelphia, PA

McInerny TK, Adam HM, Campbell DE, Kamat DM, Kelleher KJ (eds) (2009) Textbook of pediatric care. American Academy of Pediatrics, Elk Grove Village, IL

Neinstein L (2007) Adolescent health care: a practical guide, 5th edn. Lippincott Williams & Wilkins, Baltimore, MD

Potts NL, Mandleco BL (eds) (2012) Pediatric nursing: caring for children and their families, 3rd edn. Clifton Park, NY, Delmar Cengage Learning

Samour PQ, King K (2005) Handbook of pediatric nutrition, 3rd edn. Jones and Bartlett Publishers, Sudbury, MA

United States Department of Agriculture (2014) Choose My Plate.gov. Daily food plan for preschoolers. http://www.choosemyplate.gov/preschoolers/Plan/. Accessed 31 Dec 2014

29 Fifteen-Year Visit

Vishnu Bajwa is brought for his school checkup to the pediatric clinic by his mother. Vishnu weighs 56.71 kg (125 lb), and stands 169 cm tall (66.5 in.), placing him in the 50th percentile for height and weight. His BMI is 19.1, which is also in the 50 percentile. His blood pressure is 113/64. His tanner stage is 3. He lives with his parents and siblings in a three-family house, with his aunt and uncle upstairs and grandmother in the basement. Vishnu has a group of friends in school but recently had a breakup with a girlfriend and feels he will not meet another girl that he will like. Mrs. Bajwa is proud of her son's ambitions but is concerned about how to help him be resilient and self-confident and deal with stress. Vishnu is also worried about a recent outbreak of acne on his face.

- **Is Vishnu's height and weight appropriate for him?**

  Yes, he is in the 50th percentile for height, weight, and BMI—average for his age. But he is concerned about his self-image after his recent breakup with his girlfriend. The health care provider should try to ask Vishnu how he feels about the breakup and to try to validate his experience of the disappointment when a close friendship ends. Vishnu needs to be reassured that although it doesn't feel like it at the moment, other opportunities will arise for such friendships. Also the health care provider should find out who Vishnu's supports are and talk to him about his specific positive qualities and his plans for the future. This will let Vishnu know he is valued as an individual and respected for his feelings and opinions. The health care provider can see Vishnu alone for his check up and then bring in the parent if Vishnu is will. That will also boost his self-confidence.

- **Assess Vishnu's current stage of psychosocial development and how his parents can help him master this stage.**

  According to Erikson this stage is identity versus role confusion. Adolescents are usually trying to figure out their identity in the world. The health care provider can encourage Vishnu's parents to let him manage himself and make independent decisions about his health while offering a caring supportive relationship. They should

D. Kramer, *Primary Well-Being: Case Studies for the Growing Child*,
DOI 10.1007/978-3-319-56708-2_29

be showing him affection, listen to his words and feelings, help him problem solve, and praise his achievements and efforts.

Advice the parents to model the behaviors they want Vishnu to have, like speaking softly and respectfully instead of yelling. They should ask permission to enter his room or make an appointment or plan an outing.

Suggest to Mr. and Mrs. Bajwa that they set limits together with Vishnu about knowing where he is and who he is with. They should discuss the consequences of his decisions and allow him to make independent decisions. Some families have regular time each week to meet and discuss current activities and concerns. That is a good time to check in with Vishnu on how he is doing and what Mr. and Mrs. Bajwa can do to support him.

- **Assess the cognitive development of a child this age.**

  Vishnu is in Piaget's formal operations stage (Simatwa 2010). His parents should encourage Vishnu to take responsibility for completing school work, and praise positive efforts, success and achievement. They should be available to help and support Vishnu with job and college applications and other organizational issues. Vishnu should be encouraged to read a newspaper every day and read in general for pleasure as well as for school. He may need help from them in finding out about what his interests are. Teachers are also good sources of information and help about their student's interests.

- **Assess the social behaviors that Vishnu may exhibit at this age. Mrs. Bajwa is concerned about Vishnu's social life and self-image and the stresses of being a teenager in this country. What advice would you offer?**

  At this age, Vishnu is starting to couple off with girls besides hanging out in groups with boys and girls; he will break off into individual friendships and has started to date. Mr. and Mrs. Bajwa should be encouraged to get to know Vishnu's friends and girlfriends. They should know that a breakup with a girlfriend can be a real setback for a young adolescent male. It is important to watch for any changes in behavior, loss of interest, reduction in energy, or social withdrawal from friends and activities. Monitor how Vishnu is dealing with the rejection and whether he may have possible thoughts of suicide. Signs of difficulty include having trouble sleeping or eating or not being able to concentrate. Does he have a best friend or supportive adult he can talk to? The health care provider should question Vishnu about this and assess whether any signs of depression or suicide ideation are present in Vishnu (Burns et al. 2009; Dixon and Stein 2006; Hagan et al. 2008; Hockenberry and Wilson 2011; Marcdante et al. 2011; McInerny et al. 2009; Potts and Mandleco 2012; Alvardo and Richardson 2011).

- **Describe immunization needs for this age**

  For immunizations at this age, consult the CDC, ACIP, or AAP web sites for the current immunization schedule recommendations (Centers for Disease Control and Prevention 2011):

– CEC National Immunization Program (NIP): http://www.cdc.gov/vaccines
– American Academy of Pediatrics *Red Book*: http://www.aapredbook.org

- **Assess the anticipatory guidance that would be helpful for a child this age.**

The health care provider should review the changes that Vishnu is experiencing and future changes to expect in physical, cognitive, and social development. Encourage Vishnu to eat nutritious meals with healthy snacks, exercise to maintain his weight (American Academy of Pediatrics, Committee on Nutrition 2009; Samour and King 2005; American Academy of Pediatrics 2014; Hagan et al. 2008; Hockenberry and Wilson 2011; Cook and Dunifon 2012; Hammons and Fiese 2011; United States Department of Agriculture 2014), and maintain good hygiene. As his body continues to change, recommend that he shower daily. Vishnu should be getting at least 8 h of sleep at night to help him cope with this stage in his life.

He should be a member of local cultural clubs, sports teams, or other groups that reflect his interests. He may need to travel to some of these activities. The health care provider will want to counsel Vishnu with not using any alcohol or drugs or other substance abuse. It is also appropriate to discuss with him the pressures to engage in sexual activities and to give him tools to remain abstinent such as what to say, choosing friends carefully, doing things in groups, and engaging in his interests. If Vishnu is sexually active, he should have condoms with him at all times. Give Vishnu and his parents the appropriate Bright Futures patient or parent handout for 15–17-year-olds:

American Academy of Pediatrics. (2010). *Bright Futures patient handout 15 to 17 ear visits*. https://brightfutures.aap.org/pdfs/Visit%20Forms%20by%20Age%20110/15-17%20Year/D.Adol.PATH.15-17yr.pdf

American Academy of Pediatrics. (2010). *Bright Futures parent handout 15 to 17 year visits*. https://brightfutures.aap.org/pdfs/Visit%20Forms%20by%20Age%20110/15-17%20Year/D.Adol.PH.15-17yr.pdf

References

Alvardo MJ, Richardson B (2011) Fourteen to seventeen year visit (adolescent). In: Richardson B (ed) Pediatric primary care: practice guidelines for nurses. Burlington, MA, Jones & Bartlett Learning

American Academy of Pediatrics (2010) Bright Futures patient handout 15–17 year visits. https://brightfutures.aap.org/pdfs/Visit%20Forms%20by%20Age%20110/15-17%20Year/D.Adol.PATH.15-17yr.pdf. Accessed 15 Jan 2015

American Academy of Pediatrics (2014) Healthy active living for families. healthychildren.org/growinghealthy. Accessed 16 Dec 2014

American Academy of Pediatrics, Committee on Nutrition (2009) Pediatric nutrition handbook, 6th edn. American Academy of Pediatrics, Elk Grove Village, IL

Burns CE et al (2009) Pediatric primary care: a handbook for nurse practitioners, 4th edn. W.B. Saunders, Philadelphia, PA

Centers for Disease Control and Prevention (2011) Recommendations and guidelines: childhood and adolescent immunization schedules. http://www.cdc.gov/vaccines/schedules/index.html. Accessed 11 Dec 2014

Cook E, Dunifon R (2012) Parenting in context: do family meals really make a difference? (Parenting in context). Cornell University, College of Human Ecology, Ithaca, NY. http://www.human.cornell.edu/pam/outreach/upload/Family-Mealtimes-2.pdf. Accessed 2 Jan 2015

Dixon SD, Stein MT (2006) Encounters with children: pediatric behavior and development, 4th edn. Mosby, St. Louis, MO

Hagan JF, Shaw JS, Duncan P (eds) (2008) Bright futures: guidelines for health supervision of infants, children, and adolescents, 3rd edn. American Academy of Pediatrics, Elk Grove Village, IL

Hammons AJ, Fiese BH (2011) Frequency of shared family meals related to the nutritional health of children and adolescents. Pediatrics 127(6):e1565–e1574

Hockenberry MJ, Wilson DW (2011) Wong's nursing care of infants and children, 9th edn. Elsevier/Mosby, New York, NY

Marcdante KJ, Kliegman RM, Jenson HB et al (eds) (2011) Nelson Essentials of pediatrics, 6th edn. Saunders, Philadelphia, PA

McInerny TK, Adam HM, Campbell DE, Kamat DM, Kelleher KJ (eds) (2009) Textbook of pediatric care. American Academy of Pediatrics, Elk Grove Village, IL

Potts NL, Mandleco BL (eds) (2012) Pediatric nursing: caring for children and their families, 3rd edn. Delmar Cengage Learning, Clifton Park, NY

Samour PQ, King K (2005) Handbook of pediatric nutrition, 3rd edn. Jones and Bartlett Publishers, Sudbury, MA

Simatwa EMW (2010) Piaget's theory of intellectual development and its implication for instructional management at pre-secondary school level. Educ Res Rev 5(7):366–371. http://www.academicjournals.org/article/article1379610138_Simatwa.pdf. Accessed 2 Jan 2014

United States Department of Agriculture (2014) Choose my Plate.Gov. Daily food plan for preschoolers. http://www.choosemyplate.gov/preschoolers/Plan/. Accessed 31 Dec 2014

Sixteen-Year Visit

30

Marjorie is brought to the pediatric clinic for her camp check up to be a counselor in training in a local day camp by her mother Mrs. Polski, who has been a widow for many years. Marjorie weighs 55.89 kilo (123.25 pounds), stands 162.4 cm (65 in.), and is in the 50th percentile. Her BMI is 21.2, which is in the 52nd percentile. Her blood pressure is 111/66. Her tanner stage is: 4. Marjorie's best friend moved away recently and a new friend just got a tattoo and a piercing through her tongue. Mrs. Polski is concerned about the influence of peers on her daughter. Mrs. Polski is also concerned about whether Marjorie is sexually active and knows how to have safe sex. She says that Marjorie seems sad at times and withdraws from family life and at other times lashes out in anger at her mother.

- **Is Marjorie's height and weight appropriate for her?**

  At this stage, Marjorie's height and weight are in the 50th percentile and seem appropriate. It is important to assess her 24-h diet recall because of her recent sadness and loss of a friendship. The health care provider should be concerned that Marjorie may not be eating enough or eating less nutritiously because of her emotional state (Hagan et al. 2008; Dixon and Stein 2006).

- **Assess Marjorie's current stage of psychosocial development and how her mother can help her master this stage. Mrs. Polski is concerned about Marjorie's friends and their influence on her daughter, especially about tattoos and body piercing. How should she talk to her daughter about her changing attitudes? What should she be looking for?**

  The health care provider needs to be sure to use HEADSS to assess Marjorie or any adolescent. The provider should ask open-ended questions about Marjorie's feelings, activities, her life at home, in school, and socially, and any thoughts of depression or suicide. This should be done without the parent present. The health provider should speak to Marjorie and her parents in a nonjudgmental way showing respect.

D. Kramer, *Primary Well-Being: Case Studies for the Growing Child*,
DOI 10.1007/978-3-319-56708-2_30

According to Erikson, Marjorie is in the stage of identity versus role confusion. She is trying to figure out her place in the world. For Marjorie, the loss of her friend to a new community and the choice of one who may be inappropriate is a sign of her distress. The provider should ask if Marjorie is having difficulty sleeping or sleeping too much, loss of appetite or any other eating changes or weight loss or gain, or loss of menses. Has she lost interest in things she normally does? Explain to Mrs. Polski that peer group approval is very important to Marjorie at this stage as well as accepting her body image. The health provider should encourage Mrs. Polski to try to know who Marjorie's friends are and have them in the house so she can get to know them. Communication with adults is important for Marjorie and the parents should encourage it with them and other trusted adults.

Body piercings and tattoos are the subject of some health regulations but guidelines vary from state to state. Mrs. Polski is justified to be concerned as poor practices such as unsterilized needles and repeated use of needles put adolescents at risk for infection, HIV, Hepatitis C and Hepatitis B, as well as other concerns. Mrs. Polski should ask Marjorie if she has thought about doing this to her body and discuss her concerns with Marjorie and let her know there are risks involved. If Marjorie is ever considering this, Mrs. Polski should tell her daughter she would appreciate her coming to her mother to discuss it first so that it can be safely done if that is what Marjorie truly wants.

- **What would you do to address Marjorie's emotional state and advice Mrs. Polski?**

The health provider should do an assessment of the individual, family, and social/environmental factors that are associated with suicide risk. Is the family isolated; is the parent inflexible? The provider should get a good history that includes previous suicide attempts; attempts by a family member or friends; history of physical or sexual abuse or neglect; past psychiatric hospitalization; or death of a parent when child was young. The provider should assess for individual factors that include feelings of hopelessness; marked persistent depression; alcohol or drug abuse; impulsiveness; difficulty tolerating frustration; and feelings of humiliation, self-hatred, or guilt.

If there are thinking disorders, behavioral or developmental, physical or body image problems, or gender identity or sexual orientation concerns, these factors put Marjorie at increased risk for suicide. If she sees herself as a perfectionist or sees herself as totally helpless, she is also at increased risk. Family factors the health provider should look for include difficult home situations, recent or impending moves, family breakup or parental loss, and parents having especially high or low expectations. Other factors include lack of a social support system, few vocational or educational opportunities, isolation, incarceration, or exposure to another suicide (Burns et al. 2009; Dixon and Stein 2006; Hagan et al. 2008; Hockenberry and Wilson 2011; Marcdante et al. 2011; McInerny et al. 2009; Potts and Mandleco 2012; Alvardo and Richardson 2011).

- **What can Mrs. Polski do to protect Marjorie from trying to commit suicide?**

Mrs. Polski can offer Marjorie a supportive, warm, and caring environment in which Mrs. Polski listens to her daughter and provides emotional support. Mrs. Polski needs to create a cohesive family environment that shows respect for Marjorie's individuality, friendships, and school personnel. Adults she interacts with should show they care about Marjorie and foster in her high self-esteem, self-confidence, good social skills, and problem-solving abilities. They should enable Marjorie to tolerate frustration at unfavorable events, help think things through, and help her feel pleasure and celebrate good things.

Also helpful is talking to Marjorie about the importance of eating balanced meals and getting plenty of exercise, doing things she enjoys, and being with people who make her feel good. She should be selective in who her friends are and be assured that her mother is always available if Marjorie has anything to discuss.

Techniques of stress reduction can be helpful to Marjorie such as meditation, heart math, R; acupuncture, Reiki massage and reflexology; and eastern exercise regimes such as yoga, tai chi, and Qigong. Professional help can also be sought and Marjorie's guidance counselor at school should be involved in helping her. Some of these activities can be done with friends; others need a professional practitioner. The health provider should help sort these options out with Marjorie and her mother. Cost and availability may also be factors.

- **What advice would you offer on sexual behavior and to whom?**

The health care provider should talk to Marjorie separately for this part of the visit if she is not already seeing her alone.

The provider should talk about abstinence and about the fact that birth control doesn't always work. They should review the menstrual cycle and types of birth control.

Share with Marjorie current statistics on sexual intercourse for her age group. Tell her we know that nearly 40% of all teenagers ages 15–17 report having some kind of sexual contact. This statistic includes oral sex. This means teens are at risk for sexually transmitted diseases, hepatitis, and HIV, as well as getting pregnant. The US teen birth rate for girls 15–19 was 29.4, which represents a record low for this age group (Centers for Disease Control 2014).

The health care provider should ask Marjorie if she is sexually active, and if so, if she is using contraceptive protection. Review using condoms and other contraceptives correctly and discuss that abstinence is the only means of 100% birth control and protection again sexually transmitted diseases. It is important to point out that Marjorie can get sexually transmitted diseases from oral sex as well as intercourse. Research has found that parents who have a good relationship with their children have the greatest influence on them in high school to abstain from sex (American Academy of Pediatrics, Committee on Adolescence 2007; Karofsky et al. 2001; Martino et al. 2008).

Remind Marjorie that any sexual activity should be something she wants and is not being forced upon her. Point out that it has been helpful to other young adults to be careful with alcohol and drug use and to avoid risky places such as bars, night clubs, pool halls, and risky relationships (people who are abusing substances, or have a history of violence) in relation to unwanted sexual activity (American Academy of Pediatrics 2014: American Academy of Pediatrics, Committee on Adolescence 2007, Centers for Disease Control 2014).

Talk to her about being immunized with the HPV *vaccine* that can help protect against the virus that causes genital warts and may lead to some kinds of cancer. Human papillomavirus (HPV) is one of the most common sexually transmitted diseases (STDs).

- **Describe immunization needs for this age.**

  For immunizations at this age, consult the CDC, ACIP, or AAP web sites for the current immunization schedule recommendations (Centers for Disease Control and Prevention 2011):

– CDC National Immunization Program (NIP): http://www.cdc.gov/vaccines
– American Academy of Pediatrics *Red Book:* http://www.aapredbook.org

- **What anticipatory guidance can you offer Marjorie and her parents?**

  See box: Anticipatory Guidance for Adolescents in Appendix.

References

Alvardo MJ, Richardson B (2011) Fourteen to seventeen year visit (adolescent). In: Richardson B (ed) Pediatric primary care: practice guidelines for nurses. Burlington, MA, Jones & Bartlett Learning

American Academy of Pediatrics (2010a) Bright futures patient handout 15 to 17 year visits. https://brightfutures.aap.org/pdfs/Visit%20Forms%20by%20Age%20110/15-17%20Year/D.Adol.PATH.15-17yr.pdf. Accessed 15 Jan 2015

American Academy of Pediatrics (2010b) Bright futures parent handout 15 to 17 year visits. https://brightfutures.aap.org/pdfs/Visit%20Forms%20by%20Age%20110/15-17%20Year/D.Adol.PH.15-17yr.pdf. Accessed 15 Jan 2015

American Academy of Pediatrics (2014) Healthy active living for families. healthychildren.org/growinghealthy. Accessed 16 Dec 2014

American Academy of Pediatrics, Committee on Adolescence (2007) Contraception and adolescents. Pediatrics 104(5):1161

Burns CE et al (2009) Pediatric primary care: a handbook for nurse practitioners, 4th edn. W.B. Saunders, Philadelphia, PA

Centers for Disease Control (2014) About teen pregnancy. http://www.cdc.gov/teenpregnancy/aboutteenpreg.htm. Accessed 15 Jan 2015

Centers for Disease Control and Prevention (2011) Recommendations and guidelines: childhood and adolescent immunization schedules. http://www.cdc.gov/vaccines/schedules/index.html. Accessed 11 Dec 2014

Dixon SD, Stein MT (2006) Encounters with children: pediatric behavior and development, 4th edn. Mosby, St. Louis, MO

Hagan JF, Shaw JS, Duncan P (eds) (2008) Bright futures: guidelines for health supervision of infants, children, and adolescents, 3rd edn. American Academy of Pediatrics, Elk Grove Village, IL

Hockenberry MJ, Wilson DW (2011) Wong's nursing care of infants and children, 9th edn. Elsevier/Mosby, New York, NY

Karofsky PS, Zeng L, Kosorok MR (2001) Relationship between adolescent-parental communication and initiation of first intercourse by adolescents. J Adolesc Health 28(1):41–45
Marcdante KJ, Kliegman RM, Jenson HB et al (eds) (2011) Nelson essentials of pediatrics, 6th edn. Saunders, Philadelphia, PA
Martino SC, Elliott MN, Corona R et al (2008) Beyond the "big talk": the roles of breadth and repetition in parent-adolescent communication about sexual topics. Pediatrics 121(3):e612–e618
McInerny TK, Adam HM, Campbell DE, Kamat DM, Kelleher KJ (eds) (2009) Textbook of pediatric care. American Academy of Pediatrics, Elk Grove Village, IL
Potts NL, Mandleco BL (eds) (2012) Pediatric nursing: caring for children and their families, 3rd edn. Delmar Cengage Learning, Clifton Park, NY

31 Seventeen-Year Visit

Pierre comes to the pediatric clinic by himself for a physical examination for his working papers. Pierre weighs 68.8 kg (151.75 pounds) and stands 176.8 cm (69.5 in.), placing him in the 50th percentile. His BMI is 22, which is in the 52nd percentile. His blood pressure is 118/67. His tanner stage is: 4. He is planning to be a driver to deliver pizza for a local store. His parents came from Quebec to Rochester before Pierre was born for his father's job teaching engineering at the university there. The family speaks French at home. Pierre likes to be independent and wants this job to save up for college. Pierre is concerned because he has no idea what he wants to study in college and he is worried about fitting into the social scene at college.

- **Is Pierre's height and weight appropriate for him?**

Pierre's weight and height are on the 50th percentile and his body mass index is on the 52nd percentile. On the 24-h recall, Pierre's diet consists of grains, protein, vegetables, and fruits with three glasses of 1% milk daily and plenty of water. He has two to four snacks a day and eats moderate-size portions at each meal. His snacks can consist of fruit and cheese; apples and oranges are often served for dessert, and a fine pastry. A croissant pastry and an egg are served at breakfast with milk. His proteins are meat, fish, and dairy. He begins his afternoon meal usually with soup. The review of his food intake shows Pierre is eating a balanced, healthy diet diet (American Academy of Pediatrics, Committee on Nutrition 2009; Burns et al. 2009; Samour and King 2005; American Academy of Pediatrics 2014; Hagan et al. 2008; Hockenberry and Wilson 2012; Cook and Dunifon 2012; United States Department of Agriculture 2014).

- **Assess the social behaviors that Pierre may exhibit at this age and his concerns about the social scene in college. What advice would you offer?**

The health care provider should first ask Pierre what are his concerns about college and the social scene. For example, ask Pierre what his experience has been with dating and relationships and how he feels about his sexual orientation or gender

D. Kramer, *Primary Well-Being: Case Studies for the Growing Child*,
DOI 10.1007/978-3-319-56708-2_31

identity. Does he have any questions or concerns he would want to discuss with the provider (Alvarado and Richardson 2011; American Academy of Pediatrics 2010a; American Academy of Pediatrics 2010b)?

Depending on Pierre's answers, the health care provider should gently lead Pierre in a discussion about his sexuality. If he discloses his sexual orientation is male, discuss with Pierre whether he chooses to tell his family; help him make a plan in case his family does not support him. It is important to provide sensitive, nonjudgmental care to Pierre (American Academy of Pediatrics, Committee on Adolescence 2007; American Academy of Pediatrics 2013; Dixon and Stein 2006).

The health care provider should also ask Pierre whether he has or plans to obtain a driver's license. The health care provider should be aware of local laws pertaining to driving in the state. Talk to him about not texting and driving, as well as other safety precautions like not having others in the car until after the first 6 months of receiving his full license. Expand on what responsible and safe driving involves.

Ask him about his plans for applying to college, what his career interests and hobbies are, and where he sees himself in the future. Pierre should be encouraged to explore options for his future, and use the guidance counselor in his school to help him find suitable programs he should go look at. A social worker or psychologist may be an appropriate referral if Pierre is interested in exploring his options for the future and directions he could take. The health care provider should say this is a difficult time for transitioning from semi-dependence to full independence and making life choices. For some adolescents a year off of working or a gap program, such as Job Corps for those who are low income, may be an invaluable experience (Hagan et al. 2008; Hockenberry and Wilson 2011; Marcdante et al. 2011; McInerny et al. 2009; Potts and Mandleco 2012).

- **Describe immunization needs for this age.**

  For immunizations at this age, consult the CDC, ACIP, or AAP web sites for the current immunization schedule recommendations (Centers for Disease Control and Prevention 2011):

  – CEC National Immunization Program (NIP): http://www.cdc.gov/vaccines
  – American Academy of Pediatrics *Red Book:* http://www.aapredbook.org

- Identify the anticipatory guidance that would be helpful for a young man of this age.

  See box: *Anticipatory Guidance for Adolescents* in Appendix.

References

Alvardo MJ, Richardson B (2011) Fourteen to seventeen year visit (adolescent). In: Richardson B (ed) Pediatric primary care: practice guidelines for nurses. Jones & Bartlett Learning, Burlington, MA

American Academy of Pediatrics, Committee on Adolescence (2007) Contraception and adolescents. Pediatrics 104(5):1161

American Academy of Pediatrics, Committee on Nutrition (2009) Pediatric nutrition handbook, 6th edn. American Academy of Pediatrics, Elk Grove Village, IL

American Academy of Pediatrics. (2010a). Bright futures patient handout 15 to 17 year visits. https://brightfutures.aap.org/pdfs/Visit%20Forms%20by%20Age%20110/15-17%20Year/D.Adol.PATH.15-17yr.pdf. Accessed 15 Jan 2015

American Academy of Pediatrics. (2010b). Bright futures parent handout 15 to 17 year visits. https://brightfutures.aap.org/pdfs/Visit%20Forms%20by%20Age%20110/15-17%20Year/D.Adol.PH.15-17yr.pdf. Accessed 15 Jan 2015

American Academy of Pediatrics. (2013). Talking to kids and teens about social media and sexting, updated ed. http://www.aap.org/en-us/about-the-aap/aap-press-room/news-features-and-safety-tips/pages/Talking-to-Kids-and-Teens-About-Social-Media-and-Sexting.aspx#sthash.Vi05nMhk.dpuf. Accessed 15 Jan 2015

Burns CE et al (2009) Pediatric primary care: a handbook for nurse practitioners, 4th edn. W.B. Saunders, Philadelphia, PA

Centers for Disease Control and Prevention. (2011) Recommendations and guidelines: childhood and adolescent immunization schedules. http://www.cdc.gov/vaccines/schedules/index.html. Accessed 11 Dec 2014

Cook E, Dunifon R (2012) Parenting in context: do family meals really make a difference? (Parenting in context). Cornell University, College of Human Ecology, Ithaca, NY. http://www.human.cornell.edu/pam/outreach/upload/Family-Mealtimes-2.pdf. Accessed 2 Jan 2015

Dixon SD, Stein MT (2006) Encounters with children: pediatric behavior and development, 4th edn. Mosby, St. Louis, MO

Hagan JF, Shaw JS, Duncan P (eds) (2008) Bright futures: guidelines for health supervision of infants, children, and adolescents, 3rd edn. American Academy of Pediatrics, Elk Grove Village, IL

Hockenberry MJ, Wilson DW (2011) Wong's nursing care of infants and children, 9th edn. Elsevier/Mosby, New York, NY

Marcdante KJ, Kliegman RM, Jenson HB et al (eds) (2011) Nelson essentials of pediatrics, 6th edn. Saunders, Philadelphia, PA

McInerny TK, Adam HM, Campbell DE, Kamat DM, Kelleher KJ (eds) (2009) Textbook of pediatric care. American Academy of Pediatrics, Elk Grove Village, IL

Potts NL, Mandleco BL (eds) (2012) Pediatric nursing: caring for children and their families, 3rd edn. Delmar Cengage Learning, Clifton Park, NY

Samour PQ, King K (2005) Handbook of pediatric nutrition, 3rd edn. Jones and Bartlett Publishers, Sudbury, MA

United States Department of Agriculture. (2014). Choose My Plate.gov. Daily food plan for preschoolers. http://www.choosemyplate.gov/preschoolers/Plan/. Accessed 31 Dec 2014

Eighteen-Year Visit 32

Pamela Gilles is an 18-year-old female who comes to the adolescent clinic for birth control advice and to have the medical form filled out for her college application. She is stressed out about all the application details and the decisions she has to make for her future as she leaves high school. She has a core group of close girl friends and has been dating someone for the past couple of months. Pamela weighs 67 kg (140 pounds), stands 168 cm, (66 in.), and is on the 75th percentile. Her BMI is 23.7, on the 75th percentile. Her blood pressure is 113/67. Her tanner stage is: 5.

- **Is Pamela's height and weight appropriate for her?**

Yes, she is on the 75th percentile for all measurements. The health care provider asks Pamela about her health care habits: Pamela describes how she brushes her teeth at least 2× a day and flosses. She uses earplugs at concerts and other places she may be exposed to loud noises. She is eating healthy and drinking plenty of water; she is running four times a week for physical exercise (Callahan 2004; Sharma et al. 2006). When she rides her bike she uses a helmet to prevent injuries.

- **Assess Pamela's current stage of psychosocial development and how she can master this stage.**

According to Erikson this stage is identity versus role confusion (Burns et al. 2009; Dixon and Stein 2006; Hagan et al. 2008; Hockenberry and Wilson 2011; Marcdante et al. 2011; McInerny et al. 2009; Potts and Mandleco 2012). She is a young adult now, responsible for herself and facing lots of decisions about her future. It is normal for her to feel stress as she pursues the requirements for applying to college.

The health care provider should talk to Pamela about how much independence her parents give her: it should be as much as possible but they should also give their daughter guidelines about their expectations. Pamela needs her parents to be open to communication on any issue and be reassured of their trust and support.

D. Kramer, *Primary Well-Being: Case Studies for the Growing Child*,
DOI 10.1007/978-3-319-56708-2_32

- **Assess the cognitive development of a young lady this age.**

Older teens are still growing in cognitive maturity and face many transitions that they may need guidance and support for from parents and community, such as college decision-making, moving out of the parental home, obtaining employment, and entering dating relationships.

- **Assess the social behaviors that Pamela may exhibit at this age.**

As a young adult, Pamela should be encouraged to stay connected to her family even if she is not living there, especially for problem solving around difficult situations. Pamela will be meeting new people and making new friends. She may find that she drifts away from old friends. This is part of growing up. She will want to find out about her new college community and be exploring new issues that are of concern to her and finding groups in the college community that share these concerns. She will be formulating goals for the future and will want to define and stick to her values. As a young adult, the health care provider can help Pamela consider how she organizes herself, how she will be involved with community, and how she deals with up and down moods and the stress of changes in her life (Burns et al. 2009; Dixon and Stein 2006; Hagan et al. 2008; Hockenberry and Wilson 2011; Marcdante et al. 2011; McInerny et al. 2009; Potts and Mandleco 2012).

The health care provider should point out to Pamela that she will continue to need some support from trusted adults in the community and her parents and it is important to seek out their help whenever Pamela is distressed or needs guidance. She can also confide in trusted girl friends.

- **What would be included in a discussion with Pamela that would relieve her feelings of stress in anticipation of the college application process and making decisions for her future?**

The health care provider should ask Pamela if she would like some help in dealing with all these stressors and offer to give her some names of social workers and psychologists to talk to. The provider should also ask if Pamela is bored or irritable, and if she feels her stress is affecting her at home, at school, or with friends. The health care provider can offer to arrange the first appointment if Pamela would like.

Other ways to relieve Pamela's stress include complementary and alternative medicine techniques based on Eastern medicine, such as meditation, heart math, brain gym, acupuncture, Reiki, massage, and reflexology. Also exercise regimes such as yoga, tai chi, and Qigong have been found to reduce stress (Callahan 2004; Schoenfeld et al. 2013). Professional help can also be sought and the teen's guidance counselor at school should be involved in providing assistance in breaking down the application process into manageable goals and a timeline. The health provider can help sort these options out with Pamela.

- **What advice would you offer on sexual behavior and birth control?**

Pamela is coming to get birth control. The health care provider should first provide the information Pamela asks for, by reviewing the different forms of birth control and the proper way to use them. This should also include a discussion of abstinence and the fact that it is the only 100% guaranteed method of birth control. Also the provider should review the menstrual cycle and take a menstrual history of Pamela (American Academy of Pediatrics 2014; American Academy of Pediatrics 2007; Center for Disease Control 2014; Zuckerman et al. 2014; Upedhya et al. 2013).

The health care provider should also talk to Pamela about sexually transmitted infections and the fact that they can be transmitted in oral sex as well as by intercourse. Remind Pamela that any sexual activity should be something she wants and not be forced upon her. She should remember that it is ok to say "no," and that "no" needs to be listened to and respected. A healthy dating relationship includes respect and concern for one another and it is recommended that Pamela leave any relationship in which there is any sign of coercion or violence or force to do something.

Advise Pamela that if she is in a situation where any type of physical contact is forced upon her, she should go to a safe place and call for help. Also point out to Pamela that it has been helpful to other young adults to be careful with alcohol and drug use and avoid risky places such as bars, night clubs, pool halls, and risky relationships (people who are abusing substances, or have a history of violence) to prevent unwanted sexual activity.

- **Describe immunization needs for this age.**
  For immunizations at this age, consult the CDC, ACIP, or AAP web sites for the current immunization schedule recommendations (Centers for Disease Control 2011):

- CEC National Immunization Program (NIP): http://www.cdc.gov/vaccines
- American Academy of Pediatrics *Red Book:* http://www.aapredbook.org

- **Assess the anticipatory guidance that would be helpful for Pamela.**
  See the box: Anticipatory Guidance for Adolescents.

References

American Academy of Pediatrics. (2010a). Bright futures patient handout 15 to 17 year visits. https://brightfutures.aap.org/pdfs/Visit%20Forms%20by%20Age%20110/15-17%20Year/D.Adol.PATH.15-17yr.pdf. Accessed 15 Jan 2015

American Academy of Pediatrics. (2010b). Bright futures parent handout 15 to 17 year visits. https://brightfutures.aap.org/pdfs/Visit%20Forms%20by%20Age%20110/15-17%20Year/D.Adol.PH.15-17yr.pdf. Accessed 15 Jan 2015

American Academy of Pediatrics. (2014). Healthy active living for families. healthychildren.org/growinghealthy. Accessed 16 Dec 2014

American Academy of Pediatrics, Committee on Adolescence (2007) Contraception and adolescents. Pediatrics 104(5):1161

American Academy of Pediatrics, Committee on Nutrition (2009) Pediatric nutrition handbook, 6th edn. American Academy of Pediatrics, Elk Grove Village, IL

Burns CE et al (2009) Pediatric primary care: a handbook for nurse practitioners, 4th edn. W.B. Saunders, Philadelphia, PA

Callahan P (2004) Exercise: a neglected intervention in mental health care? J Psychiatr Ment Health Nurs 11(4):476–483

Centers for Disease Control. (2014). About teen pregnancy. http://www.cdc.gov/teenpregnancy/aboutteenpreg.htm. Accessed 15 Jan 2015

Centers for Disease Control and Prevention. (2011) Recommendations and guidelines: childhood and adolescent immunization schedules. http://www.cdc.gov/vaccines/schedules/index.html. Accessed 11 Dec 2014

Dixon SD, Stein MT (2006) Encounters with children: pediatric behavior and development, 4th edn. Mosby, St. Louis, MO

Hagan JF, Shaw JS, Duncan P (eds) (2008) Bright futures: guidelines for health supervision of infants, children, and adolescents, 3rd edn. American Academy of Pediatrics, Elk Grove Village, IL

Hockenberry MJ, Wilson DW (2011) Wong's nursing care of infants and children, 9th edn. Elsevier/Mosby, New York, NY

Karofsky PS, Zeng L, Kosorok MR (2001) Relationship between adolescent-parental communication and initiation of first intercourse by adolescents. J Adolesc Health 28(1):41–45

Marcdante KJ, Kliegman RM, Jenson HB et al (eds) (2011) Nelson essentials of pediatrics, 6th edn. Saunders, Philadelphia, PA

Martino SC, Elliott MN, Corona R et al (2008) Beyond the "big talk": the roles of breadth and repetition in parent-adolescent communication about sexual topics. Pediatrics 121(3):e612–e618

McInerny TK, Adam HM, Campbell DE, Kamat DM, and Kelleher KJ, Eds. (2009) Textbook of pediatric care Elk Grove Village, IL: American Academy of Pediatrics.

Potts NL, Mandleco BL (eds) (2012) Pediatric nursing: caring for children and their families, 3rd edn. Delmar Cengage Learning, Clifton Park, NY

Richardson B (ed) (2011) Pediatric primary care: practice guidelines for nurses. Jones & Bartlett Learning, Burlington, MA

Schoenfeld TJ, Rada P, Pieruzzini PR et al (2013) Physical exercise prevents stress-induced activation of granule neurons and enhances local inhibitory mechanisms in the dentate gyrus. J Neurosci 33(18):7770–7777

Sharma A, Madaan V, Petty FD (2006) Exercise for mental health. Prim Care Companion J Clin Psychiatry 8(2):106

Upadhya KK (2013) Contraception for adolescents. Pediatr Rev 34(9):384–394

Zuckerman B, Nathan S, Mate K (2014) Preventing unintended pregnancy: a pediatric opportunity. Pediatrics 133(2):181–183

Appendix: Anticipatory Guidance for Adolescents

Nutrition

- Adolescents require increased calcium and iron in their diet.
- They need three meals a day that should include protein, vegetables, fruits, and complex carbohydrates.
- See choosemyplate.gov for menu planning and suggestions by age group.
- Remind teens of the importance of eating a good breakfast every day.
- Monitor your child for eating disorders.

Sleep

- Teenagers need more sleep—about 10 h—to help them perform optimally.

Exercise

- Adolescents should exercise at least three times a week for 30 min to 1 h at a time.

Dental

- The dentist should be seen two times a year to assess for cavities, infection, and corrections to dentition.
- Twice-daily brushing and flossing are recommended.

Risky Behaviors

Drugs/substance abuse:

- Drug use is influenced by many factors. These include peer pressure, low self-image, stress, trauma, lack of positive parental communication, feeling of low value, and lack of self-confidence.
- The health care provider should find out who the adolescent's supports and friends are and talk to the patient about their specific positive qualities and plans for the future.
- The provider should let the teen know they are valued as an individual and respected for their feelings and opinions.
- The health care provider should see the teen alone to boost their self-confidence and then bring the parent in if it is all right with the teen.

D. Kramer, *Primary Well-Being: Case Studies for the Growing Child*,
DOI 10.1007/978-3-319-56708-2

- The provider can suggest that the parents set limits together with their child and discuss the consequences of decisions, allowing the teen to make an independent decision.
- Parents should set a regular time each week to meet and discuss current activities and concerns. That would be a good time to check in with your adolescent on how they are doing and what the parents can do to support them.

Sexual behavior:

- The provider should talk about abstinence and about the fact that birth control doesn't always work.
- They should review the menstrual cycle and types of birth control with the adolescent.
- Share with the adolescent the current statistics on sexual intercourse for her age group.
- Teens are at risk for sexually transmitted diseases (including from oral sex), hepatitis and HIV, as well as getting pregnant.
- The health care provider should ask the adolescent if he or she is sexually active, and if so, if he or she is using contraceptive protection. Review using condoms and other contraceptives correctly and discuss that abstinence is the only means of 100% birth control and protection against sexually transmitted diseases. It is important to point out that one can get sexually transmitted diseases from oral sex as well as intercourse. The research has found that parents who have a good relationship with their children have the greatest influence on them in high school to abstain from sex (American Academy of Pediatrics, Committee on Adolescence 2007; Karofsky et al. 2001; Martino et al. 2008).

Remind the teen that any sexual activity should be something they want and it should not be forced upon them. Point out that it has been helpful to other young adults to be careful with alcohol and drug use and to avoid risky places such as bars, night clubs, pool halls, and risky relationships (people who are abusing substances, or have a history of violence) in relation to preventing unwanted sexual activity.

Talk to the adolescent about being immunized with the HPV *vaccine* that can help protect against the virus that causes genital warts and may lead to some kinds of cancer. Human papillomavirus (HPV) is one of the most common sexually transmitted diseases (STDs).

Safety

Firearms are an important source of injury and death among adolescents, especially in suicide attempts. Ammunition and gun should be kept separately under lock and key and teenagers should not be allowed to touch them. Safety strategies need to be based on adult behavior and limiting access (American Academy of Pediatrics, Council On Injury, Violence, And Poison Prevention Executive Committee 2012).

Cars: Automobile crashes are the leading cause of adolescent death. Warn the adolescent not to get into a car with anyone who has been driving for less than 6 months. A new driver should also not have passengers for at least 6 months. Drivers should not text and drive and not be on the cell phone. Speed limit laws and signs should always be obeyed.

Body piercing and tattoos: Tattoos and body piercings are the subject of some health regulations but guidelines vary from state to state. Parents are justified in being concerned as poor practices such as unsterilized needles and repeated use of needles put adolescents at risk for infection, HIV, hepatitis C and hepatitis B, as well as other concerns. Parents should discuss with their teens any thoughts about doing this to their bodies and discuss their concerns and the risks involved. If the teenager is ever considering this, parents should tell their child they would appreciate them coming to their parents to discuss it first so that it can be safely done if that is what they truly want.

Social media and Internet safety: Parents should encourage their teenagers to talk to them when asked to do unusual things with friends or strangers. For example if your teen is on the Internet and is asked to turn on their web cam by someone they don't usually Skype with or have face-to-face computer time, the teen should refuse and tell their parents or a trusted adult. Similarly, if they are asked to allow someone else's computer to enter theirs, they should reject the offer.

Parents can talk to their teen about their use of technology and get familiar with it themselves. For example, open a Facebook profile if your teen has one and befriend them. Telling your teen about our own daily use of the social media is a good way for a parent to start a daily conversation about your teen's online habits and who has been contacting them. The parent should remind the teen that what they write on Facebook is public to everyone. Teenagers need to use discretion in what they post to their Facebook page. Parents can ask their teens if anyone has sent any disturbing chats or statements to them.

Parents can emphasize that everything sent over the Internet or a cell phone can be shared with the entire world. Remind their teen that good judgment is important in sending messages and pictures. The parent can discuss what good judgment is together with their teen and the possible consequences of poor judgment (minor punishment to legal action for sexting and bullying). Parents can help set privacy settings with their teens on social media sites appropriately.

The health care provider and the parents can talk to the teen about the dangers of chat rooms, bullying, and sexting. It is helpful to keep the computer in a public part of the household, such as the family room or kitchen, so a parent can check on what the teen is doing online and how much time they spend. The parents can also talk to other parents in their child's class about their children's use of social media.

For more guidelines on using social media and adolescence, see American Academy of Pediatrics. *Talking to kids and teens about social media and sexting.* http://www.aap.org/en-us/about-the-aap/aap-press-room/news-features-and-safety-tips/pages/Talking-to-Kids-and-Teens-About-Social-Media-and-Sexting.aspx#sthash.Vi05nMhk.dpuf. Updated May 31, 2013.

Protective gear: Adolescents should wear all required protective gear for sports as well as bike riding and skateboarding with helmets. Skiing also has gear. Always wear a seat belt in a moving car.

Emotional Behaviors:

- Review with adolescents the emotional and physical changes that are going on in their bodies and the future changes that will occur in their body during puberty.
- For older teens, teach breast self-exam or testicular self-exam.
- Review with parents the importance of accepting and respecting the adolescent and their opinions and feelings.
- Friends and the need to belong are central to adolescents as they strive to achieve independence.
- Adolescents need to feel unconditional love from their parents and friends.
- Help your teenager to stay goal directed and set limits.
- Parents should know where their teen is and who they are with and have guidelines for when their teen should come home.
- Some families have a regular meeting time to check in and discuss current activities and concerns.
- Enable your teenager to make independent decisions and feel respected.
- Monitor your child for signs of rejection and any possible thoughts of suicide.
- Always ask open-ended questions when talking to teens and be nonjudgmental.

Stress: Teenagers often experience stress as they move through puberty. The following techniques may be helpful in reducing and coping with this stress.

- Meditation.
- Heart Math.
- Brain Gym.
- Acupuncture.
- Reiki.
- Massage.
- Reflexology.
- Eastern Exercise Regimes such as yoga, Tai Chi, and Qigong.
- Professional help can also be sought and the teen's guidance counselor at school should be involved in helping them.
- Some of these activities can be done with friends; others need a professional practitioner.
- The health provider should help sort these options out with the adolescent and their parents.
- Cost and availability may also be factors.

References

American Academy of Pediatrics, Committee on Adolescence (2007) Contraception and adolescents. Pediatrics 104(5):1161

American Academy of Pediatrics, Council on Injury, Violence, And Poison Prevention Executive Committee (2012) Firearm-related injuries affecting the pediatric population. Pediatrics 130(5):e1416–e1423

Karofsky PS, Zeng L, Kosorok MR (2001) Relationship between adolescent-parental communication and initiation of first intercourse by adolescents. J Adolesc Health 28(1):41–45

Martino SC, Elliott MN, Corona R et al (2008) Beyond the "big talk": the roles of breadt and repetition in parent-adolescent communication about sexual topics. Pediatrics 121(3):e612–e618

D. Kramer, *Primary Well-Being: Case Studies for the Growing Child*,
DOI 10.1007/978-3-319-56708-2

MIX
Papier aus verantwortungsvollen Quellen
Paper from responsible sources
FSC® C105338

If you have any concerns about our products,
you can contact us on
ProductSafety@springernature.com

In case Publisher is established outside the EU,
the EU authorized representative is:
Springer Nature Customer Service Center GmbH
Europaplatz 3, 69115 Heidelberg, Germany

Printed by Libri Plureos GmbH
in Hamburg, Germany